W9-CGX-027

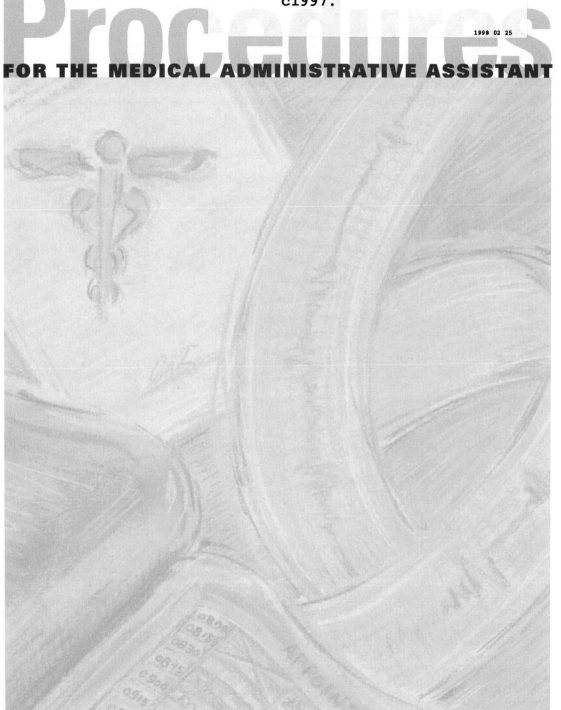

# Procedures

# FOR THE MEDICAL ADMINISTRATIVE ASSISTANT

# Procedures
## FOR THE MEDICAL ADMINISTRATIVE ASSISTANT

**LORNA PLUNKETT**
formerly of Sir Sanford Fleming

## DRYDEN

Harcourt Brace & Company, Canada

Toronto Montreal Fort Worth New York Orlando
Philadelphia San Diego London Sydney Tokyo

**Canadian Cataloguing in Publication Data**

Plunkett, Lorna, 1939–
    Procedures for the medical administrative assistant

3rd ed.
First ed. published under title: Procedures for the
medical secretary.
Includes index.

ISBN 0-03-923126-7

1. Medical assistants — Canada.   2. Medical secretaries
— Canada.   3. Office practice.   I. Title.
II. Title: Procedures for the medical secretary.

R728.8.P58   1997         651'.961         C96-930130-8

Director of Product Development: Heather McWhinney
Acquisitions Editor: Ken Nauss
Projects Manager: Liz Radojkovic
Developmental Editor: Su Mei Ku
Editorial Assistant: Martina van de Velde
Director of Publishing Services: Jean Davies
Editorial Manager: Marcel Chiera
Supervising Editor: Semareh Al-Hillal
Production Editor: Laurel Parsons
Production Manager: Sue-Ann Becker
Production Co-ordinator: Sheila Barry
Copy Editor: John Hewak
Cover Design: Sonya V. Thursby/Opus House
Cover Art: Connie Fong
Typesetting, Scanning, and Assembly: IBEX Graphic Com. Inc.
Printing and Binding: Webcom Limited

This book was printed in Canada.

1 2 3 4 5    01 00 99 98 97

# Preface

The health care field is such a dynamic environment that instructional publications must be constantly revised to keep up to date with change. It seems like four very short years since I began working on the second edition of this text and here it is time to publish the third edition.

You are embarking on a very exciting career as a medical administrative assistant, one that will present everyday challenges as well as many opportunities for change and advancement. *Procedures for the Medical Administrative Assistant* will provide you with the learning outcomes you require to be a successful contributor to health care.

The medical office is a diverse environment that requires skills and knowledge not only in office procedures but in communications, human behaviour, word processing, machine transcription, terminology, and anatomy. The focus of this text is on office procedures. All other topics require more in-depth instruction than could be integrated into the chapters of this text.

The text is divided into three parts. Part 1 discusses the most essential procedures that a medical administrative assistant is required to know. Topics include booking appointments and patient flow; records management; accounting; health care billing; hospital records, reports, and requisitioning; meeting organization; ordering procedures; and legal guidelines. Part 2 reviews appropriate formats for letters, memos, forms and requisitions, manuscripts, and financial statements. Part 3 provides timed writings and exercises to assist you in developing your keyboarding skills.

In addition, there are four useful appendices in Chapter 11. Appendix A offers a quick reference to common abbreviations used in the health care field. Appendix B lists laboratory tests and their turnaround time. In this appendix, you will also find sample forms with instructions on how to complete them. Appendix C provides names of the most commonly prescribed drugs, and Appendix D lists names of sources like medical dictionaries, handbooks, and other books on health care that you can refer to.

The assignments in the text attempt to simulate tasks that would be encountered in a medical office. Dr. J.E. Plunkett will be the physician who assigns the majority of your tasks. In reality, Dr. Plunkett was my husband's Uncle Elmer. In 1931, after graduating from Queen's University and spending nine months at the Mayo Clinic in Minneapolis, he set up his medical practice at 278 O'Conner Street in Ottawa. He was a dedicated surgeon and physician until his untimely death in 1952. The inscript on the letterhead used for the assignments was taken from one of his prescription pad pages on which his wife Marion had written a recipe. All other names and all medical information used in the book are fictitious.

Forms that are required to complete the assignments can be found in the Working Papers.

All Canadian students studying medical administrative assistant procedures will find relevant material in the text. Although Ontario is sometimes used for demonstration purposes, procedures are very similar across the country.

While every care has been taken to ensure that the information in this third edition is up to date, we cannot deny that the health care field is dynamic and is constantly evolving. Users of this text should periodically check with appropriate offices and ministries for the most current information.

After graduating, you will embark on a challenging and rewarding career. I wish you every success in all of your endeavours.

## Confidentiality

Heath care professionals have access to confidential material, and the medical administrative assistant is no exception.

You will hear, read, and observe things that are extremely confidential. It is of utmost importance that you respect the nature of the information and ensure that it is not passed on to others.

Throughout the text the importance of confidentiality will be continually reinforced.

## Acknowledgements

In order to complete the third edition of this text, many people have willingly contributed their knowledge, time, experience, and expertise. It is most rewarding to know and work with these individuals and I would like to acknowledge their contribution.

Pat Hooper, Elsbeth McCall, and Elaine Graham worked tirelessly to gather information and give advice on the revisions and revamping of the text.

Bonnie Hamilton, Carolee Awde-Sadler, and Karim Ranmal assisted in the compilation of Appendices B and C. Dr. James Mewett reviewed some of the text content to ensure that it was current. Claudette Lachance-Wykes contributed her expertise to Chapter 14.

Sandra Spencer and Cliff Pennington provided the most up to date information for the chapter on health insurance, and Luisa Giocometti co-ordinated the updates from the Workers' Compensation Board.

The comments and suggestions by those instructors who reviewed the manuscript prior to publication were invaluable to me. Those who participated in the preparation of the second edition were

Cathy Appleby (Centennial College)

Nancy Elder (Seneca College)

Christine Harris (National Training Institute)

Barb Lewis (Ontario Business College)

Toni Motone (Algonquin College)

Sylvia Taus (Canadore College)

Barbara Tanner (Assiniboine Community College)

The instructors who provided feedback for revising the third edition were

Sandie Baillargeon (Career Canada College)

Barbara Ianson (Toronto School of Business)

Marie McNeil-Rutherford (Toronto School of Business)

Agnes Seaton (Seneca College)

Several people at Dryden Canada contributed to the publication of this text. Many thanks go to Ken Nauss, Su Mei Ku, Martina van de Velde, and Laurel Parsons. Their skills and efforts are much appreciated.

Thanks also to the following organizations for the permission to print the many forms that appear in the text:

Alberta Health

The Bank of Nova Scotia

The Canadian Medical Association

Dean et fils, Inc.

Hospital and Heath Services Commission, Prince Edward Island

Manitoba Health Services Commission

Newfoundland Medical Care Commission

Department of Health and Social Services, Government of the Northwest Territories

Nova Scotia Medical Services Insurance

Peterborough County Medical Secretaries Association

The Province of British Columbia

The Province of New Brunswick

The Province of Quebec

Ontario Medical Secretaries Association

Ontario Ministry of Health

Revenue Canada Taxation

St. Joseph's Hospital, Peterborough

Workers' Compensation Board

The Yukon Territories

Without the assistance and co-operation of every person and institution, whose names I have mentioned, the publishing of this third edition would not have been possible. Many thanks for your contribution and support.

Lorna Plunkett

## A Note from the Publisher

Thank you for selecting *Procedures for the Medical Administrative Assistant*, Third Edition, by Lorna Plunkett. The author and publisher have devoted considerable time to the careful development of this book. We appreciate your recognition of this effort and accomplishment.

We want to hear what you think about *Procedures for the Medical Administrative Assistant*. Please take a few minutes to fill in the stamped reader reply card at the back of the book. Your comments and suggestions will be valuable to us as we prepare new editions and other books.

# Contents

# Part 1

# Procedures for the Medical Administrative Assistant

# Chapter 1

# Your Future As a Medical Administrative Assistant

## Learning Objectives

To identify
- potential areas of employment
- personal qualities required for employment in a medical environment
- skill requirements of the medical profession
- professional appearance for a medical administrative assistant
- the importance of customer service

A position as a health care professional is exciting and rewarding. You are embarking on a career path that will allow you, as a medical administrative assistant, to join this stimulating specialty. Historically, medicine has been a mysterious but intriguing subject; the news media frequently affords it headline status; innovations in the control of serious illnesses are happening every day. Upon completion of your training, many job opportunities will be available to you in the medical field.

# Career Opportunities

## Hospitals or Clinics

Employment opportunities exist at all stages of health care, from the admission of the patient to the discharge, or in the management of documents in the medical records department. Opportunities include the following positions:

Medical machine transcriptionist

Medical administrative assistant in doctors' offices, and in X-ray, laboratory, physiotherapy, and admissions departments

Ward secretary in emergency departments and nursing units

Operating room booking secretary

Office administrator in a health services organization or community health centre

## Government Facilities

Many opportunities exist within the public sector. A career in this environment will provide challenge and opportunity for advancement. Areas where you will be eligible for employment include the following:

Health units

Provincial laboratories

Food and drug administration offices

Nursing homes

Institutions for the physically/mentally disadvantaged

Provincial and federal health care plan offices

Medical, nursing, and research departments of universities

## Private Practices

Opportunities also abound in the private sector. Positions in this area allow employees to learn all facets of office administration:

Offices of physicians engaged in general practice or specialty services (see list of specialties in Chapter 6, pp. 65–68)

Practitioners' offices (optometrists, chiropractors, naturopaths, podiatrists)

Dentists' offices

Veterinarian hospitals and offices

Home care organizations

Medical supply companies

Medical foundations

Insurance companies

All of the above positions play a vital role in delivering quality health care.

The job turnover rate in your chosen career is surprisingly low. This would indicate that medical administrative assistants derive a great deal of satisfaction from their positions. It also indicates that those seeking employment in this field must have superior personal qualifications and skills.

**Career Qualifications**

## Personal Qualities

If you think about why you have chosen this profession, you will recognize that you possess the following qualities:

Pleasing personality
Genuine interest in people
Ability to assume responsibility
Ability to remain calm under pressure
Respect for the privacy of others
Empathy, compassion, and serenity
Honesty and reliability
Professional attitude
Dedication and loyalty
Sense of humour
Tact
Patience
Understanding and helpfulness
Efficiency

What others can you suggest?

## Skill Requirements

In order to function in a busy office environment, you must master certain job-related skills:

Effective communication skills
Good organizational ability
Fast and accurate keyboarding skills
Sound understanding of medical terminology and anatomy
Excellent medical machine transcription skills
Knowledge of word processing and software billing systems

## Personal Appearance

Professional attitude and skills are complemented by a professional personal appearance:

Neat, attractive hairstyle
Tasteful make-up (for female employees)
Clean, crisp attire appropriate for the office
Comfortable footwear suitable for a working environment
Light fragrance, if desired

## Customer Service

Never underestimate the importance of first impressions!

You are the voice of your doctor's practice. You are the first person to greet the patients when they visit the doctor. Many people judge the physician's practice by their first impression.

Gum chewing, cigarette smoking, and eating while on duty and dealing with the public are taboo.

Some doctors prefer receptionists to wear uniforms. What are your views on the pros and cons of wearing a uniform? If you had the option, would you choose to wear a uniform, or would you prefer regular business attire? Why?

It is important to be friendly and greet patients with a pleasant voice and expression. Remember that people who visit the doctor's office are usually under stress. It is your responsibility to put them at ease in order to alleviate some of their fears and concerns. Try to acknowledge them as quickly as possible and be sure to inform them of approximately how long it will be before they will be seen by the doctor.

The health care environment is very busy and demanding, often creating stressful situations for the administrative assistant. It is important that you consider situations that cause undue stress and take action to correct them, for example, by being well organized. It is equally important to get enough physical exercise, rest, and relaxation, and to eat nutritious meals — all essential ingredients for a reduced stress level.

If you encounter a difficult patient, remain calm and in control. Let angry patients talk out their frustrations, and try to be reassuring. Their anger is not usually directed at you and is usually caused by anxiety. Remain calm and do not become defensive or argumentative.

The subject of confidentiality will be stressed continually throughout the text. When patients approach your work area, it is important that you are discreet in conversing with them. Do not discuss their illness or reason for seeing the doctor in a voice that may be heard by others in the waiting area. If your conversations with patients may be overheard by others, move to an area where you can talk privately.

## Assignment 1.1

Set up a personal file (portfolio) to begin collecting evidence of your achievements, challenges, academic documents, and other relevant data. This will allow you to maintain a record of documents to be used within this program and throughout your career, for example, letters of reference, performance evaluations, work-related thank-you letters, diplomas/certificates, educational transcripts, copies of successfully completed projects/assignments.

Write a short essay (one to two pages) stating why you have chosen a career as a medical administrative assistant. Outline the personal qualities you possess that will enable you to be an effective health care professional. Be prepared to defend your ideas.

**Assignment 1.2**

Take a few moments to complete the rating sheet from the Working Papers (p. 3) as shown in Illustration 1.1. Be as objective and honest as you can. Keep the sheet in your portfolio to be used in Assignment 14.2.

**Assignment 1.3**

**Illustration 1.1   Rating Sheet**

**RATING SHEET**
**A FIRST IMPRESSION**

Place a check mark (✔) in the space that best describes your personal attributes.

**Facial Expression**
☐ Happy Smile      ☐ Serious Outlook      ☐ Blank Expression

**Voice**
☐ Loud Tone      ☐ Soft Spoken      ☐ Well Modulated

**Communication Ability**
☐ Control Conversation      ☐ Shy and Withdrawn      ☐ Outgoing and Friendly

**Language Skills**
☐ Adequate      ☐ Excellent      ☐ Poor

**Hair Style**
☐ Acceptable for Business      ☐ Unacceptable      ☐ Just Acceptable

**Make-up (for female employees)**
☐ Accentuated      ☐ Light      ☐ Heavy

**Nails**
☐ Manicured      ☐ Suitable      ☐ Rough

**Clothes**
☐ High Fashion      ☐ Comfortable      ☐ Sloppy

**Hygiene**
☐ Excellent      ☐ Good      ☐ Needs Improvement

**OVERALL FIRST IMPRESSION**
☐ Excellent      ☐ Acceptable      ☐ Poor

**Assignment 1.4**

Do you currently possess all of the skills and personal qualities required for a health care environment? Perhaps you have some of the skills and some of the personal qualities, but not at the level necessary to secure the position you are seeking.

In order to assess your current skills and personal qualities as they relate to a position as a medical administrative assistant, complete the skills and personal qualities inventory sheet found in the Working Papers (p. 4).

Be as objective as possible as you assess your skills and qualities; retain your inventory sheet in your portfolio for use in Assignment 14.2.

**Assignment 1.5**

Topic for Discussion:
Relate an experience you have had

1. When a first impression was positive. Why?
2. When a first impression was negative. Why?
3. When your first impression was inaccurate. Why?

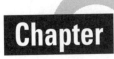

# Chapter 2

# Reception

# and Booking

# Appointments

## Chapter Outline

- Reception
- Assignment 2.1
- Booking Appointments
- Assignment 2.2
- Assignment 2.3

- Assignment 2.4
- Assignment 2.5
- Assignment 2.6
- Assignment 2.7

## Learning Objectives

To identify
- responsibilities of the medical administrative assistant regarding patient reception
- methods for scheduling patient appointments
- procedures for booking surgery
- methods of dealing with callers other than patients

Now let's take a look at some of the responsibilities you will have when you go to work, specifically, receptionist duties. You will see that these are quite different from those in a nonmedical environment. We will also discuss pertinent points concerning the doctor's appointment schedule.

## Reception

## Waiting Area

The waiting room should be a peaceful, comfortable area for patients to await their appointment. What amenities add to the atmosphere of the waiting room?

Appealing decor, comfortable chairs, interesting magazines (current issues), enjoyable music, and children's books and toys are items that should be considered. Of course, cleanliness and tidiness are the two most important features.

## Greeting Patients

A warm, friendly smile and immediate attention are two things to remember. If you are preparing a letter, adding figures, or writing a prescription note, they can wait; the most important duty you have is to attend to the patients. If you are busy with a patient and someone comes into the office, acknowledge his or her presence ("I will be with you in just a moment"). If you are on the telephone, smile or raise your hand to show you are aware someone has entered the office. Do not simply ignore the person.

Whenever possible, greet the patient by name. Initially, it is best to use the formal greeting (Mr., Mrs., Ms.) when receiving patients. Some patients will request that you refer to them by their first name after you have become acquainted. This practice is acceptable, but only after you have been instructed to take that liberty.

The majority of patients visiting the doctor are under stress. It is important for the medical administrative assistant to be considerate and caring.

## Patient Information

You are responsible for establishing and maintaining a current and accurate file of information for all new patients. To obtain the required information from a new patient, you may ask the patient to complete a patient information form as shown in Illustration 3.6. If questions are to be answered orally, move to a private place to protect confidentiality. (Note: To ensure records are always accurate and up to date, you should regularly ask if there are any changes in the patient information.)

## Assignment 2.1

**Role play** — Assume the role of a medical administrative assistant as you complete a patient information form for one of your classmates. Remember to maintain a friendly and relaxed manner. A blank form to complete the assignment is on page 5 of the Working Papers.

Your instructor may choose to evaluate your performance of this assignment. Insert the results of your evaluation in your portfolio.

## Health Card Verification

All provinces in Canada provide eligible residents with a health card (see Chapter 6, p. 62). Patients must present their health card when accessing services covered by the provincial health care system. When a patient arrives for an appointment, you must ask for the health card and verify that the card is current and belongs to the patient. If there is a question about the authenticity of the health card, it is your responsibility to report this information to the provincial ministry. Verification procedures may vary between offices, as well as provinces, ranging from manual to computerized systems.

**Illustration 2.1   Common Instruments and Supplies Used in a General Practitioner's Office**

| | | |
|---|---|---|
| Blood Pressure Cuff | Bandages | Lancets |
| Syringes | Telfa | Peak Flow Meter |
| Needles | Ear Syringe | Slides (glass) |
| Alcohol | Otoscope | Fixative (cytology) |
| Sutures | Vaginal Speculum | Forceps |
| Needle Driver | Tongue Depressors | Curette |
| Scissors | Cotton Swabs | Height and Weight Chart |
| Mosquito Forceps | Reflex Hammer | Weight Scales |
| Skin Hooks | Eye Chart | Biological Supplies |
| Scalpel (and blade) | Gowns | Ophthalmoscope |
| Cotton | Examining Table Paper | Silver Nitrate Sticks |
| Gauze | Stethoscope | Sample Bottles |
| Tensors | Hemoglobinometer | |

## Examining Rooms

The examining rooms should be prepared for the patients: instruments to be used should be readily available for the doctor; sufficient paper should be available to ensure a sterile examination table at all times; light bulbs in examining lamps must be working; and all medical supplies required for the patient should be placed in an easily accessible area (see Illustration 2.1). Of course, all areas of the medical office must be kept clean and medical instruments must be sterile.

Now that you are ready, the patients can be allocated to the examination rooms.

After each patient, you should change the paper on the examination table if necessary and ensure that all is in order.

Consider your responsibilities in preparing the patient for the doctor. Does the patient need to disrobe? If so, most doctors provide a gown or sheet. Is a urine sample required? Particulars may be required if the patient is having a Pap smear. You may be required to weigh and measure the patient. In addition, you may be required to perform such tasks as taking blood pressures and temperatures, checking pulses and respirations, and so on. These statistics are entered on the history sheet in the patient's file.

According to the Canadian Medical Protective Association, invasive procedures such as giving injections, taking blood, and other similar clinical procedures are beyond the terms of reference of a medical administrative assistant. These functions should be performed by a trained nurse or by the doctor. *Be sure to leave the patient's file readily available for the doctor.*

## Arranging for Diagnostic Testing

At the end of the doctor's consultation with the patient, you may be required to complete requisition forms for specific tests. (A more thorough outline of completion of requisition forms will be covered in Chapter 11.) It may be necessary to arrange appointments for such tests — for example, ultrasound and/or blood work. It may also be necessary to arrange an appointment with a specialist. Some points to consider when making arrangements for special tests follow:

1. Some patients who are very ill can tolerate only so much in one day. Be sure you don't overtax someone with too many tests at one time.
2. Ask about any required special preparations for the test. Ensure that instructions are clearly communicated to and understood by the patient.
3. If more than one test is required, can the patient be booked consecutively, or must the appointments be booked on separate days.
4. Inform the patient of the approximate time required to complete the test.
5. Try to be aware of your patients' comfort level with pending tests. Allay their fears, or encourage them to ask questions.
6. Discuss time availability with the patient before arranging for the testing.
7. Inform the receptionist at the testing location of any special needs of the patient.

### Topic for Discussion

Discuss with your classmates the types of special needs, or any other considerations, you may have to address.

## Booking Appointments

The scheduling system is an important component in the smooth operation of the doctor's office. A successful system depends on good decision making by the medical administrative assistant. Systems vary and can consist of a manually processed appointment book, a computerized system, or a combination of both. Not only does the system maintain a record of each day's functions in the office, but it is an official record that can be used for billing purposes or as a legal document in case of legal action. A busy doctor has many things to remember such as luncheon dates, speaking engagements, and meetings. It is the administrative assistant's responsibility to record such information as well as a full schedule of operations and/or patient visits. The doctor frequently refers to a daily diary to keep on schedule. It is, therefore, imperative that you, the administrative assistant, be exact when making entries in the appointment book. Accuracy and legibility are essential.

Illustration 2.2 is an example of a manual system appointment book. There are several variations, but most have each hour broken down into specific time segments, depending on the doctor's practice and preference. A computerized system would also have variations in format.

**Illustration 2.2   Appointment Schedule: Manual System**

DOCTOR _Plunkett_

APPOINTMENT SCHEDULE

Day_____ Month_____ Year_____

| TIME | PATIENT | PHONE | REASON FOR APPOINTMENT |
|------|---------|-------|------------------------|
| 0800 | Erik Shultz | 427-9977 | Counselling |
| 0815 | | | |
| 0830 | | | |
| 0845 | | | Surgery Assist —   Dr. Jones |
| 0900 | | | O.R. 6 St. Joseph's Hosp. |
| 0915 | | | Hemodyalisis & graft |
| 0930 | | | |
| 0945 | | | |
| 1000 | | | |
| 1015 | | | |
| 1030 | | | |
| 1045 | | | |
| 1100 | | | |
| 1115 | | | |
| 1130 | | | |
| 1145 | | | |
| 1200 | | | |
| 1215 | | | |
| 1230 | | | Kinsmen Luncheon |
| 1245 | | | |
| 1300 | | | |
| 1315 | Eliz. Green | 427-3774 | Annual Health Exam |
| 1330 | | | |
| 1345 | | | |
| 1400 | | | |
| 1415 | | | |
| 1430 | | | |
| 1445 | | | |
| 1500 | Coffee/Messages | | |
| 1515 | | | |
| 1530 | | | |
| 1545 | | | |
| 1600 | | | |
| 1615 | | | |
| 1630 | Tim Peters | 743-2525 | Boil Lanced |
| 1645 | | | |
| 1700 | Dinner Engagement | | |

REMARKS: _____

_____

Many specialists book half-hour appointments. General practitioners have ten- or fifteen-minute segments in their appointment schedule. Some books are designed to display six days on two pages, while others display a day at a time.

Walk-in clinics and some private practices do not schedule appointments. Patients are seen on a first-come, first-served basis. This, of course, could lead to long waiting periods for some patients.

Wave scheduling is another method for booking appointments (see Illustration 2.3). This method can help alleviate problems created by late arrivals. Assume that you use a schedule that books a patient every ten minutes, allowing three patients to be seen each half hour and at the time scheduled. If you changed to wave scheduling, three patients would be scheduled at the beginning of each half-hour interval and seen in order of arrival. Your initial schedule would be:

1000   Mrs. Green
1010   Mr. Shultz
1020   Ms. Smith

Your revised schedule would be:

1000   Mrs. Green
       Mr. Shultz
       Ms. Smith

If one patient were late for the appointment, it would not affect the other two, and the longest waiting interval would be twenty minutes.

We will not attempt to dictate a specific method for booking appointments. Each office varies and your doctor/employer will give you instructions about personal preferences for booking appointments. We will, however, make some suggestions.

When a patient requests an appointment, ask the reason for the visit in order to assess the time allotment required; for example, a minor sore throat or cold may need a ten-minute appointment, whereas counselling or a complete physical could require a half-hour appointment.

Always allow travel time, from hospital to office for example, when required. It is wise to leave a fifteen-minute open appointment each morning and afternoon if possible. This allows for catch-up time if the doctor is behind schedule. If the doctor is on schedule, the time could be used for a coffee break or to discuss telephone messages. However, every doctor may not want you to follow this procedure. Check with your employer before implementing such a practice in the appointment schedule.

An earache, chest pain, and high temperature are emergencies considered urgent, and *must be seen*. On the other hand, a common cold may be seen the next day. When your daily schedule is completely filled and a patient insists on seeing the doctor, tell the patient you will check with the doctor and call back with instructions. Refusing a critically ill patient could result

**Illustration 2.3  Appointment Schedule: Wave Scheduling**

APPOINTMENT SCHEDULE

DOCTOR _Plunkett_____

Day_____ Month_____ Year_____

| TIME | PATIENT | PHONE | REASON FOR APPOINTMENT |
|------|---------|-------|------------------------|
| 0930 | | | |
| 1000 | Eliz. Green<br>Erik Shultz<br>Heather Smith | 427-3774<br>427-9977<br>576-3225 | |
| 1030 | | | |
| 1100 | | | |
| 1130 | | | |
| 1200 | | | |
| 1230 | | | |
| 1300 | | | |
| 1330 | | | |

REMARKS: _____

_____

_____

in legal action against the doctor. *Never* make such a decision on your own. Remember — your responsibility is to book appointments, not to make a diagnosis.

*Never* put off an emergency patient. If the doctor should become involved in an emergency and cancellations prove necessary, always make arrangements to have urgent patients seen by another physician. Routine appointments can be booked for a later date. If time allows, contact the patient before he or she leaves for the office.

If a patient arrives at the office before you have had time to call, how would you handle the situation?

A record of the patient's telephone number (at home or work) on the appointment schedule is recommended in case it is necessary to change an appointment — this practice provides you with easy access to your patients.

## Assignment 2.2

Assume you are the administrative assistant and a patient has arrived for an appointment. Dr. Plunkett has been called to the hospital to deliver a baby — he expects to return in approximately one hour. You were unable to contact the patient. Think about how you would handle the situation, and then write a scenario.

### Additional Recommendations Concerning the Appointment Book

1. Record the date at the top of the page in pen but record all appointments in pencil. If changes are required, it is advisable to draw a line through the original entry and record the new information just above or below the crossed-out entry. Never erase an entered appointment.

2. It is wise to have preprinted appointment reminder cards (see Illustration 2.4) to give to patients who book appointments in the office. Any special instructions to the patient can be recorded on the back of the card, for instance "Bring Medication." This eliminates misunderstandings and errors. If time allows, missed appointments can be virtually eliminated by telephoning the patient the day before his or her scheduled visit. If a patient is to return for an appointment in the future, arrange the appointment time before the patient leaves the office.

#### Illustration 2.4   Appointment Reminder Card

**APPOINTMENT REMINDER**

An appointment is scheduled with

DR. J.E. PLUNKETT

Date_____

Time_____

3. Make appointments for homemakers, preschoolers, and retirees early in the day. This leaves time open for school-age children after 4 P.M. and for working patients after 5 P.M.

4. If a patient cancels an appointment and does not request a rebooking, make a notation and advise the doctor. If the missed appointment will jeopardize the patient's well-being, telephone the patient and suggest making another appointment. Draw a line through the cancelled appoint-

ment and make a notation in the remarks area at the bottom of the appointment book or in the patient's chart. If you are employed in a specialist's office and a patient cancels or misses an appointment, advise the referring/family physician.

5. Do not book several long appointments together (unless your doctor/employer does all annual health exams on a specific day).

6. When the doctor is called away from the office for an emergency and a patient arrives for an appointment:

   a.  Apologize for the inconvenience.

   b.  Explain the doctor's absence.

   c.  Tell the patient approximately how long the doctor will be detained.

   d.  If the doctor is not going to be away too long:

       i.   Suggest the patient might like to wait, and offer a magazine.

       ii.  Suggest the patient might have some errands to run and would like to come back later.

       iii. Suggest rebooking for a future date.

   e.  Offer the use of a telephone to contact children left at home, or call a taxi, and so on.

## Patients without Appointments

If a patient arrives and wishes to see the doctor without having first made an appointment, you would point out that the doctor sees patients by appointment only and that, in future, arrangements should be made before coming to the office. If you could arrange to have the doctor see the patient without inconveniencing anyone, you would then explain that there would be a waiting period (state time, for example, approximately one hour) before the patient could be seen by the doctor.

Of course, you may be faced with an emergency situation whereby a patient arrives at the office and needs to be seen immediately. In such an instance, you would usher the patient into the first available examining room.

## House Calls

The delivery of health care has changed radically over the years. If we compare health care in the early 1900s with health care delivery today, we see that early in the century the doctor came to the patient's home, while today the patient usually sees the doctor in the office or in a hospital. There are occasions, however, when it may be necessary for the doctor to visit the patient at home. If you are responsible for making arrangements for a house call, you must get explicit instructions regarding the location of the house or apartment as well as the name, telephone number, and complaint. You must also advise the patient about the approximate time of the doctor's arrival. If a doctor is making a house call, it will usually be after office hours, or before or after hospital rounds. Make a note of a house call in your appointment schedule. (Note: Remember — house calls are expensive and time consuming. Always urge patients to come to the office if at all possible.)

**Illustration 2.5   Surgical Admission Booking Card**

## SURGICAL ADMISSION BOOKING CARD

☐ PETERBOROUGH CIVIC HOSPITAL
☐ ST. JOSEPH'S HOSPITAL & HEALTH CENTRE

ADMISSION DATE: _____
                  MM      DD      YY

SURGEON: _____

PROCEDURE DATE: _____
                  MM      DD      YY

SURNAME: _____

GIVEN NAMES: _____

DATE OF BIRTH: _____
                 MM      DD      YY

PHONE NUMBER: _____

HEALTH CARD #: _____

ADMISSION DIAGNOSIS: _____

PROCEDURE: _____

COMORBID CONDITIONS: _____

IF NOT A.M. ADMIT, PLEASE GIVE REASON: _____

☐ DISCHARGE PLANNING REQUIRED
☐ HOMECARE REQUIRED

*FOR HOSPITAL USE:*
*CMG #:* _____

FORM #JF1585

## Scheduling Surgery

In most areas, hospital operating rooms are booked to capacity many weeks in advance. Procedure requirements for booking surgery will differ according to hospital and area, but the following information will be required by any operating room scheduling officer and/or admitting department:

1. Patient's sociological information (name, address, medical care plan number)
2. Is the surgery elective or urgent?
3. What type of surgery will be performed?
4. Admitting diagnosis

In order to manage more efficiently, many hospitals utilize an expected date of discharge program. If such a program is in place, the surgery registration card would include the patient's expected length of stay.

Some hospitals may accept this information by telephone; others may require the completion of a Surgical Admission Booking Card (see Illustration 2.5).

Many hospitals now have a presurgical information package to be completed prior to surgery. The package is supplied by the surgeon's secretary. Components of the required information are (may vary among institutions):

| Form | Completed by |
|---|---|
| Letter of instruction to patient | Surgeon |
| Preanaesthetic questionnaire | Patient |
| Preregistration questionnaire | Patient |
| History and physical examination form | Surgeon/Family physician |
| Consent form | Surgeon must ensure completion by patient |
| Order sheet (including pre-op testing requirements) | Surgeon |

Emergency surgery usually results after a patient has been examined in the emergency department at the hospital. The arrangements for emergency surgery would then be made within the hospital by the emergency department ward secretary and the operating room scheduling officer.

## Drug and Supply Salespersons and Nonpatient Visitors

Drug and supply salespersons often have new and innovative medicines and supplies in which the doctor is interested. They are usually aware of doctors' preferences for booking time to see them, and they arrange their appointment times well in advance of their visit.

The appearance of someone without an appointment on a very busy day may present you with a problem. Most doctors/employers will have a preference for scheduling appointments for nonpatient visitors and you will, therefore, have clear-cut guidelines on how to deal with them. If, however, there are no set rules, an efficient medical administrative assistant will tactfully, but firmly, advise all nonpatient callers that the doctor will see them only by appointment. Remember, the patients are the doctor's first priority and their appointment times should not be interrupted by those who have failed to make an appointment.

**Assignment 2.3**

Dr. Plunkett's office is very busy today. Due to an emergency, he is running behind schedule. An aggressive sales representative insists on seeing Dr. Plunkett that day because he is from out of town. He assures you he will only take five minutes of the doctor's time.

From past experience, you know that five minutes is not realistic. Dr. Plunkett has told you not to accept additional appointments today. The sales representative is very insistent.

Jot down some suggestions on how you would handle the situation.

**Assignment 2.4**

For this assignment, refer to Illustration 2.2 to complete an appointment schedule. Use the same style of form (i.e., manual system) from the Working Papers (pp. 6–9).

a.  The following appointments have been scheduled and entered in your book. Copy them from Illustration 2.2.

Dr. Plunkett and his wife have a dinner engagement at 1700.

The president of the Downtown Kinsmen Club has asked Dr. Plunkett to speak to the Kinsmen Lunch Bunch at 1200 (Dr. Plunkett agreed).

Dr. Jones, a vascular surgeon, is performing a bypass and graft for hemodialysis (synthetic) on Gary Green and has asked Dr. Plunkett to assist. Surgery will take approximately 2½ hours beginning at 0900 in O.R. 6 at St. Joseph's Hospital. (Note: When a physician is asked to assist in surgery, the surgeon's office administrator will call the physician's office administrator and advise the time, date, place, type of surgery, patient's name, and approximately length of time for surgery.)

Erik Shultz is "at the end of his rope" with his wife's drinking and needs to talk to the doctor immediately. (Note: Erik works from 0900 to 1900 and finds it difficult to arrange time off work. You feel there is some urgency in this situation. Since Dr. Plunkett usually comes into the office early in the morning, you book Erik in before Dr. Plunkett's scheduled surgery time. You discuss this with the doctor and he agrees.)

Elizabeth Green has requested an appointment for her annual health exam.

Tim Peters has a large boil on his forearm.

b.  Complete the appointment schedule by entering the following appointments, allowing appropriate time periods.

Thomas Bell (427-5327) and Heather Smith (576-3225) have requested appointments for complete physicals.

Jean Belliveau and Mary Jane Brown have requested a premarital consultation and physicals. Mary Jane is a regular patient (427-3333) and her fiancé has requested that Dr. Plunkett consider him as a patient.

Hazel Davis (427-7006) is coming in for her monthly O.B. checkup.

There is a flu epidemic and the following patients are coming in with temperatures, sore throats, and congestion: Peter John Scott (427-2245), Mel Thompson (427-5432), Amelia Jackson (748-3192), Bob Baxter (652-3179), and Lisa Basciano (742-2717).

Lois Elliott (748-3355) is coming in to have a dressing changed.

At 1 P.M. you receive a call from Mrs. Harris, whose four-month-old baby, William, has been crying and upset all morning. He is screaming in obvious pain and Mrs. Harris is very upset. What will you do?

## Daily Schedule

Many doctors prefer to have their administrative assistants produce a daily appointment schedule to have on their desks. In this way they know what patients are to be seen that day. The schedule might be formatted as follows:

DR. PLUNKETT
APPOINTMENTS FOR JANUARY 23, 19__

Morning

| | |
|---|---|
| 0900 – 1130 | Assist Dr. Jones in surgery — Gary Green — bypass |
| 1200 – 1300 | Speaking engagement — Kinsmen Lunch Bunch — Holiday Inn, Green Room |

Afternoon

| | |
|---|---|
| 1300 – 1315 | Hazel Davis, O.B. checkup |

Complete the daily schedule from your solution for Assignment 2.4.

You can use your creativity to set up a daily schedule. You may want to tabulate the time, patient's name, and reason for visit. Perhaps you would double space for readability.

**Assignment 2.5**

## 24-Hour Clock

You will notice in the appointment example that times are written in a style that is different from the norm. In the medical environment, many areas use a 24-hour schedule to identify time.

Rather than divide the day into two sections (morning and afternoon), the schedule begins at one minute after midnight and proceeds cumulatively through to midnight. At one minute after midnight, the time is written 0001 and referred to as 0-0-0-1 (pronouncing O rather than saying zero). One o'clock in the morning is written 0100 and spoken as O one hundred hours rather than 1 A.M. Twelve noon is written 1200 and spoken as twelve hundred hours. After noon hour, the time does not begin at one again but continues to be cumulative. Therefore, 1 P.M. would be written as 1300 and spoken as thirteen hundred hours, 5 P.M. would be written as 1700 and spoken as seventeen hundred hours, and so on (see Illustration 2.6).

**Illustration 2.6   Example of a 24-Hour Clock**

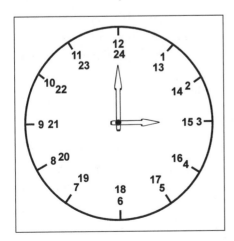

**Assignment 2.6**

Choose an appropriate scheduling system and prepare an appointment schedule (Working Papers, pp. 6–11) for the following patients. Use today's date. The doctor will see patients from 9 A.M. to 6 P.M. with lunch from 12 to 1:30.

Rosie Smythe (236-7712) has a boil on her arm.

Sara Downs (471-3327) is becoming drug dependent and requests some counselling.

Gary Groves (236-8717) has been experiencing severe dizziness when he stands up and lies down.

Annabell Ford (236-3131) has an excruciating pain in her left thigh.

George Arthur (471-3728) has large sores in his mouth.

Ryan Elder (471-3515) has oozing sores on both ankles. He thinks it might be poison ivy.

Deanna Duggan (236-4131) has had intermittent chest pains over the past few days. The pain radiates into her neck and right shoulder blade.

Brad Nichols (471-3112) is experiencing tightness in his chest and his heartbeat races periodically.

James Noris (236-3449) has a bunion on his left toe; it is causing severe discomfort.

Walter Page (471-9952) is very uncomfortable because of constipation.

Janie Packer (471-8987) has several warts on her fingers.

Chuck Leahy (236-3577) has just been fired from his job and is very depressed.

Bunni Rill (471-8338) has had a cold; she now has a fever and is having trouble getting her breath.

Kendra Hall (236-1122) is experiencing severe pain in her lower back that radiates into her left leg.

Mohamed Nasir (471-8772) is booked to have stitches removed from a laceration on his right hand.

Sue Jessup (471-5567) has a broken wrist — her cast is getting loose — she is booked for a new cast.

Cheryl Page (236-3396) has had diarrhea for almost two weeks.

Diane Stevens (236-4747) is having hot flashes and experiences occasional periods of depression.

Jack Porter (236-3991) has a cloudy film over his left eye.

John Bard (471-9988) needs to have his blood pressure checked.

Harry Duffell (236-9991) has had pains in his stomach, some blood in his stool.

Ted Lang (236-6667) needs an allergy shot.

Harold Topper (236-1112) has severe laryngitis.

**Assignment 2.7**

Your instructor will provide you with information to complete an appointment schedule for Dr. Plunkett. This assignment will be submitted for assessment.

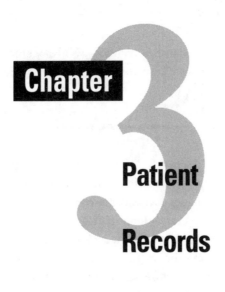

# Chapter 3

## Patient

## Records

## Management

**Chapter Outline**

- Assignment 3.1
- Assignment 3.2
- Assignment 3.3

**Learning Objectives**

To outline
- the current status of technological advancements with respect to patient files
- the procedure for preparing patient file folders (charts)
- rules for alphabetical filing
- general correspondence filing, subject and tickler filing, preparing correspondence for filing, charge-out systems, and updating files
- the purpose of colour-coding files
- points to follow for efficient filing procedures

With the advent of the computer came many progressive records management software systems. This eliminated the need for numerous file cabinets and the process of manual filing. At the time of publication, however, many medical environments dealing with patient information (private practices, hospitals) are still using manual filing systems. The reason for this is mainly the cost of the massive computer storage requirements for recording patient histories and test results, as well as government legislation (for example, the Public Hospitals Act) that requires the retention of a hard copy for all patient reports. Progress is being made in this area and facilities are moving toward or have implemented networked systems, optical disk storage, and/or voice recognition. Some facilities have been more progressive than others in the move toward an electronic record system.

## Assignment 3.1

In order to determine the status of technology advancement in your community, research this topic with your local health care facilities. Your instructor will direct this project.

---

In this chapter we will discuss the importance of good filing procedures, the typical patient file or chart, the most common filing system (alphabetical) used in private practice, the tickler file, and the charging-out of files.

The patient's chart is a legal document, and maintenance of this record is extremely important. Information concerning transferring of files, release of information from files, and the length of time files must be retained is covered in a later chapter. Medical records management in a hospital setting will also be discussed in Chapter 11.

The doctor generally maintains a personal file folder (chart) for each patient. The folders are usually filed in alphabetical order and colour-coded for easy reference.

Since files are the backbone of the physician's practice, the administrative assistant must be precise when handling the files. Here are a few important things to keep in mind when you are handling files:

1. A lost file could cause a disaster — be very careful to accurately file all documents. When files have been removed, be sure you promptly return them to their proper place when they are no longer needed.
2. Do not leave files in open view of others in the office — remember confidentiality. If you leave your desk, even for a moment, cover the files or turn them face down.
3. When colour-coding is used, a periodic scan for misplaced files is quick and ensures that each chart is in the correct location.
4. Be sure to put all relevant material in the correct patient's file.

Each doctor has preferences for the set-up of individual patient files. The outside and/or inside cover of the file folder can be utilized to provide patient information, thereby saving time when looking up patient details. (A rubber stamp can be designed and ordered to suit the physician's requirements or a computerized label maker may be used — see Illustration 3.1.)

**Illustration 3.1   Rubber Stamp/Label Format**

| | |
|---|---|
| NAME _____ | D.O.B. _____ |
| HEALTH CARD # _____ | VERSION CODE _____ |
| PHONE # (HOME) _____ | WORK _____ |
| ALLERGIES _____ | |
| EMERGENCY CONTACT _____ | |

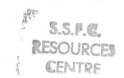

Patient allergies may be written in red pen, or a coloured sticker may be placed beside the word "allergies" in order to alert the doctor that a patient has allergies. Each page that is added to the patient's history should also include an allergy notation.

In Quebec, patient charts must include a woman's maiden name — Mary Jane Belliveau (Brown).

A typical file may include:

1. A family medicine chart (see Illustration 3.10) of information giving all the details about the patient's past history up to the most recent illness. (This sheet should have the patient's medical billing number displayed at the top.)
2. Other relevant forms the doctor requires (for example, infant and child progress record forms [see Illustrations 3.11 and 3.12], results of tests, X-rays, and so on). These forms should be filed after the family medicine chart.
3. Correspondence, which would be filed behind all pertinent medical information.
4. Special notations regarding allergies, medications, or serious illnesses may be made on a form and attached to the left inside cover of the folder so that they will be immediately noticeable.

Items (1), (2), and (3) would be filed on the right side of the folder with the history sheet on top, followed by reports in date order and then correspondence in date order.

Small requisition forms such as biochemistry (Illustrations AB.1, AB.2, and AB.3) and urinalysis (Illustration 11.23) should be taped or stapled to a full-size (8½ inch × 11 inch) sheet of paper in order to avoid misplacement. All records concerning a specific illness may be stapled together. Paper clips are not recommended because papers can pull away from the clip and become mixed with unrelated documents, or the clip may catch onto other documents.

## Cabinets

The most popular types of file cabinets used in medical offices are the four- or five-drawer upright steel cabinets and the open-shelf file cabinets. "Hang-a-file" systems are often used for easy access to each file. Although open-shelf files save floor space and provide quicker access than drawer-type cabinets, their one drawback is that they are not fireproof. The five-drawer cabinet unit will hold approximately 720 files and the open-shelf unit with seven 90-cm (36-inch) shelves will hold approximately 1000 files. A lock is essential on any type of medical record holder in order to maintain confidentiality.

## Folders

Letter-size manila file folders with ⅕, ½, or full cut tabs are generally used. The tab is the projection at the top or side of the folder. Fifth and half cuts would appear in a file drawer as shown in Illustrations 3.2 and 3.3.

**Illustration 3.2    ⅕ Cut Folders**

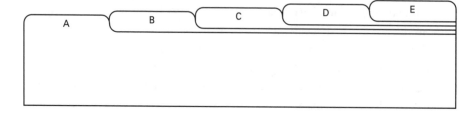

**Illustration 3.3    ½ Cut Folders**

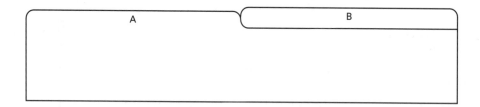

## General Rules for Alphabetical Filing

The following general rules should be applied when filing patient file folders:

1. A person's name is divided into separate indexing units, using the surname as the first unit, first given name as the second unit, and so on.

| Unit 1 | Unit 2 | Unit 3 |
|---|---|---|
| BASCIANO | Lisa | |
| BAXTER | Robert | T. |
| ★BELL | Thomas | William |
| BELLIVEAU | Jean | Etienne |
| BROWN | Mary | Jane |

★When identical names occur, the next consideration may be town or city, province, followed by street address. For example, Thomas Bell, 175 Park Street, Ottawa; Thomas Bell, 134 King Street, Ottawa; and Thomas Bell, 283 King Street, Ottawa, would be indexed as follows:

| Unit 1 | Unit 2 | Unit 3 | Unit 4 | Unit 5 |
|---|---|---|---|---|
| BELL | Thomas | Ottawa | King Street | 134 |
| BELL | Thomas | Ottawa | King Street | 283 |
| BELL | Thomas | Ottawa | Park Street | 175 |

In some medical offices, when identical names occur, the next consideration may be date of birth.

2. Always remember the rule "nothing before something" when considering *all* alphabetizing; for example, N & S would precede Nothing & Something.

3. Surname prefixes and hyphenated names are considered to be one indexing unit; for example, St. John, MacDonald, and MacKenzie-King would all be indexed under Unit 1.

4. Abbreviated names should be considered in full; for example, Jas. is James, Chas. is Charles, and Wm. is William.

5. Titles and degrees such as Dr. or M.D. are not considered when indexing names.

6. When filing correspondence for medical facilities and other businesses, names are filed as they are written (introductory and connecting words such as "the," "and," and "A" are not considered when indexing. If a business name consists of a person's given name and surname, follow rule 1.

| Unit 1 | Unit 2 | Unit 3 |
|--------|--------|--------|
| Arbrook | Industries | |
| Ottawa | General | Hospital |
| Parke (&) | Davis | |
| Parker | James | Limited |

7. When a name consists of a title and either a given name or a surname, do not transpose the name; make the title an indexing unit:

| Unit 1 | Unit 2 |
|--------|--------|
| Reverend | Mulhaney |
| Sister | Veronica |

| Unit 1 | Unit 2 |
|--------|--------|
| Mulhaney | Robert (Rev.) |
| O'Neill | Veronica (Sister) |

## General Correspondence

A doctor's private practice is classified as a small business. As a result, you will be dealing with records other than patient charts. Some general correspondence files would be kept separate from patient charts. Examples of files your general correspondence requirements may include are:

Drug suppliers
Travel agents
Building and equipment maintenance
Insurance companies
Utilities, heat, and telephone
Office supplies
Medical supply companies

You may choose to file your general correspondence alphabetically, or you may use a subject filing system.

## Subject Filing

In a subject filing system, the main subject (for example, drug suppliers) is typed on the divider tab and all drug suppliers' files are placed in alphabetical order in the drug suppliers' section. The main sections are also filed in alphabetical order.

The order of your general correspondence file system would appear as follows:

BUILDING AND EQUIPMENT MAINTENANCE — Main Subject Index

> Adams Carpentry Service
> Brintnell General Maintenance ⎫ Subsidiary Files
> Dynamic Maid Service ⎭

DRUG SUPPLIERS
> Best Buy Drugs
> Medicare Drug Company
> Zanzibar Clinical Supplies

INSURANCE COMPANIES
> Component Property Insurance
> Friendly Automobile Insurance
> Jackson Life Insurance

TRAVEL AGENCIES
> Fly Safe Travellers
> Plan-a-Trip Agencies
> Quiet Vacations Limited

UTILITIES, HEAT, AND TELEPHONE
> Bell Canada
> Public Utilities Ltd.
> Research Gas Company

## Numeric Filing

Hospitals and large group practices generally use a numeric filing system. Doctors may choose to file by number for reasons of confidentiality. Each patient chart is assigned a special number and filed in numeric order. A cross-reference file is required where the patients' names are listed with their assigned numbers and filed in alphabetical order. The cross-reference system may be on cards (see Illustration 3.4), on paper, or stored in a computer.

**Illustration 3.4 Cross-Reference File**

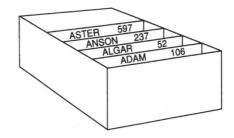

## Soundex Filing

Soundex filing is generally used to overcome the problem of names that sound similar but are spelled many different ways, for example, Bare, Bear, Baher, and Bayer. The soundex system incorporates six basic phonetic sounds with coded numbers. Although not widely used, it is efficient and allows for rapid filing. Because it is fairly complex, it will not be discussed further in this text.

## Tickler File

Every efficient medical administrative assistant has some type of reminder system. In a busy medical office, it is impossible to remember all the details for efficient patient health care. A reminder system is often referred to as a "tickler file," because the system is designed to "tickle" your memory. There are several ways to implement a tickler system. You may choose simply to record reminder notes on your daily calendar and asterisk them with a red pen. A more complex system is to have a small file box with twelve divisions for each month of the year. A subdivider for each day of the month is placed behind the month divider. Reminders are recorded on cards and placed behind the appropriate month/day division.

If you have a calendar messaging system on your computer, you could use it to "tickle" your memory.

It is important to refer to your tickler file each day, as soon after your arrival in the office as possible.

## Filing Preparation

Offices use various methods to prepare documents for filing. Some routines include:

1. Indicating by a code number, check mark, or other means that action, as required by the document, has been taken and it is ready for filing.
2. Using a coding system to indicate where the material is to be filed; e.g., John T. Parker — this indicates the document will be filed as PARKER, JOHN T.
3. Preparing a cross-reference page to be filed with material that may be filed under a different heading. Cross-reference sheets should be coloured (for easy identification) and lightweight (to conserve space). Here are some situations that would require cross-referencing:

a. When names sound the same but are spelled differently; e.g., Thompson and Thomson.

b. When it is difficult to distinguish between a given name and surname; e.g., Lloyd George (George is the surname).

c. When a woman retains her maiden name after marriage and you want to have a cross-reference to her husband's name.

4. Sorting all material in preparation for filing. The documents to be filed are sorted in the order (alphabetical, numerical, by subject) of the system that is being used. This procedure generally takes place on a desk or by means of a collating rack. The sorted documents are then taken to the file area for quick and easy insertion into the appropriate file folders.

## Charge-Out Systems

If a file is removed, an "out" card may be inserted in its place (see Illustration 3.5). The card is generally made of heavy coloured cardboard and has lines on which to write the date of removal, the name of the person who has removed the file, and its present location. However, it would be very time consuming for a medical administrative assistant to "charge-out" the files of patients visiting the office each day. So, for regular patient visits, you would not insert an "out" card in place of the patient's file because it should either be on your desk or with the doctor. Removal of a patient's chart from the files for any other reason, however, would require a "charge-out."

Some offices may use a computerized chart location system to eliminate the need for a manual charge-out system.

**Illustration 3.5   Charge-Out Card**

| FILE LOCATION | | | | |
|---|---|---|---|---|
| Date Removed | By | Can Be Found | Date Returned | Initial When Ret. |
| Dec. 20/94 | Jane Smith | In Business Office | Dec. 23/94 | J.S. |
| Jan 11/95 | Dr. Plunkett | My Desk | Jan 15/95 | JEP |
| Mar. 18/95 | Dr. Pelham | at my home | Mar. 22/95 | C.J.P. |
| | | | | |
| | | | | |
| | | | | |
| | | | | |
| | | | | |
| | | | | |
| | | | | |

## Purging Files

In order to maintain an efficient filing system, it is necessary to perform periodic purging of your records. This task may be done when the physician is absent from the office and your workload is not as heavy as usual. Files of patients who have moved out of town, have transferred to another physician, or are deceased would be removed from your active files and stored as inactive files in a storage area. (Note: An accurate and current list of stored files and their location must be maintained.)

It is important that you scan your files regularly in order to detect any charts or folders that may have been misfiled. It is often necessary to secure patient information on a moment's notice; misfiled charts may result in serious problems.

## Colour-Coded Files

The use of colour-coded files is a very efficient system for identifying file folders and is used extensively in the medical environment. It is easy to find misplaced files in a colour-coded system: if a purple label is mixed in with the red labels, it is easily spotted. Colour-coding also makes filing records faster and easier.

There are many colour-coding systems produced by office supply companies. They consist of adhesive coloured tabs, with each colour stamped with a letter of the alphabet. However, if these tabs are not affordable, file folders may be colour-coded with coloured pencils or coloured file labels. The first two letters of the last name are identified with colours. For example, if your colour-coded system stipulated that the letter "A" would be red, the letter "G" would be blue, and the letter "U" would be pink, then the folder for "Agar" would have a red tab and a blue tab, and the folder for "Austin" would have a red tab and a pink tab. The folder tab would still have the full name typed on it, last name first.

## Suggestions for Efficient Filing

1. File *behind* the guides. This is common practice because it is more efficient.
2. The miscellaneous folder is placed behind its matching primary guide and is the last folder before the next primary guide. For example, the miscellaneous folder for accounting documents would be filed as the last folder in the "accounting" section. That section's primary guide is the divider at the beginning of the section labelled "accounting."
3. Five items for one firm or customer are the maximum that should collect in a miscellaneous file. Miscellaneous files are not usually used in a patient file system. However, the doctor would have miscellaneous files in his or her business files.
4. Letters and other material in individual folders should be arranged in order of date, the most recent at the front. Generally, you are dealing with current information, and using this system allows easier access.

5. Allow four to five inches of working space in drawers to prevent jamming and tearing material.

6. When removing folders from the file, always grasp them by the side or centre, never by the tab. When filing or removing papers, lift up the folders part way and rest them on the side of the drawer to avoid inserting papers between folders.

7. All headings of papers should be to the left as you face the file to facilitate correct placement and easy finding.

8. In order to prevent injuries to staff, it is important that you keep all file drawers closed when not in use.

9. To locate misplaced files, charts, or documents:
   a.  Look immediately in front of and behind the place of the file folder — materials may not have been put in the folder.
   b.  Look under names that have similar spelling or that sound alike.

## Assignment 3.2

For this assignment you will be required to purchase sixteen file folders.

Prepare file folders using the information found on the patient information forms (Illustrations 3.6 and 3.7). Use age, birthday, and current year to calculate each patient's year of birth. Code the folders using coloured pencils and the following colour key (see Illustration 3.8). Also prepare a miscellaneous folder for documents that do not pertain to your regular patient files.

| | |
|---|---|
| A = red | J = dark blue |
| B = light green | L = gold |
| C = light blue | M = dark green |
| D = orange | P = mauve |
| E = yellow | R = purple |
| G = black | S = pink |
| H = brown | T = tan |

Blank stamp forms (as shown in Illustration 3.1) are included in the Working Papers (pp. 12–15) and can be pasted on the front of each file folder. Alternatively, you can type the stamp form directly onto each file folder, or your instructor may have an ink stamp prepared for this assignment.

Print the patient's name (or place a file folder label with the name) on the tab of the folder, last name first in capitals, for example, BASCIANO, Lisa. Insert a family medicine chart and a record form for allergies and medications in the appropriate place in each file. These, and any other forms your instructor wishes inserted in the file, will be provided. Extra forms are available in the Working Papers, pp. 16–23. Samples of these forms include a patient information form (Illustration 3.6), prescription record (Illustration 3.9), family medicine chart (Illustration 3.10), infant progress record (Illustration 3.11), and child progress record (Illustration 3.12). It is your responsibility to file all information pertaining to each patient in the appropriate folder and in the order indicated in this chapter.

**Illustration 3.6   Patient Information Form**

---

PATIENT INFORMATION

(Please Print Clearly)                    Date _____

NAME _____ AGE _____ SEX _____

ADDRESS _____

CITY _____ PROV. _____ CODE _____

_____ ☐ Mar.   ☐ Sing.   ☐ Wid.   ☐ Div.
Date of Birth

PHONE: Home _____ Work _____

EMPLOYED BY _____

CITY _____ PROV. _____

OCCUPATION _____

SPOUSE'S NAME _____

EMPLOYED BY _____

CITY _____ PROV. _____

PHONE _____ OCCUPATION _____

REFERRED BY _____

---

HEALTH CARD NO. _____ VERSION CODE _____

ALLERGIES _____

SERIOUS ILLNESS _____

EMERGENCY CONTACT _____ _____ _____
                        Name              Relation          Phone

**Illustration 3.7    Patient Information Forms**

### Form 1 (Robert Baxter)

PATIENT INFORMATION

(Please Print Clearly)                           Date _July 30 -_

NAME _Robert (Bob) Baxter_    AGE _37_    SEX _M_

ADDRESS _24 Stapleton Road_

CITY _Manotick_    PROV. _Ont_    CODE _K6Y 3T7_

Date of Birth _Oct 7_    ☑ Mar.  ☐ Sing.  ☐ Wid.  ☐ Div.

PHONE: Home _652-3179_    Work _652-6643_

EMPLOYED BY _Town of Manotick_

CITY _Manotick_    PROV. _Ont_

OCCUPATION _Township Clerk_

SPOUSE'S NAME _Sylvia_

EMPLOYED BY _Self_

CITY _Ottawa_    PROV. _Ont_

PHONE _652-6643_    OCCUPATION _Boutique Owner_

REFERRED BY _____

HEALTH CARD NO. _4892608532_    VERSION CODE _____

ALLERGIES _____

SERIOUS ILLNESS _____

EMERGENCY CONTACT _Sylvia_    _Wife_    _652-6643_
                    Name      Relation      Phone

### Form 2 (Lisa Basciano)

PATIENT INFORMATION

(Please Print Clearly)                           Date _Aug. 31, 19 -_

NAME _Lisa Basciano_    AGE _42_    SEX _F_

ADDRESS _2796 Waycross Cres._

CITY _Ottawa_    PROV. _Ont._    CODE _J7X 2X9_

Date of Birth _Nov. 19_    ☑ Mar.  ☐ Sing.  ☐ Wid.  ☐ Div.

PHONE: Home _742-2717_    Work _743-7776_

EMPLOYED BY _Government of Canada_

CITY _Ottawa_    PROV. _Ont._

OCCUPATION _Accountant_

SPOUSE'S NAME _Dino_

EMPLOYED BY _Government of Canada_

CITY _Ottawa_    PROV. _Ont._

PHONE _743-7776_    OCCUPATION _M.P._

REFERRED BY _____

HEALTH CARD NO. _2719278836_    VERSION CODE _____

ALLERGIES _____

SERIOUS ILLNESS _Rheumatoid Arthritis_

EMERGENCY CONTACT _Dino_    _Husband_    _243-7776_
                    Name      Relation      Phone

**Illustration 3.7　Patient Information Forms (continued)**

## PATIENT INFORMATION

Date **June 23, 19-**

(Please Print Clearly)

NAME **Melville Thompson**　AGE **75**　SEX **M**

ADDRESS **22 Edward Road**

CITY **Ottawa**　PROV. **Ont**　CODE **J7X 2t6**

Date of Birth **Nov. 8**　[✓] Mar.　[ ] Sing.　[ ] Wid.　[ ] Div.

PHONE: Home **427-5432**　Work _____

EMPLOYED BY **Retired**

CITY _____　PROV. _____

OCCUPATION _____

SPOUSE'S NAME **Laura**

EMPLOYED BY _____

CITY _____　PROV. _____

PHONE _____　OCCUPATION _____

REFERRED BY _____

HEALTH CARD NO. **6448417672**　VERSION CODE _____

ALLERGIES _____

SERIOUS ILLNESS **Emphysema**

EMERGENCY CONTACT **Laura** Name　**wife** Relation　**427-5432** Phone

## PATIENT INFORMATION

Date **JULY 12, 19-**

(Please Print Clearly)

NAME **AMELIA JACKSON**　AGE **57**　SEX **F**

ADDRESS **13 CROSS ST.**

CITY **KEMPTVILLE**　PROV. **ONT**　CODE **KON 2L0**

Date of Birth **APR. 29**　[ ] Mar.　[ ] Sing.　[ ] Wid.　[✓] Div.

PHONE: Home **748-3192**　Work **748-5532**

EMPLOYED BY **KEMP HOSPITAL**

CITY **KEMPTVILLE**　PROV. **ONT**

OCCUPATION **NURSE**

SPOUSE'S NAME _____

EMPLOYED BY _____

CITY _____　PROV. _____

PHONE _____　OCCUPATION _____

REFERRED BY **DR. JAMES**

HEALTH CARD NO. **8806773712**　VERSION CODE _____

ALLERGIES _____

SERIOUS ILLNESS _____

EMERGENCY CONTACT **STEVEN** Name　**SON** Relation　**427-0098** Phone

**Illustration 3.7    Patient Information Forms (continued)**

---

**PATIENT INFORMATION**

(Please Print Clearly)                Date  April 12, 19—

NAME  Hazel Davis    AGE  30    SEX  F

ADDRESS  539 Cherryhill Lane

CITY  Ottawa    PROV.  Ont.    CODE  K0W 3S5

Feb 2.    ☑ Mar.  ☐ Sing.  ☐ Wid.  ☐ Div.
Date of Birth

PHONE: Home  427-7006    Work  —

EMPLOYED BY _____    PROV. _____

CITY _____    —

OCCUPATION  —

SPOUSE'S NAME  Brent

EMPLOYED BY  Ottawa College

CITY  Ottawa    PROV.  Ont.

PHONE  426-0001    OCCUPATION  Maint. Mech.

REFERRED BY _____

HEALTH CARD NO.  178 105 0552    VERSION CODE _____

ALLERGIES  —

SERIOUS ILLNESS  —

EMERGENCY CONTACT  Brent    Husband    426-0001
                    Name    Relation    Phone

---

**PATIENT INFORMATION**

(Please Print Clearly)                Date  March 12, 19—

NAME  Mary Jane Brown    AGE  21    SEX  F

ADDRESS  731 Hampole St.

CITY  Ottawa    PROV.  Ont.    CODE  J8X 4X9

Jan. 1    ☐ Mar.  ☐ Sing.  ☑ Wid.  ☐ Div.
Date of Birth

PHONE: Home  427-3333    School  427-5566
                          Work

EMPLOYED BY _____    PROV. _____

CITY _____

OCCUPATION  Student

SPOUSE'S NAME _____

EMPLOYED BY _____

CITY _____    PROV. _____

PHONE _____    OCCUPATION _____

REFERRED BY _____

HEALTH CARD NO.  3820703795    VERSION CODE _____

ALLERGIES  Sulpha, Aspirin

SERIOUS ILLNESS  —

EMERGENCY CONTACT  Bert    Father    Work 456-9321
                    Name    Relation    Phone

**Illustration 3.7    Patient Information Forms (continued)**

## PATIENT INFORMATION

(Please Print Clearly)

Date _MARCH 11, 19 —_

NAME _BELLIVEAU, JEAN_    AGE _22_    SEX _M_

ADDRESS _729 UPPERHILL DRIVE_

CITY _OTTAWA_    PROV. _ONT._    CODE _J8Z 4X7_

_DECEMBER 26_    ☐ Mar.    ☑ Sing.    ☐ Wid.    ☐ Div.
Date of Birth

PHONE: Home _427-3899_    School _427-9987_    ~~Work~~

EMPLOYED BY _____

CITY _____    PROV. _____

OCCUPATION _STUDENT_

SPOUSE'S NAME _____

EMPLOYED BY _____

CITY _____    PROV. _____

PHONE _____    OCCUPATION _____

REFERRED BY _____

HEALTH CARD NO. _691 004 7635_    VERSION CODE _____

ALLERGIES _____

SERIOUS ILLNESS _____

EMERGENCY CONTACT _BARB_    _MOTHER_    _427-3665_
                   Name      Relation    Phone

---

## PATIENT INFORMATION

(Please Print Clearly)

Date _Feb 13, 19 —_

NAME _HEATHER SMITH_    AGE _18_    SEX _F_

ADDRESS _BEAVER CRES._

CITY _MANOTICK_    PROV. _ONT_    CODE _K6Y 3T7_

_APRIL 4_    ☐ Mar.    ☑ Sing.    ☐ Wid.    ☐ Div.
Date of Birth

PHONE: Home _576-3225_    Work _____

EMPLOYED BY _GOVERNMENT OF CANADA_

CITY _OTTAWA_    PROV. _ONT_

OCCUPATION _FILE CLERK_

SPOUSE'S NAME _____

EMPLOYED BY _____

CITY _____    PROV. _____

PHONE _____    OCCUPATION _____

REFERRED BY _DR. JOHNSTON_

HEALTH CARD NO. _908 182 038_    VERSION CODE _____

ALLERGIES _____

SERIOUS ILLNESS _____

EMERGENCY CONTACT _CHRISTINE_    _MOTHER_    _576-3225_
                   Name          Relation    Phone

**Illustration 3.7 Patient Information Forms (continued)**

## PATIENT INFORMATION

(Please Print Clearly)

Date June 18, 19—

NAME Peter John Scott AGE 14 SEX M

ADDRESS 16 Binn St.

CITY Ottawa PROV. Ont. CODE J7X 2X6

Aug. 18 — Mar. ☐ Sing. ☑ Wid. ☐ Div. ☐
Date of Birth

PHONE: Home 427-2245 Work

EMPLOYED BY

CITY PROV.

OCCUPATION

SPOUSE'S NAME

EMPLOYED BY

CITY PROV.

PHONE OCCUPATION

REFERRED BY

HEALTH CARD NO. 9191801099 VERSION CODE

ALLERGIES Morphine

SERIOUS ILLNESS Epilepsy

EMERGENCY CONTACT Glen Father
Name Relation

work 372-7687
Phone

---

## PATIENT INFORMATION

(Please Print Clearly)

Date MAY 3, 19—

NAME ROBERT ERIK SHULTZ AGE 55 SEX M

ADDRESS 17 BOND STREET.

CITY OTTAWA PROV. ONT. CODE J8Z 4H3

MAY 26 — Mar. ☑ Sing. ☐ Wid. ☐ Div. ☐
Date of Birth

PHONE: Home 427-9977 Work 427-3456

EMPLOYED BY TEXTILES LIMITED

CITY PERTH PROV. ONT.

OCCUPATION PERSONNEL DIRECTOR

SPOUSE'S NAME MARY.

EMPLOYED BY

CITY PROV.

PHONE OCCUPATION HOMEMAKER

REFERRED BY

HEALTH CARD NO. 7819749313 VERSION CODE

ALLERGIES

SERIOUS ILLNESS CANCER, RIGHT THIGH —ON CHEM.

EMERGENCY CONTACT MARY WIFE
Name Relation

427-9977
Phone

**Illustration 3.7    Patient Information Forms (continued)**

## PATIENT INFORMATION

(Please Print Clearly)    Date _Sept. 26, 19—_

NAME _LOIS ELLIOTT_    AGE _51_    SEX _F_

ADDRESS _RR3_

CITY _Kars_    PROV. _ONT._    CODE _W9U4W9_

Date of Birth _MARCH 19_    ☐ Mar.  ☐ Sing.  ☑ Wid.  ☐ Div.

PHONE: Home _748-3355_    Work _427-3478_

EMPLOYED BY _GLOUCESTER CLOCK WORKS_

CITY _OTTAWA_    PROV. _ONT._

OCCUPATION _EXECUTIVE SECRETARY_

SPOUSE'S NAME _____

EMPLOYED BY _____

CITY _____    PROV. _____

PHONE _____

REFERRED BY _DR. CARL ROLLINGS_

HEALTH CARD NO. _L954154S092_    VERSION CODE _____

ALLERGIES _____

SERIOUS ILLNESS _____

EMERGENCY CONTACT _LORRAINE_    _DAUGHTER_    _799-5473_
  Name    Relation    Phone

---

## PATIENT INFORMATION

(Please Print Clearly)    Date _OCT 3. 19—_

NAME _TIMOTHY PETERS_    AGE _36_    SEX _M_

ADDRESS _10 LORD ST._

CITY _KEMPTVILLE_    PROV. _ONT._    CODE _KDW 2W_

Date of Birth _JAN 1_    ☑ Mar.  ☐ Sing.  ☐ Wid.  ☐ Div.

PHONE: Home _743-2525_    Work _743-5550_

EMPLOYED BY _SMITH AND SMITH LIMITED_

CITY _OTTAWA_    PROV. _ONT._

OCCUPATION _LABOURER_

SPOUSE'S NAME _KRISTA_

EMPLOYED BY _KEMPTVILLE COLLEGE_

CITY _KEMPTVILLE_    PROV. _ONT._

PHONE _743-7557_    OCCUPATION _TEACHER_

REFERRED BY _____

HEALTH CARD NO. _7031381135_    VERSION CODE _____

ALLERGIES _____

SERIOUS ILLNESS _____

EMERGENCY CONTACT _KRISTA_    _WIFE_    _WORK OR HOME ABOVE_
  Name    Relation    Phone

**Illustration 3.7   Patient Information Forms (continued)**

## PATIENT INFORMATION

(Please Print Clearly)

Date: Jan. 20, 19

NAME: Thomas Bell   AGE: 82   SEX: M

ADDRESS: 321 Adelaide St.   PROV.: Ont.   CODE: J3Z 5X3

CITY: Ottawa   PROV.: Ont.

Date of Birth: Sept. 25   ☑ Mar. ☐ Sing. ☐ Wid. ☐ Div.

PHONE: Home 427-5327   Work 427-3227

EMPLOYED BY: Self

CITY: Ottawa   PROV.: Ont.

OCCUPATION: Free Lance Writer (Retired)

SPOUSE'S NAME: Janet

EMPLOYED BY: —

CITY: _____   PROV.: _____

PHONE: _____   OCCUPATION: House Wife

REFERRED BY: _____

HEALTH CARD NO.: 6875231059   VERSION CODE: _____

ALLERGIES: Penicillin

SERIOUS ILLNESS: _____

EMERGENCY CONTACT: Janet (Name)   Wife (Relation)   427-5327 (Phone)

## PATIENT INFORMATION

(Please Print Clearly)

Date: Jan. 16, 19-

NAME: Elizabeth Green   AGE: 36   SEX: F

ADDRESS: 72 Hillcrest St.   PROV.: Ont.   CODE: J3Z 5X4

CITY: Ottawa   PROV.: Ont.

Date of Birth: Aug. 12   ☑ Mar. ☐ Sing. ☐ Wid. ☐ Div.

PHONE: Home 427-3774   Work _____

EMPLOYED BY: _____

CITY: _____   PROV.: _____

OCCUPATION: _____

SPOUSE'S NAME: Gary

EMPLOYED BY: ABC Deliveries

CITY: Ottawa   PROV.: Ont.

PHONE: 427-4545   OCCUPATION: Manager

REFERRED BY: _____

HEALTH CARD NO.: 3777220777   VERSION CODE: _____

ALLERGIES: Nil

SERIOUS ILLNESS: Hypertension

EMERGENCY CONTACT: Gary (Name)   Husband (Relation)   427-4545 (Phone)

**Illustration 3.7   Patient Information Forms (continued)**

PATIENT INFORMATION

(Please Print Clearly)                    Date __Nov 1, 19—___

NAME __William Harris___ AGE _2 month_ SEX _M_

ADDRESS __362 BlueJay Cres.___

CITY __Ottawa___ PROV. _Ont_ CODE _J7K 2X9_

__Sept. 5___ ☐ Mar. ☑ Sing. ☐ Wid. ☐ Div.
Date of Birth

PHONE: Home __778-2367___ Work _____

EMPLOYED BY _____

CITY _____ PROV. _____

OCCUPATION _____

SPOUSE'S NAME _____

EMPLOYED BY _____

CITY _____ PROV. _____

PHONE _____ OCCUPATION _____

REFERRED BY _____

HEALTH CARD NO. __2722575673___ VERSION CODE _____

ALLERGIES __Sulphas, milk, Penicillin___

SERIOUS ILLNESS _____

EMERGENCY CONTACT __Brad___ __father___ __427-0009___
                    Name        Relation        Phone

**Illustration 3.8    File Folders**

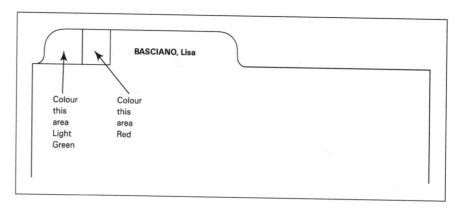

**Illustration 3.9    Prescription Record**

NAME

| # OF PRESCRIPTION | LONG TERM MEDICATION AND TREATMENT | DATE FILLED |
|---|---|---|
| | | |
| | | |
| | | |
| | | |
| | | |
| | | |
| | | |
| | | |
| | | |
| | | |
| | | |
| | | |
| | | |
| | | |
| | | |
| | | |
| | | |
| | | |
| | | |
| | | |

**Illustration 3.10    Family Medicine Chart**

| FAMILY MEDICINE | | | | | | |
|---|---|---|---|---|---|---|
| Name | | | Insurance # | | | S  M  W  D |
| Address | | | Phones (H) | | (O) | |
| Occupation | | | Date of Birth | | | Age |
| Medical Data | HT | WT | BP | PULSE | RESP | TEMP |
| Allergies | | | Drug Allergies | | | |

| DATE | HISTORY & PHYSICAL |
|---|---|
| | |
| | |
| | |
| | |
| | |
| | |
| | |
| | |
| | |
| | |
| | |
| | |
| | |
| | |
| | |
| | |
| | |
| | |
| | |
| | |
| | |
| | |
| | |
| | |
| | |
| | |
| | |
| | |
| | |
| | |
| | |

**Illustration 3.11    Infant Progress Record**

# INFANT PROGRESS RECORD
## 0 – 24 Months

Name _____

Date of Birth _____ Sex M/F

B.Wt. _____ Kg _____ lb. Length _____ cm. Head _____ cm. Chest _____ cm. D.Wt _____ Kg _____ lb.

Maturity _____ wks. Apgar _____ / _____ Blood Gp. _____ Rh _____ P.K.U. _____ Thyroid _____

Problems: Prenatal _____ Labour _____ Neonatal _____

Defects: _____ Marks _____ Circ. _____

Breast until _____ Bottle until _____        Started juice _____ Started solids _____

**Landmarks — 25th Percentile – 90th Percentile in months**

| Motor | Date | Mo |
|---|---|---|
| Prone lifts head 1.3 – 3.2 | | |
| Follows light 1.8 – 4.0 | | |
| Rolls over 2.3 – 4.7 | | |
| Grasps 2.5 – 4.2 | | |
| Reaches out 2.9 – 5.0 | | |
| Sits unsupported 4.8 – 7.8 | | |
| First tooth | | |
| Stands holding 5.0 – 10.0 | | |
| Stands alone 9.8 – 13.9 | | |
| Walks 11.3 – 13.3 | | |
| Kicks ball 15.0 – 24.0 | | |

| Social | Date | Mo |
|---|---|---|
| Blinks to clap | | |
| Smiles back – 1.9 | | |
| Laughs 1.4 – 3.3 | | |
| Sleeps through night 6 + hours | | |
| Turns to voice 3.8 – 8.3 | | |
| Things to mouth | | |
| Feeds self 4.7 – 8.0 | | |
| Says Dada or Mama 5.6 – 10.0 | | |
| Drinks from cup 10.0 – 14.3 | | |
| Uses spoon 13.3 – 23.5 | | |
| Combine 2 words 14 – 23 | | |

DPTp: 1 _____ 2 _____ 3 _____ 4 _____

O.T.T. _____ M.M.R. _____ Reactions _____ Allergies _____

| Months | 1 | 2 | 3 | 4 | 6 | 9 | 12 | 15 | 18 | 24 |
|---|---|---|---|---|---|---|---|---|---|---|
| Date | | | | | | | | | | |
| Wt. kg. | | | | | | | | | | |
| Length/cm. | | | | | | | | | | |
| Head circ. | | | | | | | | | | |
| Heart sounds | | | | | | | | | | |
| Breath sounds | | | | | | | | | | |
| Abdomen | | | | | | | | | | |
| Skin | | | | | | | | | | |
| Legs | | | | | | | | | | |
| Other | Hips | Hearing | PKU | Hips | Babbling | Hb | | | | |

**Illustration 3.12   Child Progress Record**

# CHILD PROGRESS RECORD
## 2 – 15 Years

Name _____

Date of Birth _____ Sex   M/F

INFANT & HEREDITARY PROBLEMS _____

_____

| LANDMARKS 25-90%ile in Yrs. | Date | Age |
|---|---|---|
| Testes Descended | | |
| Clean at night | | |
| Dry at night | | |
| Throws ball 1.4 – 2.6 | | |
| Gives own name 2.0 – 3.8 | | |
| Does up buttons 2.6 – 4.2 | | |
| Recognizes 3 colours 2.7 – 4.9 | | |
| Hops on one foot 3.0 – 4.9 | | |
| Catches ball 3.5 – 5.5 | | |
| Ties shoelaces | | |
| First menstruation | | |
| Voice breaks | | |
| Axillary hair | | |

| ILLNESSES | Date | Age |
|---|---|---|
| Eczema | | |
| Croup | | |
| Bronchitis | | |
| Allergies | | |
| Tonsillitis | | |
| Ear infections | | |
| Pyrexia over 40°C | | |
| Convulsions | | |
| Chicken Pox | | |
| | | |
| | | |
| | | |

**IMMUNIZATIONS:**

**Pre School**
DPTp x 3 + 1 _____
M.M.R. _____
DPTp _____
O.T.T. _____

**10 Years**
DPT _____
O.T.T. _____
Hb _____
Rubella Titre _____

**15 Years**
DPT _____
O.T.T. _____
Hb _____
ASOT _____

| Years/Months | 2 | 3 | 4 | 5 | 6 | 7 | 8 | 9 | 10 | 11 | 12 | 13 | 14 | 15 |
|---|---|---|---|---|---|---|---|---|---|---|---|---|---|---|
| Height cm. | | | | | | | | | | | | | | |
| Height %ile | | | | | | | | | | | | | | |
| Wt. kg. | | | | | | | | | | | | | | |
| Wt. %ile | | | | | | | | | | | | | | |
| Vision   Right | | | | | | | | | | | | | | |
| Left | | | | | | | | | | | | | | |
| Near | | | | | | | | | | | | | | |
| Urine Albumin | | | | | | | | | | | | | | |
| Glucose | | | | | | | | | | | | | | |
| Blood Pressure | | | | | | | | | | | | | | |
| Ears | | | | | | | | | | | | | | |
| Eyes | | | | | | | | | | | | | | |
| Nose | | | | | | | | | | | | | | |
| Throat | | | | | | | | | | | | | | |
| Teeth | | | | | | | | | | | | | | |
| Neck | | | | | | | | | | | | | | |
| Lungs | | | | | | | | | | | | | | |
| Heart sounds | | | | | | | | | | | | | | |
| Abdomen | | | | | | | | | | | | | | |
| Legs | | | | | | | | | | | | | | |
| Back | | | | | | | | | | | | | | |
| Posture | | | | | | | | | | | | | | |
| Other | | | | | | | | | | | | | | |

**PUBERTY STATUS**

**Female**
1. Flat
2. Breast buds
3. Enlargement – Slight raising
4. Separate breast contour

**Male**
1. Infantile
2. Testes enlarging, scrotum & coarse
3. Penis lengthening
4. Penis enlarging, scrotal skin pigmented

**Pubic Hair**
1. None
2. Sparse, downy
3. Pigmented, coarse, curling
4. Adult

**Assignment 3.3**

a. Index the following list of names.
b. Prepare an alphabetized list.

Indexing may be keyed or handwritten. Submit both the indexing exercise and the alphabetized list. For the purposes of this assignment *only*, consider all shortened names to be abbreviations of the full name; for example, Nick would be Nicholas.

Mary Shier-Sorrie
Don Bruce, 156 Park St., Ottawa
Dr. Rob T. Durin
Mrs. John L. Kingston (Rena)
Masie Shierman
Nicholas Maziotti, 223 George St., Virgil, B.C.
Delbert J. McCall
Robbin Durin
Nick Mazzioti, 107 George St., Virgil, N.S.
Jamie Dickens
Connato DiCarlo
Michael Terry Masters
Wm. Ainsworth
John Kingston
Mike T. Masterson
Nicholas Mazziotti, 372 George St., Virgil, Alta.
Wilma Ainsworth
Nick Mazziotti, 315 George St., Virgil, Ontario
Donald Bruce, 101 Park St., Ottawa
D.J. MacCall
Mrs. Donalda Bruce, 96 Park St., Ottawa, Ont.

# Chapter 4

# The Telephone

## Chapter Outline

- Types of Calls
- Answering Services
- The Telephone Directory
- Equipment
- Assignment 4.1
- Assignment 4.2

## Learning Objectives

To learn
- effective telephone usage including answering, screening, holding, and making outgoing calls
- how to handle calls regarding appointments, house calls, prescription requests, and emergencies
- how to use the telephone directory as a reference source
- the types of telephone equipment

The telephone is the link between the physician and the patient. Do not let the phone ring while you finish adding a column of figures or chat with another patient. Answer it immediately (at least within three rings). Your voice should sound pleasant and friendly; identify the doctor's office and then yourself: "Good morning. Dr. Pelham's office, Ann speaking." Then determine if you can accommodate the patient's needs, or answer a question. If not, inform the patient you will speak to the doctor and either you will return the call or have the doctor do so.

If you put a smile on your face, you will put a smile in your voice.

One of the most important aspects of telephone usage in a medical practice is to *record all incoming patient requests and inquiries.* You should have a notebook and pencil beside the telephone at all times. When a patient calls, record the time, date, patient's name and telephone number, and message. After you have noted details of the call, it is good practice to repeat the message to the caller. This ensures that the information is correct. Most offices use message pads similar to that in Illustration 4.1. (Note: If you receive an urgent message, highlighting "urgent" will indicate to the doctor that the message requires immediate attention.)

**Illustration 4.1    Telephone Message**

```
┌─────────────────────────────────────────────────────────┐
│ MESSAGE                                                   │
│                                                           │
│  ┌──────────────────────┬──────────────────────────────┐ │
│  │       (Urgent)       │  Yes ☑    │    No ☐            │ │
│  └──────────────────────┴──────────────────────────────┘ │
│                                                           │
│  To  Dr. Plunkett                                         │
│  Time  10:30 A.M.              Date  Oct. 16, 19 –        │
│  Mrs.  Hazel Davis                                        │
│  of                                                       │
│  Phone no.  427-7006                                      │
│                                                           │
│  ☑ Telephoned            ☑ Please call back               │
│  ☐ Called to see you     ☐ Will call again                │
│  ☐ Returned your call    ☐ Left the following message     │
│                                                           │
│  Is having some low back pain                             │
│  -- wonders if she is starting                            │
│  in labour                                 GG             │
│                                                Operator   │
└─────────────────────────────────────────────────────────┘
```

Computer networks are a part of today's modern offices. If you work in an office where you have the responsibility of answering the telephone, and you have a computer network system in your office, you will no longer have to write telephone messages on paper. Your system will likely be equipped with electronic messaging capabilities. You will call up a preprogrammed message form (see Illustration 4.2) on your screen, key in the details of the call, and forward the message using the computer. The terminal of the message recipient will display the message for perusal.

Be patient and courteous at all times. Remember, the people you are dealing with usually have problems. They are not like customers coming to buy a product. You must be sympathetic and empathetic; let them know you are listening to what they are saying and that you will do whatever is necessary to help. Your voice should be friendly, interested, expressive, calm, and natural. If the patient is in distress, be sympathetic and, most important, be reassuring.

How you listen is also very important. Be sure to get the caller's name and use it during the conversation to show that you are attentive. Do not allow your mind to wander while a patient talks to you. Some patients may want to discuss their problems at length. Because you work in a busy environment, it is important, without being rude, to encourage patients to be specific about their needs. You may say, "Do you wish to make an appointment, Mrs. Davis?"

**Illustration 4.2    Preprogrammed Message**

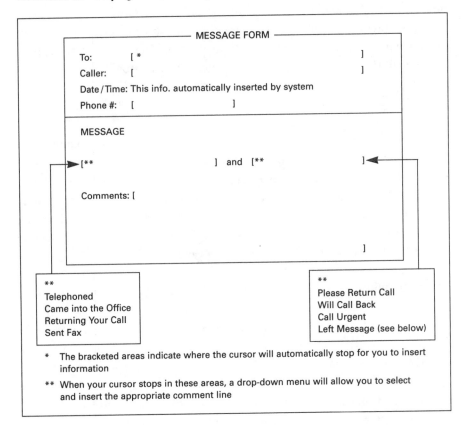

## Screening

You are the barrier between the doctor and interruptive calls. Screen all calls. Do not interrupt the doctor unless absolutely necessary. Be careful not to give the impression that the doctor is never available. If the doctor is with a patient, relate that to the caller. Don't say, "The doctor is busy"; say, "The doctor is with a patient. May I give him a message, or will I have him return your call?" Discuss with your doctor/employer the preferences regarding callback times, and what calls will be accepted during the day.

Many of the phone calls that come into the office can be handled by you without referring to the doctor. However, the Canadian Medical Protective Association recommends that you *do not give any medical advice at any time.*

Patients often explain their symptoms and then ask, "What do you think I should do?" Your only answer is to ask the patient to come in for an appointment or have the patient speak to the doctor. If the doctor is not available, make complete and accurate notes concerning the patient's call; this will save time when the doctor makes the return call.

The administrative assistant should use discretion when relaying test results over the phone. If you receive a call requesting tests results, it is absolutely essential that you know the caller; otherwise ask for the person's name and number and discuss the situation with the doctor. Of course, you should never release any results without checking first with the doctor. If test results indicate medical problems, you should make an appointment for the patient to see the doctor.

Many physicians will not renew prescriptions over the telephone — they will ask you to make an appointment for the patient. In some provinces, pharmacies will take telephone prescriptions from physicians only.

### "Holding" Callers

Do not answer the phone and say, "Dr. Plunkett's office, will you hold please?" and then immediately leave the line. In today's busy office, it is not uncommon to have two or three lines engaged at one time. If another line rings, make certain before you place the caller on hold that it is not an emergency. It is common courtesy to wait for an answer to the "will you hold?" question. If the call is not an emergency, and you cannot handle the call immediately, give the caller a choice of holding or being called back.

### Outgoing Calls

In the course of your working day, you will have many occasions to make calls on behalf of your employer. Ensure that you have all pertinent information organized before placing the call. For example, if you are scheduling a test, have available all the patient's sociological information, as well as the types of tests required, and the days and times the patient is available to have the tests performed. It would be helpful if you had some information about related tests previously performed and the names of the facilities where these tests were administered.

## Types of Calls

### Appointments

Be sure to get all the necessary information in order to book the appointment properly: name, reason for appointment, time frame (how soon if urgent), and best time for the patient. After booking a date and time, repeat this back to the patient and give any further instructions, such as urine sample required or diet restrictions prior to lab tests.

### Prescriptions

If a prescription renewal is required, ask the patient for the name and/or number of the medication and at what pharmacy the prescription was purchased. If this information is not available from the patient, you can refer to the file. Of course, you must record the patient's name; ask for the telephone number as well to save time in case you have to call back.

At a convenient time, prescriptions should be transferred to a separate record. A steno pad is ideal if using a manual system, or you may utilize a computerized database. This information must also be recorded in the patient's file. All drug orders must be kept as part of the physician's records. Ensure that hard copy or backed-up computer files are stored safely and securely.

Before calling the prescription to the pharmacy, *you must always have approval from the doctor.* He or she should place his or her initials beside the entry in your book that lists the patient's name, date of order, medication name and/or number, and name of the pharmacy where the prescription is ordered.

Please note that the above information regarding prescriptions is for your consideration. In today's health care environment, from a risk management and quality care perspective, few physicians will consider renewing prescriptions over the telephone. They prefer to have the patient come into the office for an assessment.

## Cancellations

If a patient calls to cancel an appointment, make a note in the patient's chart and/or on the appointment record. Often the patient will arrange another appointment. If this does not happen, and you feel it is important for the patient to be seen, discuss it with the doctor.

## Ordering Supplies

You will be responsible for keeping sufficient stock of all office supplies. Before calling your supplier, ensure that you have an accurate list of your requirements and follow your telephone order with a formal purchase order.

## Emergencies

You will at times be faced with panic situations or emergencies. Use *common sense* and *keep calm.* First determine if it is a real emergency or just a patient overreacting. Get all the necessary information: the type of emergency, duration, and whether an ambulance is required. Where possible, the ambulance should be arranged by the person calling the doctor's office. If that person is unable to make the call, be sure to get all necessary information, such as location and directions, and call for the ambulance yourself. If you have more than one line, inform the caller that you will put the call on hold and then call the ambulance. After you have the instructions from the ambulance service, go back to the patient and report when the ambulance will arrive. In some areas, dialling 911 will give you immediate access to emergency services.

## Answering Services

There are two types of answering services. One is a separate number (usually listed after the office number in the telephone directory), where messages can be left for after-hours callback. The most common type, however, is a direct connection with the doctor's office telephone so that when a call is made to the office, it is picked up by the answering service.

Answering services can be used after hours, at lunch time, or at peak periods to relieve the administrative assistant. If a service is used, you must check first thing every morning for all messages, and last thing before you leave to advise the service where the doctor may be reached and when the office will be open again. In areas where telephone answering services are not available, many physicians use answering machines.

## The Telephone Directory

Your best reference source is the local telephone directory. Take time to go through it and note the wide variety of information available, not only about telephone services — local areas, long-distance charges, area codes, business hours — but for other available services such as government offices, the yellow pages listings, and so on.

You should also set up your own office telephone directory, listing in it numbers you call frequently such as drug stores, hospitals, laboratories, other doctors, ambulance and emergency services, the Victorian Order of Nurses or other home nursing services, social service/community agencies, and family and close friends (the doctor's — not yours!).

A Cardex or Rolodex system is an efficient way to keep reference information such as referring physicians' names, addresses, identification numbers, and telephone numbers.

If you are using a computer, you can access alphabetized lists of frequently used information with one or two keystrokes.

If you have a speed dial feature on your telephone system, store the most frequently called numbers. Have an index of the stored numbers in a convenient location.

## Equipment

There are several companies that offer sophisticated telephone equipment for business and industry. If you work in a private-practice setting with one or two physicians, you will probably have a telephone system with three or four incoming lines. A hospital, clinic, or medical centre generally employs a receptionist/switchboard operator, and the equipment used in this type of setting is generally a multiline device. The use of voice mail is increasing in popularity and can provide many conveniences related to incoming calls.

Modern telephones are programmed to allow you to do such things as dial a second number if the first number you called is busy; when the number you have called is free, your telephone will ring, at which time you can complete your call. Call waiting, redial, speed dial, caller identification, and call forwarding are other telephone features that assist in the operation of an efficient office.

The following situations are designed for role play. Choose a partner, decide how you would handle the situation, and write the script. If possible, you should have a prop telephone for authenticity. You and your partner will then act out the scene, with one student playing the role of the administrative assistant and the other the role of the patient. The remainder of the class will observe, and a session to evaluate your performance should follow.

**Assignment 4.1**

1. Mrs. Scott calls to inform you that Peter John has just rammed his head into a brick wall while pushing his brother on his bicycle. His head is bleeding profusely, and she thinks the child needs stitches. It is 4:30 P.M., and the doctor has just left to do rounds at the hospital.

2. Mary Shultz, who is extremely inebriated, calls and insists on speaking to the doctor. The office is full of patients, and the doctor is running behind schedule.

3. A woman calls and tells you her husband has locked himself in the bathroom and is threatening suicide. The doctor is out of town at a convention.

4. Thomas Bell calls and tells you his wife has just collapsed on the floor. He thinks she has had a stroke because her mouth seems to be twisted.

5. The doctor has asked you to take all calls because he is having a consultation with a patient who is on the verge of a nervous breakdown. Amelia Jackson calls and insists on speaking to the doctor.

6. Julie Harris calls and is at the point of hysteria. Her son William has a very high temperature and is convulsing. She lives two miles outside the city, her husband has taken the car to work, and she does not know any of the people who live in her neighbourhood. The doctor is not in the office.

7. The doctor's wife is on the phone wishing to speak with her husband. You know that she often calls without good reason, but she insists on speaking with the doctor.

8. Mr. and Mrs. Chang have recently arrived from Korea and their sponsor has asked Dr. Plunkett to take them into his practice. Mrs. Chang calls you to book an appointment; however, she is not fluent in English and you are having trouble understanding her.

9. A new patient (Rosa Geary) called two weeks ago and you booked her for an appointment. She did not come to the office for her appointment. She called the next day with an excuse and you booked her again. Again, she did not arrive for her scheduled appointment. She is now calling with an excuse and a request for another appointment.

10. Lori Brier (a single parent) was injured at work. Dr. Plunkett examined and treated her and sent the required forms to the Workers' Compensation Board. Mrs. Brier calls. She is very anxious. She hasn't any money for rent and groceries. She has called WCB and they have informed her that they haven't received the required documents from her doctor. You tell Mrs. Brier that you have sent the forms, but she doesn't believe you — she NEEDS MONEY NOW!

11. Dr. Plunkett has agreed to cover emergencies for Dr. Moore, who is going on vacation. Dr. Plunkett is doing rounds at the hospital when you receive a call from Tiffany Black, one of Dr. Moore's patients. (You don't know anything of her history.) She tells you she has attempted suicide twice in the past and is considering it again.

12. Gary Brown is schizophrenic and has been receiving treatment in the psychiatric ward of Ottawa Civic Hospital. You received a call from the hospital last week informing you that Gary had left the hospital and had not returned. Today you receive a call from Gary. He is in Florida. He doesn't have any money and he seems very confused.

## Assignment 4.2

Appoint two members of your class to arrange to have a telephone equipment supplier in your area visit your classroom; or you may prefer to arrange a class tour of a telephone equipment supply office.

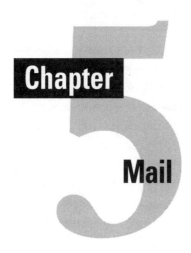

# Chapter 5

## Mail

**Chapter Outline**

- Incoming Mail
- Outgoing Mail
- Postal Services
- Courier Services

- Electronic Equipment
- Assignment 5.1
- Assignment 5.2

**Learning Objectives**

To learn
- how to handle incoming mail
- how to handle outgoing mail
- the varieties of delivery services

One of your responsibilities as administrative assistant will be the handling of both incoming and outgoing mail. It is essential that you become familiar with postal services, delivery services such as couriers, and electronic mailing equipment.

Incoming mail consists of the following:

## Incoming Mail

1. Correspondence (reports from consultants, legal claims, insurance claims)
2. Circulars
3. Magazines and medical journals
4. Medical information (from medical associations)
5. Cheques
6. Health insurance plan documents (supplies, remittance advice information, or medical consultants' inquiries)
7. Confidential mail
8. Laboratory, diagnostic imaging, and consultation reports
9. Hospital reports
10. Advertisements and drug samples

On receipt of the mail, you should open all correspondence with the exception of envelopes specifically marked "confidential" or "personal." If any letters refer to previous correspondence, retrieve the relevant documents from the file and attach. The administrative assistant should date stamp each piece of mail, organize it in order of importance, and place it in the doctor's incoming mail tray.

Prioritizing or sorting should be done according to the importance or urgency with which the information should be handled. For example:

1. Patient information (lab, X-ray, and consultation reports)
2. Correspondence (special delivery or telegrams first)
3. Cheques and health insurance plan information
4. Medical information
5. Drug samples
6. Medical journals, magazines, circulars

All cheques must be stamped "For Deposit Only." (See Illustration 7.7 in Chapter 7.) Magazines (with the exception of the doctor's professional journals) can be placed in the waiting room, and inconsequential unsolicited mail in the wastebasket.

If a return address does not appear on the letter, check the envelope before discarding it.

Loose enclosures should be attached to the appropriate correspondence.

Enclosed cheques should be safely stored and a notation made on the accompanying letter to this effect.

After the doctor has read the mail, documents should be initialled to indicate they have been read and a notation made to indicate what action is required, for example, file, discard, or reply.

## Outgoing Mail

Outgoing mail consists of the following:

1. Doctor's correspondence (replies to requests, doctor's inquiries, information reports)
2. Health insurance plan cards, computer tapes, or diskettes
3. Insurance information forms (Workers' Compensation Board, accident reports)
4. Referral requests
5. Supply requisitions and purchase orders
6. Statements of account ("opted-out" doctors)
7. Files of transferred patients (a photocopy of the complete chart or a résumé dictated by the doctor should be sent "confidential" by courier)

After the document is prepared, it should be appropriately assembled. A general rule of thumb is to place the original and enclosure, if any, on top of all copies together with an envelope. The completed mail pack should then be secured with a paper clip and placed on the doctor's desk for signature. After it has been read and signed, the completed correspondence will be returned to you for mailing.

Remember, it is essential that you retain a *dated copy* of *all* documents. It may be useful to keep general correspondence in a correspondence file or binder. All patient-related documents would be filed in the patient's chart.

Fold and insert documents in the appropriate size envelope and seal. Make sure that if an enclosure is part of the package, you remember to include it before sealing the envelope.

Stamps should be available in the office for regular mail (some larger offices may use a postage meter). Larger packages may require a visit to the post office. If you are in doubt about the mailing of any correspondence, consult your local postal authorities.

Pickup time at the nearest mailbox (or by internal mail in a large organization) should be investigated. It is your responsibility to ensure that urgent mail reaches the box or the internal mail room in time to be collected that day.

## Postal Services

Canada Post offers many types of mail-handling services. Important letters and other documents can be sent "registered" or by Priority Post, which gives overnight delivery; valuable parcels can be "insured"; sealed letters and postcards are sent "first class"; parcels may be sent "parcel post"; "second class" mail is used for some newspapers and periodicals; small parcels and printed matter would be sent "third class." Because Canada Post's services and rates are extensive, and subject to frequent change, we will not elaborate any further. Most administrative assistants, if they are uncertain about the method to use in forwarding material by mail, will consult the local postal authorities.

## Courier Services

To ensure prompt and safe delivery of special letters and parcels, many businesses use courier services. Although using a courier is more expensive than regular mail services, it guarantees prompt delivery — often overnight. Courier services are listed in the yellow pages of the telephone directory. It is important for the efficient administrative assistant to be aware of the cost of courier services and to use them with discretion.

Most communities have intercity courier services that will pick up samples and drugs to be transported between physicians' offices and laboratories and hospitals. Medical administrative assistants should know the names and scope of service of such courier services in their locality. If it is necessary to send samples or drugs by mail, there are specific rules that must be followed. Check with your local postal authorities before placing such materials in the mail.

## Electronic Equipment

Many large businesses have computer networks that allow communication from branch to branch by computer. Letters, memos, and reports are keyed into a computer terminal and sent on-line to branches within the same area, from city to city, or country to country. Messages are relayed in the time it takes to key the information and have it transmitted to the receiving terminal — a matter of minutes.

More and more medical professionals are utilizing computer network systems that allow communication among offices and hospitals.

Most hospitals and doctors' offices are also equipped with, or have access to, fax machines. This technology allows the speedy transmission of such documents as preoperative notes from the doctor's office to the hospital.

The postal service provides an electronic mail (e-mail) service called Telepost, which promises delivery in 24 hours. Intelpost is a similar service provided by Canada Post/Teleglobe Canada/CNCP Telecommunications.

## Assignment 5.1

This assignment is designed as a group project. Choose one of these three delivery services — the post, electronic mail, or courier — and write a report outlining all aspects of the service. Assign specific duties to each student: for example, two students may be responsible for gathering the material, two may be responsible for organizing and writing the information, and one or two may be responsible for keying. Prepare the information in an attractive form and have copies produced for each member of the class. Students responsible for gathering the information will contact a courier service or visit the post office to determine details of regular mail and electronic mail services. Prepare a summary of the service, including points such as the name of the service, how it is provided, where the service extends (intercity/country to country), the cost of the service, preparations necessary before using the service, and so on.

## Assignment 5.2

Research how medical environments in your community handle incoming and outgoing mail, and prepare a report on your findings.

In order to accomplish this, form into groups, develop a simple questionnaire, and distribute it to your target audience.

Don't forget to request information on the current use of mail technology, such as e-mail and fax.

Insert your report in your portfolio.

## Chapter

# 6

# Health

# Insurance Plans

## Chapter Outline

- Introduction
- Eligibility
- Health Card
- Billing Options
- Bill 94
- Provider Registration
- Explanation of Providers' Specialty Codes
- MOH Schedule of Benefits
- Introduction to Claims Submission
- Submission Dates and Payment Dates
- Health Service Claim Cards
- The Billing Process
- Service Codes
- Diagnostic Codes
- Coding Examples
- Supporting Documentation
- Returned Claims
- Remittance Advice
- Remittance Advice Inquiries
- Nonpayment of Claims
- Appeals

- Northern Health Travel Grant
- Visitors from Outside Ontario
- Out-of-Province Benefits
- Machine-Readable Input
- Purchasing Computer Hardware and Software
- Using a Microcomputer System to Submit Claims
- MOH Specifications for Claim Submission
- Source Documentation Requirements
- After the Switch to Diskettes
- Who to Call When Help Is Required
- How the MOH Communicates with Medical Administrative Assistants
- Conclusion
- Assignment 6.1
- Assignment 6.2
- Workers' Compensation
- Making a Claim
- Assignment 6.3
- Third-Party Insurance
- Assignment 6.4

## Learning Objectives

To
- outline eligibility for a health care plan
- explain premium assistance
- list criteria for dependent eligibility
- understand different billing options
- explain the procedure for physician registration and learn the significance of registration number units
- identify specialty codes and the appropriate specialization
- give a basic interpretation of the Schedule of Benefits and knowledge of how to use it
- identify significant parts of a claims card and gain thorough knowledge of its completion, either by regular submission, precoded submission, or both
- identify supporting documentation for specific services

- understand reprocessing of returned claims
- give an interpretation of the remittance advice form
- understand the processing of remittance advice inquiries
- explain nonpayment of claims and appeals
- explain out-of-province claim submissions
- explain out-of-province benefits
- summarize advantages of submitting claims on machine-readable input
- outline considerations for purchasing software and hardware for use in a medical environment
- outline specific procedural benefits of machine-readable input
- outline what to do when you need assistance

Adequate medical care can be very costly, especially for accident victims, the chronically ill, and those needing surgery. In order to minimize these expenses, Canada has instituted a universal health care plan. This protection came about through the enactment of the Medical Care Act, introduced by Prime Minister Lester B. Pearson during the 1966/67 session of Parliament. This Act was replaced by the Canada Health Act of 1984.

Each province has its own government-sponsored plan, for example, Nova Scotia's Medical Services Insurance (MSI) program, British Columbia's Medical Services Plan, the Alberta Health Care Insurance Plan (AHCIP), and Ontario's Ministry of Health Plan.

If you were to read through the brochure that describes the health care plan for each province, you would note that there are minor differences in each plan. Most features — eligibility and enrollment, out-of-province benefits, payment options, and the fact that the plan pays only for *medically necessary* services — are almost identical.

Complete information on processing of claims, physician and subscriber registration, and eligibility can be obtained through your provincial Ministry of Health office.

Illustrations 6.1a, b, and c show examples of billing cards from Nova Scotia, Alberta, and British Columbia. They show that the information required for claim submissions is identical in each province; only the card format is different. Pertinent information required to complete a billing card includes physician identification, patient identification (including registration number), date of service (health number), service and diagnostic fee schedule codes, the admission date, cost of service, and whether or not the patient is hospitalized. If the patient has been referred by another physician, that physician's registration number is also included.

**Illustration 6.1a Nova Scotia Medical Services Insurance (MSI) Billing Card**

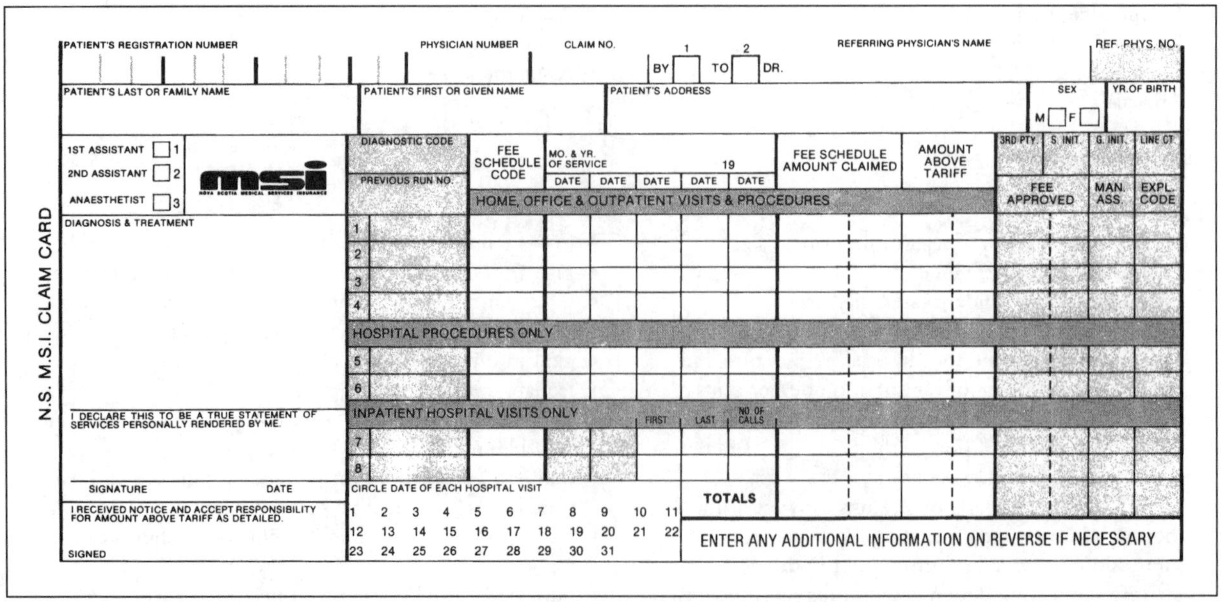
N.S. M.S.I. CLAIM CARD

PATIENT'S REGISTRATION NUMBER | PHYSICIAN NUMBER | CLAIM NO. | 1 BY | 2 TO | DR. | REFERRING PHYSICIAN'S NAME | REF. PHYS. NO.

PATIENT'S LAST OR FAMILY NAME | PATIENT'S FIRST OR GIVEN NAME | PATIENT'S ADDRESS | SEX M F | YR. OF BIRTH

1ST ASSISTANT 1
2ND ASSISTANT 2
ANAESTHETIST 3

DIAGNOSTIC CODE | FEE SCHEDULE CODE | MO. & YR. OF SERVICE 19 | FEE SCHEDULE AMOUNT CLAIMED | AMOUNT ABOVE TARIFF | 3RD PTY. | S. INIT. | G. INIT. | LINE CT.

PREVIOUS RUN NO. | DATE | DATE | DATE | DATE | DATE | FEE APPROVED | MAN. ASS. | EXPL. CODE

DIAGNOSIS & TREATMENT

HOME, OFFICE & OUTPATIENT VISITS & PROCEDURES
1
2
3
4

HOSPITAL PROCEDURES ONLY
5
6

INPATIENT HOSPITAL VISITS ONLY | FIRST | LAST | NO. OF CALLS
7
8

I DECLARE THIS TO BE A TRUE STATEMENT OF SERVICES PERSONALLY RENDERED BY ME.

SIGNATURE DATE

CIRCLE DATE OF EACH HOSPITAL VISIT
1 2 3 4 5 6 7 8 9 10 11
12 13 14 15 16 17 18 19 20 21 22
23 24 25 26 27 28 29 30 31

TOTALS

I RECEIVED NOTICE AND ACCEPT RESPONSIBILITY FOR AMOUNT ABOVE TARIFF AS DETAILED.

SIGNED

ENTER ANY ADDITIONAL INFORMATION ON REVERSE IF NECESSARY

**Illustration 6.1b   Alberta Billing Card**

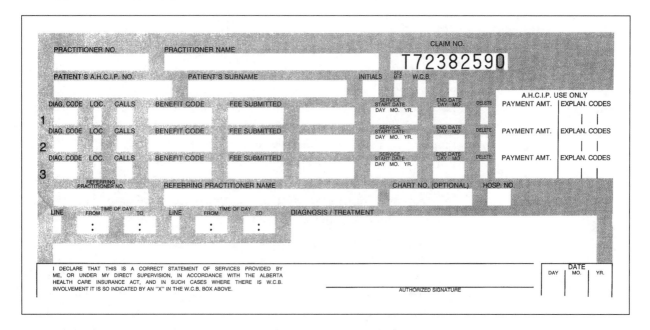

**Illustration 6.1c   British Columbia Billing Card**

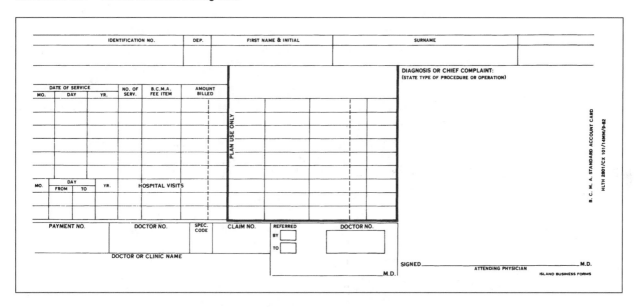

To demonstrate the intricacies of a provincial health insurance plan, we will use the Ontario Ministry of Health format.

In order to complete the service code and service fee portions of the health insurance billing card, you must refer to the provincial Schedule of Benefits. Schedules may be obtained from the Ontario Government Book Store, 880 Bay St., Toronto, Ontario, M7A 1N8.

Ontario's health insurance program is a comprehensive provincial government-sponsored plan of health coverage for Ontario residents. It provides

## Introduction to Health Care Billing

a wide range of benefits for medical, hospital, and certain other health care provider services.

This chapter contains information about the program that you will need to know when you become a medical administrative assistant in Ontario.

## Eligibility

All residents of Ontario, regardless of age, state of health, or financial means, are entitled to participate. A resident is a person who is legally entitled to remain in Canada and whose home is in Ontario. Tourists, transients, and visitors to Ontario are not eligible to enrol.

Patients from another province or territory who require treatment before their coverage comes into effect are usually covered by their previous provincial or territory health plan.

## Health Card

The Ministry of Health (MOH) has converted from a family-based OHIP number to a new individual health number for each eligible resident of the province of Ontario. The health number appears on a plastic health card (see Illustration 6.2), which contains embossed and magnetic stripe information.

There are several versions of the Ontario Health Card in use at present. Illustration 6.2 depicts the new photo health card.

Ontario residents who were issued cards prior to July 1, 1991, have their old OHIP number printed in the bottom corner of their new health card. Health cards issued after this date no longer contain the old number. The province of Ontario is now in the process of reregistration using the new photo health card. Children under 16 years of age will not have a photo on their health card.

Other provinces in Canada also issue health cards. Examples of these appear at the end of this chapter (see Illustration 6.26).

### Illustration 6.2    Ontario Photo Health Card

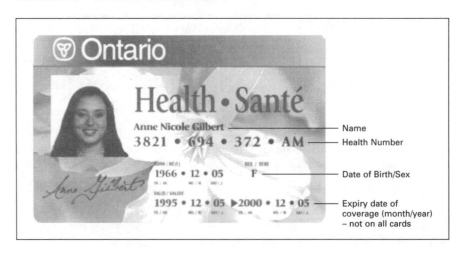

## Registration

Health care providers must submit a registered health number for each patient in order to receive a fee for service. Every patient must provide a health number at the time of service. In order to register for a health number, a Registration for Ontario Health Coverage form must be completed by the patient and submitted in person to the Ministry of Health (see Illustration 6.3).

### Illustration 6.3 Registration for Ontario Health Coverage Form

Ministry of Health
Ontario

**Registration for Ontario Health Coverage**

Microfilm use only

Health Number | Version

**1 General Information** *Tourists, transients and visitors to Ontario are not eligible for health coverage.*

*You can only apply while present in Ontario. There may be a three (3) month waiting period for coverage.*

Last name | First name | Middle name

Sex ☐ M ☐ F | Birth date Year Month Day | Language preference ☐ English ☐ French | *Previous Ontario Health number, if any* Health Number Version

**2 Address** *If you are moving in the next 4–6 weeks, please check* ☐ *and indicate your new address on a separate sheet.*

**Mailing Address**
Current mailing address (street no. & name or R.R., P.O. Box, General Delivery)

Apt. | Street no. & name, R.R., P.O. Box, General Delivery

City

Province | Country | Postal Code

**Residence Address** *Provide exact residence location if mailing address is a R.R., P.O. Box or General Delivery.*

Apt. | Lot, Concession, Township or Street no. & name

City

Province | Country | Postal Code

**3 Residence in Ontario** *Supporting documents are required to prove residence in Ontario.*

**A** **Have you lived in Ontario since birth?** ☐ Yes ☐ No *If no, please complete the remainder of section A.*

**Most recent arrival date in Ontario?** Year Month Day

**Where did you move from?** Province/Territory/State | Country

**Date you left previous province/territory** Year Month Day

**If you came from another province or territory did you have government health insurance?** ☐ No ☐ Yes, **provide your health number:**

Former address:

**B** **If you have left the Canadian Forces, RCMP or federal penitentiary, please provide the date of discharge and enclose ORIGINAL discharge document.** Year Month Day

**4 Citizenship Status** (Only **ORIGINAL** documents will be accepted)

*Check one of the following and attach* ***original*** *required documents.*

☐ Returning Canadian ☐ Canadian Citizen (Canadian birth, citizenship, or baptismal certificate (Quebec or Newfoundland only) or Canadian Passport)

☐ Aboriginal People (Birth certificate, certificate of Indian status – band identification)

☐ Landed Immigrant ☐ Convention refugee (Immigrant Visa/Record of Landing)

☐ Returning Immigrant (Returning Resident Permit)

☐ Others (Canadian Immigration document)

**MINISTRY OF HEALTH USE ONLY**

Residence effective date

Arrival date

Document issued date

Document expiry date

Cit. type | Doc. type | Issued by

Document Serial number

Client ID

W. P. E.? | Original documents verified?

Clerk no. | Date

**5 Signature** *(Please sign below.)*

I am a resident of Ontario and declare the information provided to be true. I agree to allow the Ministry of Health to verify all information given in this application.

Signature or signature of guardian | Date | Home phone number ( ) – | Business phone number ( ) –

Collection of the information on this form is for the assessment and verification of eligibility for Health Insurance and Drug Benefit and administration of the Health Insurance and Ontario Drug Benefit Acts, and for health planning and coordination. It is collected/used for these purposes under the authority of the Ministry of Health Act, section 6(1,2), Health Insurance Act, section 4(2) (b,f), 10, 11(1), and Regulation 689/86 under the Ontario Drug Benefit Act, section 2. For information about collection practices contact the Director, Registration and Claims Branch at 613–548–6559, or by mail, through the addresses listed for local Ministry of Health offices.

7530–4480

0265–82 (94/06)

### Newborn Registration

When a child is born in an Ontario hospital, hospital staff and the child's parents complete and submit an Ontario Health Coverage Infant Registration form to the Ministry of Health. This is to ensure that newborns are registered under their own individual health number and not under their parents' numbers, as was the practice under OHIP.

### Confidentiality of the Health Number

Bill 24 became law on April 4, 1991. The Act prohibits anyone from registering your health card number or asking you to show your health card for any purpose unrelated to the provision of provincially funded health services.

### Premium Payment

Residents of Ontario no longer pay premiums for their health coverage. Premiums have been replaced with a payroll tax, which is paid by employers.

## Billing Options

Providers may bill for insured services by choosing one of two methods:

1. Providers who are "opted-in" to the plan will bill the Ministry of Health for eligible services rendered to the patient. The patient does not receive a bill from the physician for these services.
2. Providers who are "opted-out" of the plan will bill the patient directly for services rendered. Claims for eligible services will then be submitted to the Ministry of Health on the patient's behalf, and payment for insured services is made to the subscriber by the ministry. However, as stated in Bill 94, a patient is not required to make a payment for insured services to an opted-out physician, optometrist, or dentist until the patient has been reimbursed.

## Bill 94

Since Bill 94 became law on June 20, 1986, "a physician, optometrist, or dentist shall not charge more or accept payment for more than the amount payable under the plan for rendering an insured service to an insured person."

## Provider Registration

Every provider and group registered with the Ministry of Health is assigned an identification number. This is a twelve-digit number: the first four digits identify the group, the following six digits identify the provider, and the last two digits identify the specialty. This number is used to determine the payment of claims to providers.

## Examples

1. Registration number 0000-123456-00

   | | |
   |---|---|
   | 0000 | The provider is not in a group practice. |
   | 123456 | Indicates the provider's identification number. This number is unique and belongs to the provider for a lifetime. (It does not change if the provider changes option type or specialty.) This number should be quoted on any correspondence with the Ministry of Health. |
   | 00 | The specialty is general practice. |

2. Registration number 9999-123456-13

   | | |
   |---|---|
   | 9999 | This is the identification number of the group with which the provider is affiliated. A provider may be affiliated with more than one group, each of which will have a unique four-digit identification number. |
   | 123456 | Individual identification number as above. |
   | 13 | The specialty is internal medicine. |

Providers who wish to register with the Ministry of Health must obtain an application form from their nearest Ministry of Health office. Once registered, they will receive a supply of Ministry of Health computer diskettes. The location of the practice will determine the Ministry of Health district office to which claims should be submitted. An introductory kit will be sent by the district office to each newly registered provider.

Any changes to registered information (such as option or specialty changes) must be submitted to the Ministry of Health in writing.

The following is a list of specialty services recognized by the Royal College of Physicians and Surgeons of Canada relevant to services covered by the Ministry of Health.

## Explanation of Provider's Specialty Codes

## Physicians

| Specialty Code | Explanation |
|---|---|
| 00 | Family practice and practice in general<br>This provider is not a specialist in any field, although he or she may limit his or her practice to a particular field. |
| 01 | Anaesthesia<br>Specialist in anaesthetics. |
| 02 | Dermatology<br>Specialist in diseases of the skin. |

03       General surgery
Specialist in general surgery.

04       Neurosurgery
Specialist in surgery of the nervous system.

06       Orthopedic surgery
Specialist in the preservation and restoration of the skeletal system.

07       Geriatrics
Specialist in all problems peculiar to old age and aging.

08       Plastic surgery
Specialist in repair of skin and underlying tissues.

09       Cardiovascular and thoracic surgery
Specialist in surgery of the heart and chest.

12       Emergency Medicine
Specialist in emergency department medicine.

13       Internal medicine
Specialist in diseases of the internal structures of the body.

18       Neurology
Specialist in diseases of the nervous system.

19       Psychiatry
Specialist in mental and emotional problems.

20       Obstetrics and gynecology
Specialist in two fields: pregnancy and childbirth, and the female genital organs.

23       Ophthalmology
Specialist in diseases of the eye.

24       Otolaryngology
Specialist in diseases of the ear, nose, and throat.

25       Pediatrics
Specialist in child care and diseases of children.

28       Pathology
Specialist in structural and functional changes in tissues of the body caused by disease.

29       Microbiology
Specialist in study of micro-organisms.

30       Clinical biochemistry
Specialist in the practice of chemical pathology.

31          Physical medicine
            Specialist in the field of diagnosis and treatment of disease by
            physical methods (manipulation, massage, exercise).

33          Diagnostic radiology
            Specialist in the taking and interpretation of X-rays.

34          Therapeutic radiology
            Specialist in the treatment of disease by radiotherapy (radium,
            X-ray therapy).

35          Urology
            Specialist in the urinary system (kidneys and bladder) in both
            male and female, and genital organs in the male.

41          Gastroenterology
            Specialist in the field of diseases of the gastrointestinal tract.

47          Respiratory disease
            Specialist in the field of diseases of the respiratory system.

48          Rheumatology
            Specialist in the field of rheumatic disease.

60          Cardiology
            Specialist in the field of heart and circulatory disease.

61          Haematology
            Specialist in the field of blood disease.

62          Clinical immunology
            Specialist in the field of immunity (producing immunity by
            natural or artificial stimulation).

63          Nuclear medicine
            Specialist in the clinical evaluation of a patient diagnosed or
            treated by unsealed sources of radionuclides.

64          General thoracic surgery
            Specialist in surgery of the chest.

## Dentists

| Specialty Code | Explanation |
| --- | --- |

49          Dental surgery
            The dentist in general practice; not a specialist.

50          Oral surgery
            Surgical specialist (the surgical treatment of diseases of, and
            injuries to, the teeth, jaws, and associated structure).

51          Orthodontics
            Specialist in the field of malocclusion of the teeth, including
            developmental abnormalities of the jaws.

52          Pedodontics
            Specialist in the field of dentistry for children.

53          Periodontics
            Specialist in the field of treatment of the diseases of the
            supporting tissues of the teeth.

54          Oral pathology
            Specialist in identification and diagnosis of diseased tissue after
            it has been removed from its normal site.

55          Endodontics
            Specialist in treating diseases involving the pulp of teeth and
            periradical tissues.

70          Oral radiology
            Specialist at interpreting X-rays of the teeth.

71          Prosthodontist
            Specialist in the making of crowns, bridges, and dentures.

## Other Providers

Chiropractors, chiropodists, osteopaths, optometrists, and physiotherapists are
not certified in specialties. However, to avoid including these health care
providers' statistical data with that of general health care providers, individual
specialty codes have been assigned.

| Specialty Codes | Explanation |
| --- | --- |
| 56 | Optometrist |
| 57 | Osteopath |
| 58 | Chiropodist (Podiatrist) |
| 59 | Chiropractor |
| 80 | Private physiotherapy facilities approved to provide home treatment only. |
| 81 | Private physiotherapy facilities approved to provide office and home treatment. |

A specialty code is also assigned to the nonmedical laboratory director:

27          59993
            Nonmedical laboratory directors are always registered under
            this number.

The Ontario Ministry of Health publishes the Schedule of Benefits, which lists the fees established through negotiations between the profession and the Minister of Health. The Ministry of Health Schedule of Benefits is similar to, but separate from, the Ontario Medical Association Schedule of Fees.

As a medical administrative assistant, you will require an extensive knowledge of the schedule and will be required to pay close attention to the regulations and definitions contained in the preamble. Complete familiarity with the preambles is a prerequisite for accurate billing.

Whenever new fees are negotiated, providers routinely receive updated schedules. Additional copies may be available from your local Ministry of Health office or, for a nominal fee (to cover printing and handling), from the Ontario Government Book Store, 880 Bay Street, Toronto M7A 1N8, or call toll free 1-800-668-9938.

Currently, there are four media used to submit claims for insured services to the Ministry of Health. These are claim cards, magnetic tape, 5¼-inch diskettes, and 3½-inch diskettes.

As other media become available, the Ministry of Health will investigate each for possible future implementation.

Claims submitted on cards by opted-in providers and received at the local Ministry of Health office by the tenth day of each month will be paid by the middle of the following month. Magnetic tapes or diskettes must be received by the eighteenth day of each month for payment by the middle of the following month.

In order to encourage providers to make submissions on magnetic media, a charge is levied for any manual submissions made on claim cards.

Opted-out (pay subscriber) claims are normally paid two to four weeks after receipt by the Ministry of Health.

All claims must be submitted to the Ministry of Health within six months of the service date. **Only under extreme circumstances will the Ministry of Health consider making payments for claims submitted six months after the date of service.**

Each resident of Ontario is issued an individual health number consisting of ten digits. This number is used on the health claim card to identify the patient. The card may or may not contain a version code (for further explanation of the version code, please see p. 72).

There are two types of claim cards:

1. *The Health Claim Card* — (See Illustration 6.4.) This card is used for health claims for services rendered by Ontario providers to residents of Ontario who are covered by the Ministry of Health and by the Workers' Compensation Board. The card can be identified by the red stripe on the upper left corner.

## MOH Schedule of Benefits

## Introduction to Claims Submission

## Submission Dates and Payment Dates

## Health Service Claim Cards

**Illustration 6.4    Health Claim Card**

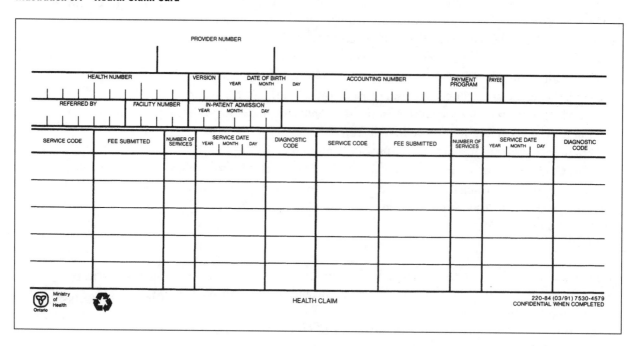

2.  *The Reciprocal Claim Card* — (See Illustration 6.5.) This card is used for health claims for services rendered by Ontario providers to residents of other provinces (except Quebec). This card can be identified by the purple stripe on the upper left corner.

**Illustration 6.5    Reciprocal Claim Card**

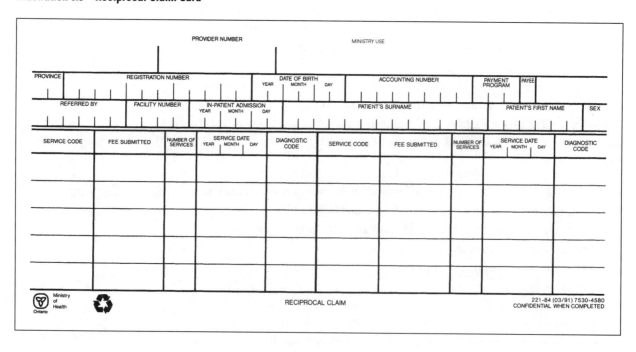

By way of patient identification, the health claim card requires the patient's ten-digit health number, plus version code if applicable, and complete birth date (year, month, day). The reciprocal claim card requires the name of the insuring province and the patient's provincial health registration number, complete with date, full name, and sex.

Claim cards, if used, can be obtained on request of the provider from the Ministry of Health through Data Business Forms. A claim card order form (see Illustration 6.6) must be completed and mailed to Data Business Forms. After completion, fold and seal the form. The mailing address is printed on the reverse side. If the cards are in duplicate, one copy is submitted to the ministry for payment and one is retained by the provider to facilitate reconciliation of payment.

**Illustration 6.6 Claim Card Order Form**

Ministry of Health / Ministère de la Santé
Ontario

**CLAIM CARD ORDER FORM**
**BON DE COMMANDE DE CARTE DE DEMANDE DE RÈGLEMENT**

Registry No. 1234-23456-01 N° d'inscription

**Shipping Address/Adresse d'expédition**

Provider's name and address

**Alternate Shipping Address/Autre adresse**

Name/Nom

Address/Adresse

Postal Code/Code postal | Signature

**Claim Cards will be sent to the Shipping Address above unless an Alternate Address is supplied.**
**Les cartes de demande de règlement seront envoyées à l'adresse d'expédition ci-dessus à moins que vous n'ayez fourni une autre adresse.**

Fold Here / Pliez ici — 952-84 (02-91) — Fold Here / Pliez ici

**1**

**Please check (✓) which forms you would like sent to the above address.**
**Veuillez cocher (✓) les formules que vous souhaitez voir envoyées à l'adresse ci-dessus.**

- [X] HEALTH CLAIM / DEMANDE de RÈGLEMENT (220-84)
- [ ] RECIPROCAL CLAIM / DEMANDE de RÈGLEMENT HORS PROVINCE (221-84)
- [X] LABORATORY REQUISITION / DEMANDE du LABORATOIRE (300-84)

**2**

**Please check (✓) if you want the cards printed with your Registration Number.**
**Veuillez cocher (✓) si vous souhaitez que les cartes soient imprimées avec votre n° d'inscription.**

YES [X] OUI NO [ ] NON

**3**

**In the event that we need to contact you, please provide your telephone number.**
**Veuillez nous fournir votre n° de téléphone au cas où nous devions vous joindre.**

Telephone No. 613-376-5433 Numéro de téléphone

MOISTEN AND SEAL/HUMECTER ET SCELLER

**Illustration 6.7    Health Claim Card Components**

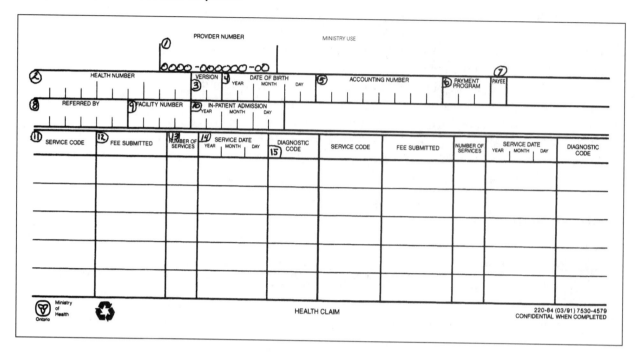

## Health Claim Card

This card is used by the provider to submit claims for payment of medically necessary services. Providers include physicians, health care providers, and private medical laboratories. Payment is made either by the Ministry of Health or the Workers' Compensation Board. Components of this card are shown in Illustration 6.7.

1. **Provider Number** — Identifies the provider and includes the three components of the provider identification explained on page 64 under "Provider Registration." The initial section (four digits) identifies the group/solo status of the provider; the middle section (six digits) identifies the provider; the last section (two digits) indicates the provider's field of specialization (a list of specialty codes appears on pp. 65–68).

2. **Health Number** — The ten-digit number issued by the Ministry of Health to each individual who is a permanent resident of Ontario.

3. **Version** — The initial plastic health card issued by the ministry did not have a version number. Replacement cards will include a version code. This version code *must* be included on submission claims.

4. **Date of Birth** — The patient's date of birth is required in year/month/day format with two digits for each component and *no* punctuation (e.g., 85 09 25).

5. **Accounting Number** — Can consist of eight alphanumeric characters. This component is optional but recommended. It is used by the provider for accounting purposes and for comparing claims submitted with payments made.

6. **Payment Program** — Identifies payment to be made either by the Ministry

of Health or the Workers' Compensation Board and is entered "HCP" (Health Claim Payment) or "WCB" (Workers' Compensation Board).

7. **Payee** — If the provider is to be paid, enter "P"; if the patient is to be paid, enter "S."

8. **Referred by** — Here you enter the provider's six-digit identification number. The provider is the health care provider/physician who has referred the patient for the service. This section must be completed for *all* types of consultations in any location, for *all* physiotherapy services, and for any referred diagnostic or laboratory services.

9. **Facility Number** — This is a four-digit number identifying the facility where the service is performed. This component must be completed for all in-patient, out-patient, and emergency services performed in hospitals and long-term-care facilities (including special-visit premium) and for all insured dental services.

10. **In-Patient Admission** — When a patient is admitted to and seen in the hospital, the date of admission is entered on the claim card in year/month/day format. The services include all hospital services (except any consultations) and special-visit premiums to a patient who has been admitted to the hospital (referred to as a hospital in-patient).

11. **Service Code** — Codes for all insured services are listed in the Ministry of Health Schedule of Benefits. They consist of five alphanumeric characters (e.g., A001A). A broader explanation of this code will be given later in this chapter.

12. **Fee Submitted** — This is the amount the provider claims for the service rendered. Write figures only, with no dollar or cent signs, decimals, or spaces (e.g., if the fee is $102.50, enter the charge as 10250).

13. **Number of Services** — Use numerals 01 to 99. Two-digit numbers are required. If the number of services is below ten, the number should be preceded by a zero (e.g., five services would be entered as 05). If the number of services exceeds 99, it should be entered on two lines (e.g., for 108 services, enter 99 on one line and 09 on the next line).

14. **Service Date** — Enter the date the service was provided in year/month/date format.

15. **Diagnostic Code** — Consists of three or four characters and identifies the diagnosis of the patient's complaint (e.g., 460 is the diagnostic code for a common cold). If more than one diagnosis is involved, use the code for the primary diagnosis. Most, but not all, services require diagnostic codes. Some of the visits or procedures that do not require a diagnostic code are newborn baby care in hospital and home, all immunizations and vaccinations, as well as several others. A list of diagnostic codes can be obtained from your Ministry of Health district office.

## Reciprocal Claim Card

This card is used to submit claims for services rendered by providers to patients who reside in another province. All areas of the reciprocal claim card are identical to the health claim card except for the additional required information identified in Illustration 6.8.

**Illustration 6.8   Reciprocal Claim Card Components**

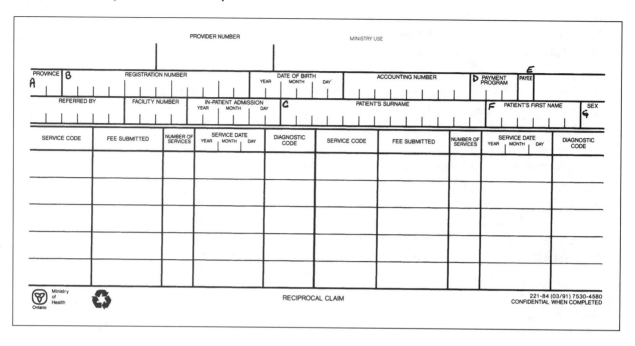

A. **Province** — The province where the patient resides is identified by a two-letter code (e.g., AB=Alberta, MB=Manitoba, BC=British Columbia, NS=Nova Scotia, NF=Newfoundland, etc.).

B. **Registration Number** — Patients have a health care number unique to their resident province. These numbers range from six to twelve digits in length and will be given to you by the patient.

C. **Patient's Surname** — Enter up to thirteen letters of the patient's last name (e.g., for Smith enter "SMITH"; for Mountainpayneski enter "MOUN-TAINPAYNE").

D. **Payment Program** — For *all* reciprocal billing claims enter "RMB" (reciprocal medical billing).

E. **Payee** — The payee *must* be the provider; enter "P."

F. **Patient's First Name** — Enter up to six letters of the patient's first name (e.g., for Elizabeth enter "ELIZAB").

G. **Sex** — Enter "F" for female and "M" for male.

# The Billing Process

The Schedule of Benefits and a list of diagnostic codes are required to complete the health claim card. Familiarity with the format of the schedule is important to the medical office administrator. Preambles that precede the various sections in the schedule contain pertinent information necessary to the accurate process of medical billing. This information includes special-visit premium payments and service codes, calculation of time unit, and fees for anaesthetists and assistants. Be sure to read the preamble and highlight all information that pertains to the completion of the billing process.

**Service Codes**

The service code consists of five alphanumeric characters, for example, A001A.

1. The first character is alpha and is an indicator of the service: Prefix alpha A indicates services listed under the general listing (consultations, assessments) or special visits to the office; B is for special visits to the patient's home; G is for diagnostic and therapeutic procedures; P is for obstetrical care; X is for radiology services; and so on.
2. The three middle characters are numeric service identifiers: for example, 001 is for a minor assessment.
3. The last character is alpha and identifies who renders the service.

   A = Provider rendered the service
       Combination of hospital technical and professional components

   B = Assistant rendered the service
       Hospital technical component

   C = Anaesthetist rendered the service
       Professional component

The most common service codes used in general practice follow:

1. **General Assessment** (A003) — The patient presents the provider with a complaint and the provider investigates all systems to make a diagnosis.
2. **General Reassessment** (A004) — The patient returns within one year with the same complaint (two per year per diagnosis may be charged).
3. **Intermediate Assessment/Well Baby Care** (A007) — The provider examines a specific system for a diagnosis (less time than a general assessment), or sees an infant for periodic health assessment and progress up to two years.
4. **Annual Health Examination** (K017=child after two years; A003=adolescent, adult) — The patient visits the doctor for a yearly review of physical well-being with no complaint (one visit per year can be charged).
5. **Minor Assessment** (A001) — The diagnosis is fairly simple and less time-consuming than for an intermediate assessment.

The above service codes would have the alpha suffix "A" (A003A) because a provider renders the service.

**Diagnostic Codes**

The provider diagnoses the patient's condition after performing an examination. For the purposes of health care billing, the diagnosis is identified by a three- or four-digit numeric code (e.g., 110 identifies athlete's foot, 850 identifies concussion, 303 identifies alcoholism, and 917 is the diagnostic code used for adolescent and adult annual health examinations). A complete listing of all diagnostic codes is available from your Ministry of Health district office.

**Illustration 6.9   Completed Health Claim Card**

| PROVIDER NUMBER | | | | | | MINISTRY USE | | | | |
|---|---|---|---|---|---|---|---|---|---|---|

0000-123456-00

| HEALTH NUMBER | VERSION | DATE OF BIRTH | | | ACCOUNTING NUMBER | PAYMENT PROGRAM | PAYEE | |
|---|---|---|---|---|---|---|---|---|
| | | YEAR | MONTH | DAY | | | | |
| 3 8 2 0 7 0 3 7 9 5 | | – | – 01 | 01 | | HCP | P | |
| REFERRED BY | FACILITY NUMBER | IN-PATIENT ADMISSION | | | | | | |
| | | YEAR | MONTH | DAY | | | | |

| SERVICE CODE | FEE SUBMITTED | NUMBER OF SERVICES | SERVICE DATE | | | DIAGNOSTIC CODE | SERVICE CODE | FEE SUBMITTED | NUMBER OF SERVICES | SERVICE DATE | | | DIAGNOSTIC CODE |
|---|---|---|---|---|---|---|---|---|---|---|---|---|---|
| | | | YEAR | MONTH | DAY | | | | | YEAR | MONTH | DAY | |
| A001A | 1510 | 01 | – | 01 | 16 | 110 | | | | | | | |
| | | | | | | | | | | | | | |
| | | | | | | | | | | | | | |
| | | | | | | | | | | | | | |
| | | | | | | | | | | | | | |

Ministry of Health Ontario

HEALTH CLAIM

220-84 (03/91) 7530-4579
CONFIDENTIAL WHEN COMPLETED

# Coding Examples

## Example 1

Mary Jane Brown came to Dr. Plunkett's office on January 16, 19__, with a rash on her toes. The diagnosis was "athlete's foot." The completed health claim card is shown in Illustration 6.9. Fee for services is from the April 1989 Schedule of Benefits and will change as subsequent schedules are issued.

The procedure for completing the health claim card is as follows:

1. Generally, the provider number is preprinted at the ministry district office.
2. Mary Jane's health number and date of birth would be extracted from her chart and entered in the appropriate area.
3. The payment program is the health care plan (enter HCP), and the provider is to be paid (enter "P").
4. Because the complaint is isolated and fairly simple to diagnose, Dr. Plunkett would charge for a minor assessment. The service code and fee would be obtained from the Schedule of Benefits under "Family Practice and Practice in General (00)" because Dr. Plunkett is a general health care provider.
5. The service fee is found in the schedule opposite the service code.
6. One service has been performed.
7. The service date is the day Mary Jane presented her complaint — enter year, month, and day (__ 01 16).
8. The diagnostic code would be extracted from the MOH diagnostic code listing.

**Illustration 6.10   Completed Health Claim Card**

| SERVICE CODE | FEE SUBMITTED | NUMBER OF SERVICES | SERVICE DATE YEAR MONTH DAY | DIAGNOSTIC CODE | SERVICE CODE | FEE SUBMITTED | NUMBER OF SERVICES | SERVICE DATE YEAR MONTH DAY | DIAGNOSTIC CODE |
|---|---|---|---|---|---|---|---|---|---|
| A185A | 10245 | 01 | – 01 22 | 850 | | | | | |
| C994A | 3160 | 01 | – 01 22 | 850 | | | | | |
| C182A | 5010 | 03 | – 01 23 | 850 | | | | | |

PROVIDER NUMBER: 0000-345678-18
HEALTH NUMBER: 1892608532  DATE OF BIRTH: – – 07 30  PAYMENT PROGRAM: HCP  PAYEE: P
REFERRED BY: 123456  FACILITY NUMBER: 98716  IN-PATIENT ADMISSION: – – 01 22

HEALTH CLAIM

220-84 (03/91) 7530-4579 CONFIDENTIAL WHEN COMPLETED

Ministry of Health Ontario

## Example 2

While Bob Baxter was cleaning windows, he fell off the ladder, banged his head on a rock, and was knocked unconscious. His wife called an ambulance to take him to the hospital. Dr. Plunkett admitted Bob and then called in a neurologist, Dr. R.T. Schmidt, for consultation. Dr. Schmidt's diagnosis was concussion. He visited Bob on three consecutive days after the admitting date. The accident happened on Saturday, January 22, 19__.

The completed health claim card for Dr. Schmidt is shown in Illustration 6.10.

The procedure for completing the health claim card is as follows:

1. The provider number is usually preprinted.
2. Patient's health number and birth date would be taken from the patient's chart.
3. Because Dr. Plunkett referred Baxter to Dr. Schmidt, Dr. Plunkett's personal registration number would be entered in the space "Referred By."
4. Because Baxter was admitted to hospital, the "Facility Number" and "In-Patient Admission" spaces must be completed.
5. The service codes are as follows:
   a. A185A — The service is a consultation performed in the hospital by a specialist in neurology. When a provider makes a special trip, the billing code for the assessment component of the visit is taken from the general listing for the applicable specialty. In the fee schedule

under neurology (18) you will find A185 — Consultation. Service codes used for special trip billings *must be* taken from general listing's *Office Service Codes*. A consultation can only be charged when the provider is seeing a patient who has been referred by another provider.

The suffix for each service code is "A" because the service was rendered by the provider.

b. C994A — Providers can charge a premium if they respond to calls outside of office hours, on weekends and holidays, or if they sacrifice office hours. The appropriate codes are listed in the preamble under "Premiums." If the special visit is to the emergency department, the alpha prefix would be "K"; for a visit to a patient's home, the alpha prefix would be "B." However, in this instance, the alpha prefix is "C" because Dr. Schmidt rendered the service to a non-emergency hospital in-patient.

c. C182A — This is the code used when a neurologist makes subsequent hospital visits to a patient; it is found just below the C185 consultation code.

6. The appropriate service fees are found in the schedule beside the relevant service codes.

7. Note that, under "Number of Services," the number "03" is entered opposite "C182A." This is because Dr. Schmidt visited the patient for three consecutive days. The service date entered is the date of the first visit. (If the visits run consecutively without a break, you can put them together.)

8. The diagnostic code for concussion is 850.

## Supporting Documentation

Certain services must include supporting documentation.

1. Independent consideration (IC) — Independent consideration may be given when a set fee is not listed in the fee schedule. Claims rendered under this heading should contain an explanation of the fee claimed. It is helpful to the medical consultant if claims for IC include an operative or consultation report and a comparison of the scope and difficulty of the procedure with other procedures in the schedule. (Note: The medical consultant is a provider assigned to each Ministry of Health district office to provide advice and guidance on medical and payment policy.)

2. Preauthorized and reconstructive surgery — Services mentioned in preamble D of the Ministry of Health Schedule of Benefits require ministry preauthorization. Request forms are available from your local Ministry of Health office (see Illustration 6.11).

## Returned Claims

### Claim Cards

Ministry of Health claims clerks will return cards to you if the information is missing or incorrect. Since this will delay payment, always check your submissions for completeness and accuracy before submission.

## Illustration 6.11 Request for Approval of Payment for Proposed Surgery

Ministry of Health / Ministère de la Santé
Ontario

### Request for Approval of Payment for Proposed Surgery
### Demande d'approbation de réglement de frais d'actes chirurgicaux proposées

Confidential when completed
Les renseignements portés sur la formule sont confidentiels

**PATIENT IDENTIFICATION/IDENTIFICATION DU MALADE**

PATIENT'S LAST NAME & INITIALS / NOM DE FAMILLE ET INITIALES DU MALADE — ☐ MR. / M. ☐ MRS. / Mme ☐ MISS / Mlle

PATIENT'S ADDRESS / ADRESSE DU MALADE

HEALTH NUMBER / NUMÉRO DE CARTE SANTÉ

VERSION CODE

PATIENT'S FIRST NAME PRÉNOM DU MALADE

PATIENT'S SEX / SEXE DU MALADE — ☐ MALE / MASCULIN ☐ FEMALE / FÉMININ

PATIENT'S BIRTHDATE / DATE DE NAISSANCE DU MALADE — YEAR ANNÉE MONTH MOIS DAY JOUR

POSTAL CODE / CODE POSTAL

**SURGERY DETAILS/RENSEIGNEMENTS SUR L'INTERVENTION CHIRURGICALE**

NAME AND ADDRESS OF HOSPITAL / NOM ET ADRESSE DE L'HÔPITAL

DATE OF ADMISSION (IF KNOWN)/DATE D'ADMISSION (SI CONNUE)

PROPOSED FEE / HONORAIRES ENVISAGÉS

DIAGNOSIS AND PROPOSED PROCEDURE / DIAGNOSTIC ET ACTE ENVISAGÉ

MEDICAL INDICATION FOR SURGERY / RAISONS MÉDICALES JUSTIFIANT L'INTERVENTION CHIRURGICALE

REASON FOR REFERRAL OUTSIDE ONTARIO / RAISONS DE LA RECOMMANDATION D'UN SPÉCIALISTE À L'EXTÉRIEUR DE L'ONTARIO

SURGEON'S AND/OR REFERRING PHYSICIAN'S NAME IN FULL / NOM ET PRÉNOMS DU MÉDECIN QUI ADRESSE LE MALADE OU/ET DU CHIRURGIEN

SURGEON'S AND/OR REFERRING PHYSICIAN'S ADDRESS / ADRESSE DU MÉDECIN ET/OU DU CHIRURGIEN NOMMÉS

SURGEON'S AND/OR REFERRING PHYSICIAN'S MINISTRY OF HEALTH IDENTIFICATION NUMBER / NUMÉRO D'IDENTIFICATION OHIP DU MEDECIN ET/OU DU CHIRURGIEN NOMMÉS

SURGEON'S AND/OR REFERRING PHYSICIAN'S SIGNATURE / SIGNATURE DU MÉDECIN ET/OU DU CHIRURGIEN NOMMÉS

DATE / DATE

POSTAL CODE / CODE POSTAL

**MINISTRY OF HEALTH ASSESSMENT/ÉVALUATION PAR MINISTERE DE LA SANTE**

1 & 2 PERTAIN ON CONDITION THAT HEALTH INSURANCE COVERAGE IS IN EFFECT ON DATE OF SERVICE
1 ET 2 NE SONT À CONSIDÉRER QUE SI L'ASSURANCE -SANTÉ EST EN VIGUEUR À LA DATE OU LES SOINS SONT DISPENSÉS

☐ 1 APPROVED FOR BENEFITS AS SUBMITTED / RÈGLEMENT APPROUVÉ SANS MODIFICATIONS

☐ 2 APPROVED AS AMENDED / APPROUVÉ AVEC MODIFICATIONS

☐ 3 NOT AN ELIGIBLE BENEFIT / INTERVENTION NON COUVERTE

COMMENTS / REMARQUES

N.B.: This authorization is valid for one year after date of approval
La presente autorisation est valide pour un an à compter de la date d'autorisation

SIGNATURE FOR MINISTRY OF HEALTH/ SIGNATURE AU NOM DE MINISTÈRE DE LA SANTÉ

DATE / DATE

*Instructions to surgeons/physicians/Instructions au chirurgien/médecin*

*1. Forward all copies of this form to Medical Consultant c/o your district office./Envoyez toutes les copies de cette formule au médecin-conseil, aux soins du bureau de district.*

*2. Please advise Assistant and Anaesthetist of status of claim.(that approval has to be requested)./Veuillez aviser l'assistant et l'anesthésiste qu'une demande d'approbation est en cours.*

*3. Return your copy of this form with your claim card if request is approved./Si la demande est approuvée, renvoyez votre copie de la formule avec votre carte de demande de règlement.*

*4. Please print or type — you are making 3 copies./Veuillez datylographier ou écrire en lettres moulées — il y a trois copies.*

691-84 (91/01) *(See reverse / Au verso)* 7530-4239

SURGEON

**Illustration 6.12    Missing/Incorrect Information**

| | Missing/Incorrect Service |
|---|---|
| ☐ Health Number is missing/invalid | |
| ☐ Invalid version code | |
| ☐ Date of Birth missing/incorrect | ☐ Referring Provider #   ☐ Fee |
| ☐ Date of Birth/Health Number mismatch | ☐ Facility Number   ☐ Number of Services |
| ☐ Health Number not registered with Ministry of Health | ☐ Admission Date   ☐ Service Date |
| ☐ Payment Program is missing/invalid | ☐ Service Code   ☐ Diagnostic Code |
| ☐ Payee is missing/incorrect | ☐ Missing/incorrect information as highlighted on front of card |
| ☐ OHIP # required for this service date (submit using OHIP Claim Card) | DATE:   STATION: |
| ☐ Health Number required for this service date | |
| ☐ Please resubmit as Reciprocal Claim | |

The error may be indicated with a highlighter pen if the submission is made on a claim card. Do not complete a new card unless the original is illegible. Simply correct the error and return the card to your district office.

The MOH claims clerks indicate an error by highlighting it or they complete the reverse side of the card by checking the appropriate box as in Illustration 6.12.

## Remittance Advice

The Remittance Advice (see Illustration 6.13) is an itemized statement of the individual payments made by the Ministry of Health for insured services. Payments made for WCB-related services will be identified with an asterisk located next to the accounting number field.

The Remittance Advice for opted-in providers lists patients for whom payment was made in their monthly cheque.

Opted-out providers receive a Remittance Advice detailing the payments made to the patients for insured services.

The Remittance Advice has three basic divisions:

1. Header information
2. Claim information
3. Total payment information

### Header Information

The header information appears at the top of the form and includes:

A. Provider's name.
B. District office — the name of the district to which the group/provider has been allocated. And a district identification code, a one-letter identifier where:

**Illustration 6.13   Remittance Advice**

Page 3

| MINISTRY OF HEALTH (Ontario) | ① | Dr. J.J.Jones | Ⓐ | Oshawa (I) B | 0000-123456-01 Ⓑ | Ⓒ | Ⓓ |

REMITTANCE ADVICE FOR 10 MAY 91

| | ACCT'G NUMBER | PATIENT'S NAME LAST | FIRST | PROV INCE | REGISTRATION NUMBER | VER-SION | CONVERTED HEALTH NO. | PAY PGM | CLAIM NUMBER | SERVICE DATE | NO. OF SERV'S | SERV. CODE | ELIG IND | FEE SUBMITTED | AMOUNT PAID | EX CD |
|---|---|---|---|---|---|---|---|---|---|---|---|---|---|---|---|---|
| 01 | 57079111 | Shaw | Olga | On | 1234567899 | L | | HCP | B9876543342 | 910320 | 01 | G310A | | 6.55 | 6.55 | |
| 02 | 78956624 | Bradford | John | On | 9877779933 | Q | | HCP | B1234577772 | 910620 | 01 | G303A | | 8.80 | 8.80 | |
| 03 | 57085125 | Andrews | Geof | On | 8933340421 | M | | HCP | B1440823495 | 910326 | 01 | G700A | | 4.60 | 4.60 | |
| 04 | 57009812 | Arnold | Anit | On | 9725356729 | | | HCP | B1440701277 | 910408 | 01 | J201A | | 103.00 | 103.00 | |
| 05 | 57092378 | Kline | Robe | On | 8945990023 | | | HCP | B1356788841 | 910218 | 01 | 0310A | | 6.55 | 6.55 | |
| 06 | 57081321 | Altas | Keit | On | 7779356211 | | | HCP | B5668932195 | 910421 | 01 | J201A | | 103.00 | 103.00 | |
| 07 | 56912355 | Quick | Glen | On | 9921456144 | Q | ② | HCP | B4162889211 | 910506 | 01 | G313A | | 8.80 | 8.80 | |
| 08 | 57092264 | Jones | Ralp | On | 7753219432 | M | | HCP | B6132115664 | 910423 | 01 | G310A | | 6.55 | 6.55 | |
| 09 | 57699022 | Bland | Sus | On | 5558210036 | | | HCP | B4442172561 | 910302 | 01 | G313A | | 8.80 | 8.80 | |
| 10 | 55532144 | Night | Zera | On | 8832921443 | | | HCP | B1440823178 | 910318 | 01 | G310A | | 6.55 | 6.55 | |
| 11 | 57082166 | Archibal | Marg | On | 9727315693 | | | HCP | B1663233997 | 910222 | 01 | J210A | | 103.00 | 103.00 | |
| 12 | 59011125 | Anthony | Edwi | On | 7772457123 | | | HCP | B1992123339 | 910210 | 01 | G313A | | 8.80 | 8.80 | |
| 13 | 57781234 | Crisp | Har | On | 4321145679 | | | HCP | B2133451677 | 910108 | 01 | J201A | | 103.00 | 103.00 | |
| 14 | 53334891 | Brown | Gai | On | 7899332145 | | | HCP | B1992347892 | 910307 | 01 | G310A | | 6.55 | 6.55 | |
| 15 | 51782311 | Lake | Gwe | On | 9342322431 | | | HCP | B2347891234 | 910523 | 01 | G313A | | 8.80 | 8.80 | Ⓢ |
| | Ⓕ | Ⓖ | Ⓗ | Ⓘ | Ⓙ | Ⓚ | | Ⓛ | Ⓜ | Ⓝ | Ⓞ | Ⓟ | | Ⓠ | Ⓡ | |

| | | PAGE TOTALS Ⓣ | 493.35 | 493.35 |
| | | ③ Ⓤ | 4,096.50 | 4,045.60 |

Ⓥ CHEQUE # 301

INQUIRES REGARDING OVER-PAYMENTS, UNDER-PAYMENTS OR NON-PAYMENT MUST BE MADE WITHIN 6 MONTHS OF SERVICE DATE.
FOR LABORATORIES ONLY, FEE SUBMITTED IS TOTAL FEE PAID PER CLAIM

| | |
|---|---|
| A   is Mississauga | L   is London |
| B   is Oshawa | M   is Toronto (Metropolitan Toronto) |
| C   is Ottawa | S   is Sudbury |
| H   is Hamilton | T   is Thunder Bay |
| K   is Kingston | |

C.  Group/provider's registration number.

D.  Payment date.

E.  Page number.

## Claim Information

The claim information is the main part of the form and relates all data relevant to each card claim submission as follows:

F.  Provider accounting number — the number assigned by a provider to the patient for accounting purposes. Maximum of eight alphanumeric characters. May or may not be present according to whether the allotted space was filled on the original claim.

G. Patient's last name — maximum of fourteen alpha characters.

H. Patient's first name — maximum of three alpha characters.

I. The patient's province of residence.

J. Ministry of Health ten-digit number.

K. Version code. Each time a patient's registration card is revised, one alpha character is added beside the ten-digit number on the registration card.

L. The type of payment identification, e.g., HCP, WCB, or RMB.

M. The Ministry of Health claim number — a unique number assigned by the Ministry to identify each claim, eleven characters in length.

N. Initial service date — the date the service was performed.

O. Number of services.

P. Fee schedule code — obtained from the Ministry of Health Schedule of Benefits.

Q. Fee submitted — the fee submitted by the provider, regardless of whether this fee is lower than, the same as, or greater than that shown in the Schedule of Benefits.

R. Amount paid — the amount actually paid to the provider for the service. The fee allowed is usually 100 percent of that specified in the Schedule of Benefits.

S. Explanatory codes — the explanatory code will appear in cases where zero payment, or payment less than 100 percent of the fee allotted, is being issued. The remittance advice explanatory codes are given in Illustration 6.14. More complete or detailed descriptions may be obtained from your Ministry of Health claims clerk.

## Total Payment Information

T. Page totals — the total amounts billed and paid per page.

U. An aggregate total of previous pages.

V. Cheque number — for opted-in providers only; a cheque number is given if payment is made by cheque.

The last page will state the total claims payable to the provider and any accounting adjustments or interim payments.

**Illustration 6.14    Remittance Advice Explanatory Codes**

Explanatory Codes:

| Code | Description | Code | Description | Code | Description |
|------|-------------|------|-------------|------|-------------|
| C6 | Allowed as type 2 admission assessment. | E5 | Service date is not within an eligible period. | RD | Duplicate, paid in RMBS. |
| EA | Service date is not within an eligible period — services provided on or after the 20th of this month will not be paid unless eligibility status changes. | FF | Additional payment for the claim shown. | S4 | Procedure fee reduced when paid with related surgery. |
| | | G1 | Other critical/comprehensive care already paid. | T1 | Fee allowed according to surgery claim. |
| EF | Incorrect version code — service provided on or after the 20th of this month will not be paid unless current version code is provided. | HF | Concurrent or supportive care already claimed in period. | 48 | Paid as submitted — clinical records may be requested for verification purposes. |
| | | I2 | Service is globally funded. | 49 | Interim payment — clinical records/operative reports are required for final adjudication of claim. |
| EV | Check Health Card for current version code. | I3 | FSC is not on the IHF licence profile for the date specified. | | |
| E1 | Service date is prior to start of eligibility. | | | 60 | Not a benefit of the reciprocal medical billing agreement. |
| E2 | Incorrect version code for service date. | I4 | Records show this service has been rendered by another practitioner, group, or IHF. | | |
| E4 | Service date is after the eligibility termination date. | I5 | Service is globally funded and FSC is not on IHF licence profile. | | |

## Remittance Advice Inquiries

Ministry of Health staff attempt to minimize the necessity for inquiries concerning claims payment. However, sometimes discrepancies do occur.

If, after examining the Remittance Advice, you find a discrepancy, the first step is to verify that you have submitted the claim correctly. If this is the case, and you feel that you have been incorrectly paid for the service(s), the next step is to complete a Remittance Advice Inquiry form.

Two types of these inquiry forms are available: single inquiry and multiple inquiry.

The single inquiry form is usually used by opted-out providers on behalf of the patient (see Illustration 6.15).

**Illustration 6.15 Remittance Advice Inquiry Form — Single Inquiry**

| Provider no. | Provider's accounting number | Pymt. prg. | Payee |
|---|---|---|---|

| Province | Registration no. | Version | |
|---|---|---|---|

| Patient's last name | Patient's first name | Patient's birthdate (Year / Month / Day) | Pat's. sex (M / F) |
|---|---|---|---|

Patient's address

City | Province | Postal Code

**Instructions**

*1. Inquiries on claim payments should be made within one month of receipt of remittance advice.*
*2. Use this form to itemize under- or over-payments.*
*3 Claims outstanding for two payment cycles (remittances) after submission should be resubmitted if no advice received.*

| Service date Year | Service date Month | Service date Day | Claim number | Fee submitted | Date paid Year | Date paid Month | Date paid Day | Amount paid |
|---|---|---|---|---|---|---|---|---|
| | | | | | | | | |
| | | | | | | | | |
| | | | | | | | | |

Remarks

| Date of inquiry | Provider's telephone no. |
|---|---|

*For Ministry of Health use only*

1. Claim under review – ☐ You will be advised further.
2. Claim indicated to – ☐ Pay patient directly.
3. Adjustment – ☐ Under payment – will credit your account in the amount of $
   – ☐ Overpayment – will debit your account in the amount of $
   – ☐ No Adjustment – amount paid correctly according to available information.
4. Remarks:

Ministry of Health
Ontario

White and Yellow copy to Ministry of Health Office. Retain Pink copy.

| Date | Station number | Signature |
|---|---|---|

0588–84 (90/12) 7530–4256

The multiple inquiry form is normally used by opted-in providers when several inquiries are made (see Illustration 6.16).

**Illustration 6.16 Remittance Advice Inquiry Form — Multiple Inquiry**

Ontario | Ministry of Health | Ministère de la Santé

**REMITTANCE ADVICE INQUIRY**
**DEMANDE DE RENSEIGNEMENTS (AVIS DE RÈGLEMENT)**

**IMPORTANT:**

A. State your Provider and Group Number.
B. State your name and address.
C. Retain **pink** copy for your records.
D. Send white and yellow copies to your **MINISTRY OF HEALTH OFFICE.**

A. Inscrivez votre numero de fournisseur et votre numéro de groupe.
B. Inscrivez votre nom et adresse.
C. Gardez la copie **rose** pour vos dossiers.
D. Envoyez les copies blanche et jaune à votre **BUREAU DU MINISTÈRE DE LA SANTÉ.**

| | |
|---|---|
| Provider/Group name - Nom du fournisseur groupe | |
| Address - Adresse | |
| | |
| Postal Code - Code postal | Telephone Number - Nº de téléphone |
| Date of Remittance Advice<br>Date de l'avis de règlement | Provider/Group number<br>Numéro du fournisseur groupe |

**INSTRUCTIONS:**

1. Use this form to itemize **under** or **over**-payments. **ONLY**
2. Claims outstanding for two payment cycles (remittances) after submission should be re-submitted if no advice received.
3. Inquiries on claim payments should be made within **one** month of receipt of remittance advice.
4. Submit all inquiries from one remittance advice at the same time.

1. **N'utilisez** cette formule **QUE** pour dresser la liste des paiements **insuffisants** ou **excédentaires**.
2. Les paiements qui n'ont pas été effectués au bout de deux périodes de paiement suivant la date de la soumission de la demande de règlement doivent faire l'objet d'une nouvelle demande si l'on n'a reçu aucun avis.
3. Les demandes de renseignements sur les paiements doivent être faites moins d'**un** mois après réception de l'avis de règlement.
4. Soumettre en une seule fois toutes les demandes de renseignements relatives à un avis de règlement.

| | |
|---|---|
| **Under Review - you will be advised.**<br>**À l'étude - on vous avisera.** | **U.R.** |
| **Paid Correctly according to our records.**<br>**Payé correctement selon nos dossiers.** | **P.C.** |
| **Adjustment Required - being processed.**<br>**Redressement requis - présentement en cours.** | **A.R.** |

DATE OF INQUIRY / DATE DE LA DEMANDE

UP.-underpayment OP.-Overpayment
P.I.-paiement insuffisant P.E.-paiement excédentaire

| PAGE NO. Nº DE PAGE | LINE NO. Nº DE LIGNE | CLAIM INFORMATION RENSEIGNEMENTS (DEMANDE DE RÈGLEMENT) | U.P. O.P. P.I. P.E. | PROVIDER GROUP REMARKS OBSERVATIONS DU FOURNISSEUR GROUPE | OFFICE USE ONLY RÉSERVÉ AU BUREAU | CODE CODE |
|---|---|---|---|---|---|---|
| | | Health No./Nº de carte sante | | | | |
| | | Claim No./Nº de la demande de règlement | | | | |
| | | Payment Program/Programme de paiement | | | | |
| | | Surname/Nom de famille | | | | |
| | | Date of Birth/Date de naissance Y/A M/M D/J | | | | |
| | | Accounting No./Nº de compte | | | | |
| | | Health No./Nº de carte sante | | | | |
| | | Claim No./Nº de la demande de règlement | | | | |
| | | Payment Program/Programme de paiement | | | | |
| | | Surname/Nom de famille | | | | |
| | | Date of Birth/Date de naissance Y/A M/M D/J | | | | |
| | | Accounting No./Nº de compte | | | | |
| | | Health No./Nº de carte sante | | | | |
| | | Claim No./Nº de la demande de règlement | | | | |
| | | Payment Program/Programme de paiement | | | | |
| | | Surname/Nom de famille | | | | |
| | | Date of Birth/Date de naissance Y/A M/M D/J | | | | |
| | | Accounting No./Nº de compte | | | | |
| | | Health No./Nº de carte sante | | | | |
| | | Claim No./Nº de la demande de règlement | | | | |
| | | Payment Program/Programme de paiement | | | | |
| | | Surname/Nom de famille | | | | |
| | | Date of Birth/Date de naissance Y/A M/M D/J | | | | |
| | | Accounting No./Nº de compte | | | | |

| | | |
|---|---|---|
| NAME OF CLERK (PRINT):<br>NOM DU COMMIS<br>(LETTRES MOULÉES): | TELEPHONE | DATE RETURNED TO PROVIDER/GROUP<br>RETOURNÉE AU FOURNISSEUR GROUPE LE: |

918-84 (90/02) 7530-4240

Both forms, however, may be used by either opted-in or opted-out providers depending on the medical administrative assistant's preference.

The forms are self-explanatory. Assistance in completing the forms may be obtained from your Ministry of Health claims clerk. Forms may be ordered from your local Ministry of Health office.

The Remittance Advice Inquiry form contains three copies: white, yellow, and pink. The white and yellow copies are sent to the Ministry of Health. The pink is retained for your records. The yellow copy will be returned to you with the Ministry's reply.

**Claims that do not appear on the Remittance Advice after two successive months should be resubmitted.** If a large volume of claims has not been paid, a phone call to your Ministry of Health claims clerk is advisable. If you resubmit a claim, ensure that you mark it "resubmission" in the diagnosis area of the card and show the date of first submission. Claims submitted six months after service date will not be considered for payment.

## Nonpayment of Claims

If the provider still disagrees with the payment of a claim after submitting an inquiry form, the unit supervisor should be consulted. Appeals of complicated claims may be directed to the ministry's medical consultant in a district office.

## Appeals

The Northern Health Travel Grant is an Ontario Ministry of Health program that helps northern residents of the province pay for travel to receive medically necessary care that is unavailable locally. The program provides grants to help reimburse the transportation costs of residents who must travel more than 300 kilometres (one way) from their residence to visit a medical specialist or receive a medical specialist's services at a hospital in Ontario or Manitoba.

The amount of the grant is based on the distance travelled to the closest appropriate medical specialist, as determined by the referring provider.

Application forms and booklets detailing who is eligible and how the grant works are available for your patients at Northern Ontario Ministry of Health offices or by contacting the closest office of the Ministry of Northern Development.

## Northern Health Travel Grant

While working as a medical administrative assistant in Ontario you may encounter patients who are visitors from outside Ontario. As discussed earlier in this chapter, for Canadian residents (excluding Quebec) you will complete a reciprocal claim card and submit it to the Ministry of Health.

Claims for visitors from outside Canada are to be billed directly to the patient.

## Visitors from outside Ontario

## Out-of-Province Benefits

The Ministry of Health pays for insured medical and hospital services received in any part of the world by Ontario residents who have a valid health number. Providers' services are paid at the rates listed in the Ministry of Health Schedule of Benefits for comparable services performed in Ontario. Hospital charges are reimbursed based on the level of care received. For example:

- $400 (Canadian) per day is paid for intensive out-of-country hospital care such as invasive surgery, high-technology treatment, and frequent monitoring of a patient's condition.
- $200 (Canadian) per day is paid for rehabilitative and other less intense care, such as treatment for substance abuse, psychiatric illness, and eating disorders.

An itemized bill should be sent by the patient to the local Ministry of Health office. To avoid delays in payment, the bill should also state the patient's name, address, and health number.

## Machine-Readable Input

Submitting claims to the Ministry of Health on machine-readable input (MRI) is becoming increasingly popular. As mentioned earlier, the ministry is currently accepting machine-readable data on magnetic tape, 5¼-inch, and 3½-inch diskettes.

There are some major advantages to submitting claims on one of these media:

1. Reconciliation of payments is easier.
2. Less handling, especially of large volumes of cards.
3. All claims on diskettes are accounted for; only a slight chance of a claim going "missing."
4. All diskettes, both input and output, are supplied by the ministry free of charge.
5. Creation of a database eliminates entry of repetitive information.
6. Claim records occupy minimal storage space.
7. Emergency cash-flow procedures are in place in the event of a data crash.
8. Reduces incidence of rejected claims.
9. Reduces accounting costs.
10. Saves time; increases staff productivity.
11. All claims can now be submitted by MRI. (Printed cards are not required.)

## Purchasing Computer Hardware and Software

If you are involved in purchasing computer hardware and software for your medical office, there will be many things for you to consider. The following information has been compiled to assist you in your investigation of computers and to familiarize you with the ministry's capacity for accepting automated billing and delivering reconciliation data on magnetic media.

It is very important to determine your *software* needs before you purchase computer *hardware*. Since computer software is the driving force of a micro-computer system, it should be selected with much care and consideration. Software packages are not always compatible with all the computer hardware offered on the market. By making a software selection first, you can eliminate many computer hardware brands from your list of considerations. Purchasing incompatible hardware and software is a costly mistake.

Before you actually purchase a software package you should have a good idea of what you are looking for. There is a wide variety of packages with diverse applications and considerable differences in cost.

You should begin your market research by looking closely at the way your office is currently operating. What office tasks and activities could be stream-lined? How could your time be better spent? Do you spend hours or even days carrying out routine clerical and administrative tasks? These are the types of questions that you may wish to review.

It can be of tremendous help in your search for the right software if you prepare a checklist of the functions or activities that you are interested in see-ing demonstrated on a computer. A sample checklist is provided below.

## Office Functions and Activities

Appointment scheduling          _____
Medical billing          _____
Word processing          _____
Accounting          _____
Financial reporting          _____
Medical records          _____
Patient registration          _____
Telecommunications          _____
Research and analysis          _____
Other: _____          _____

## Selection Considerations

With such a wide variety of software packages available, providers and medi-cal administrative assistants should be armed with a number of key questions that will make the selection process much easier.

1. Does the system keep basic demographic information on patients (age, sex, health number, address, telephone number)? Can this information be easily retrieved and updated (as in a change of address)?
2. Can it maintain patient medical histories (X-rays, allergies, surgery)?
3. Does it meet your needs for an accounting and billing system with an audit trail? Does it provide an accounts payable system?
4. Can it store referring provider information? Ministry of Health procedure codes? Diagnostic code information?
5. Are there features that will make it easier to manage active and inactive files?

6. How well will the system meet Ministry of Health billing and reconciliation needs? Is it compatible with ministry specifications? What financial summaries can the system provide?

The answers to some of these questions should help you identify those systems that clearly do not meet your needs and those that would be suitable for your office.

### Other Selection Criteria

Once the functional requirements for a new system have been determined, a number of other key questions should be considered:

1. What reputation does the vendor have?
2. What reputation does the manufacturer have?
3. What is the cost of purchasing a complete system?
4. How much staff training will be provided? Is it included in the purchase price?
5. How is equipment maintenance covered in the contract?
6. How long will it take to get the system "up" if there is a breakdown?
7. Is there a consultant and repair service in your area?

## Using a Microcomputer System to Submit Claims

In terms of providing machine-readable claims to the Ministry of Health, microcomputers offer a number of benefits.

### Validity Rejects

You can use a microcomputer to check the validity of a claim *before* sending it to the ministry to identify many of the input errors that would otherwise result in a claim that cannot be processed. Some of the errors that can be detected and corrected before submitting follow:

1. Missing information, such as date of birth or a diagnostic code.
2. Invalid health numbers, referring provider numbers, service codes, diagnostic codes, facility numbers, region codes, specialty indicators, fees, and dates.
3. Incorrect use of numbers, letters, or special characters (such as punctuation in the service date).

### Input Control

With an automated system, you have control over the accuracy of all billing data submitted to the Ministry of Health. The software checks the validity of information as it is being entered, eliminating many of the common errors that cause claims to be rejected. When a claim is rejected by the ministry's mainframe computer, a claims error report (Illustration 6.18) is mailed to the health care provider. This report will identify the claim and explain why it was rejected. The corrected claim may be re-entered as a new claim on your next automated submission or on a claim card.

## Reconciliation of Remittance Advices

The remittance advice provided by the Ministry of Health in a machine-readable form makes it easier for you to reconcile payments with billings. You can use your system to run diskette remittance advices against your billing input files to provide only a printout of the variances. In a manual system, this reconciliation process can take days, whereas with an automated system, it can be done in minutes!

Whether the provider has decided to buy prepackaged software or is a technology enthusiast who wishes to develop individual application programs, there are specifications that must be met for claim submissions (see Illustration 6.17). The Ministry of Health has published a *Technical Specifications Manual* for media on which machine-readable data can be submitted. This manual provides an essential guide for the development of an effective computer system and includes details on the following:

**MOH Specifications for Claim Submission**

1. The *conditions* governing the plan's acceptance and processing of claims data in machine-readable form (magnetic tape, $5\frac{1}{4}$-inch, and $3\frac{1}{2}$-inch diskettes).
2. The *technical criteria* that apply to the processing of claims data received in machine-readable form.
3. The *output documents* produced after claims data are processed.
4. The specifications related to *remittance advice* (payments) data supplied by the plan in machine-readable form.

Health care providers are responsible for the accuracy and validity of all described and coded services submitted to the Ministry of Health for payment. Source documentation must be maintained in hard copy or photographic form for seven years and must be kept available for review by the ministry (upon reasonable notification).

**Source Documentation Requirements**

## Payment Cycle

**After the Switch to Diskettes**

Although diskette input may be submitted anytime prior to the cutoff date, providers may choose to submit input weekly or biweekly. This procedure would limit the potential consequences of a processing problem should one occur (due to difficulty in reading the diskette, for example). It would also enable you to change incorrect data for resubmission during the current processing cycle.

**Illustration 6.17   Switching to Diskettes**

SWITCHING TO DISKETTE INPUT

CALL OR VISIT THE COMPUTER DROP-IN CENTRE AT YOUR
LOCAL MOH DISTRICT OFFICE

MOH Technical Services staff will demonstrate a computerized medical billing system and provide
the provider and his or her staff with an opportunity to try it out. Other literature such as the
Self-Teaching Guide and the Specifications Manual will be made available.

SUBMIT TO MOH:
– APPLICATION FORM
– LETTER OF UNDERSTANDING
– DESCRIPTION OR SAMPLE OF
  SOURCE DOCUMENTATION

After MOH has confirmed that this documentation is in order, you will be asked to prepare test
data on your system. Your software supplier should be able to assist you in preparing the data for
submission to MOH for testing and specification checks.

SUBMIT TEST DATA

The results will be returned to you within a few days. Once this system verification has been
completed, MOH will notify you of the start date for "live" data submissions and provide you with
a free supply of diskettes.

BEGIN "LIVE" SUBMISSION OF CLAIMS ON DISKETTES

Payment for claims received up to and including the cut-off date of the "start" month can be
returned on a diskette prepared on or before the payment date of the following month, if
requested.

RECEIVE REMITTANCE ADVICE ON DISKETTE
(OPTIONAL)

## Diskettes Are Supplied

An initial supply of diskettes will be provided free of charge to you upon
approval of your "live" data submission system. Additional diskettes will be
provided as needed and replaced as they become worn out. The Ministry of
Health performs quality-control checks and preformats all diskettes before
giving them to you.

## Delivery of Diskettes

To minimize the risk of damage or accidental erasure, you should make sure
that your diskettes are securely packaged. They may be delivered in person or
by courier service directly to any MOH office. Remittance advices on
diskettes will be mailed to you.

## Remittance Advice Format

Claims submitted on claim cards will receive remittance advice in paper format. Machine-readable submissions will receive remittance advice in machine-readable format.

## "Y" Indicator Capability

For machine-readable input, all software packages should have a "Y" indicator capability. This "Y" indicator will flag a claim that must have supporting documentation. The supporting documentation should accompany the diskette to the Ministry of Health district office.

## Error Reports

When an input error prevents the processing of a claim, a Claims Error Report will be generated and sent to you (see Illustration 6.18). The error report identifies the claim and provides an error message to explain why the claim was rejected.

## Error Codes

The Claims Error Report contains error codes to explain why the claim has not been accepted. In Illustration 6.18, the second claim (d) error code is V22. The V22 explanation is "Diagnostic Code is not a valid code." A *Computer User Information* booklet has been produced by the ministry and is available at your district office. This booklet contains a list of all error codes as well as useful information about provider submissions.

**Who to Call When Help Is Required**

A claims clerk will be assigned by the ministry to handle your claims input and to answer questions regarding billing and payment of claims.

The medical consultant and the adjudication support section are available to answer questions regarding complicated claims.

The registry clerk will assist you in matters regarding changes in the provider's registration information. Changes in registration information (e.g., change of address, banking change) should be in writing.

For more information regarding machine-readable input, the technical services section will answer any questions you may have.

The customer service section will answer your patient's questions regarding enrollment and eligibility.

Of course, management and supervisors of Ministry of Health offices are also accessible to you.

**Illustration 6.18    Claims Error Report for Machine-Readable Input**

### CLAIMS ERROR REPORT FOR MACHINE-READABLE INPUT

|  | (1) |  | (2) |  | (3) |
|---|---|---|---|---|---|
| RUN DATE | – MAR 26,1993 | CLINIC-PRACTITIONER # | : 0000–144436 | BILLING AGENT # | : D00999 |
| REPORT-ID | – MCDR 13–R1 | CLINIC | : DOE | NAME AND ADDRESS | : DR. JOHN DOE |
| DISTRICT | – OSHAWA | PRACTITIONER | : |  | 1234 ANY STREET |
| CODE | – F |  |  |  | TESTVILLE, ONTARIO |
| STATION NO | – 554 |  |  |  | A1A 1A1 |

| RECORD TYPE * | GROUP/LABORATORY LICENCE NUMBER | OHIP #/ VERSION CODE | PROVIDER/PHYSIO FACILITY/ LABORATORY DIRECTOR'S NUMBER | | | | | | | | | | ERROR CODES |
|---|---|---|---|---|---|---|---|---|---|---|---|---|---|
|  |  |  | PATIENT'S LAST NAME | PATIENT'S FIRST NAME | PATIENT'S BIRTHDATE | SERVICE DATE | No. OF SERVICES | DIAG. CODE | SPECIALTY | ACCOUNTING NUMBER | PAYMENT PROGRAM | PAYEE | SEX |
| | | | | | | | | | REFER/REQUIS PROVIDER NUMBER | PROVINCE CODE | FACILITY NUMBER | IN-PATIENT ADM DATE | REFER LAB LICENCE NUMBER |

| | RECORD TYPE | HEALTH NUMBER | VERSION CODE | REGISTRATION | FEE SUBMITTED | SERVICE CODE | No. OF SERVICES | SERVICE DATE | DIAG. CODE | PAYMENT PROGRAM | PAYEE | SEX | PROVINCE CODE | ERROR CODES |
|---|---|---|---|---|---|---|---|---|---|---|---|---|---|---|
| (4) | BTCH | | | | | 0000 | | | 14436 | | 00 | | | |
| a) | HDR1 | 0102030400 | | | | 581103 | 01 | D0017177 | HCP | P | | | | |
| b) | ITM | A007A | | 002450 | | | | 930314 | 072 | | 00 | | | EH2 |
| d) | BTCH | | | | | 0000 | | | 14436 | | | | | |
| | HDR1 | | | | | | | | | | | | | |
| | HDR2 | 123456789012 | | | | | | 00000003 | RMB | P | | | | |
| c) | ITM | | | | SOMEONE | | | | PERSON | | 1 | | BC | |
| d) | ITM | A007A | | 002450 | | | 01 | 930315 | 705 | | | | | V22 |
| (5) | TOTAL REJECTS FOR CLINIC/PRACTITIONER 0000–144436 : | | | | | | | | | | | | 2 | |

\* RECORD TYPE : "BTCH" – BATCH, "HDR1" – HEADER 1, "HDR2" – HEADER 2, "ITM" – ITEM

THIS FORM IS MAILED FROM THE MINISTRY ADVISING YOU OF THE CLAIMS ON YOUR SUBMISSION THAT CANNOT BE ACCEPTED FOR PAYMENT AS BILLED. *THESE CLAIMS MUST BE CORRECTED AND RESUBMITTED FOR PAYMENT.*

## EXPLANATION:

1.  The RUNDATE is the date your claims were processed through the Ministry's computer.

2.  CLINIC-PRACTITIONER is your registered number and name for billing with the Ministry of Health.

3.  BILLING AGENT is the unique number and address for your machine readable billing to the Ministry.

4.  RECORD TYPE – these are the headings for the layout of your claim on your submission for easy identification.
    a)  BTCH – group/provider/specialty number on the batch header record on your submission.
    b)  HDR1 – is a header record for all claims giving basic patient information needed to process your claims.
    c)  HDR2 – is an additional header record needed for reciprocal medical claims only.
    d)  ITM – is an item record that shows what has been claimed. On the right hand side you will find the error code for the rejection. In the first example, EH2 is the rejection code which means a version code is required for this health number. In the second example, V22 is the rejection code which means the diagnostic code is not a valid code; the diagnostic code used is 705 which must be corrected.

5.  This is the total number of claims rejected per run date.

*(Error Codes can be found in your HEALTH CARE PROVIDER'S MANUAL, Pages W1 to W7).*

Rev. 0693–JW/ms

The Ministry of Health communicates with medical administrative assistants in various ways. The following is a list of some of these ways:

1. Schedule of Benefits — sent to the provider whenever ministry fees are renegotiated.
2. Bulletins — sent whenever updates in rules or fees are required.
3. Brochures/Posters/Forms — available for a variety of subjects. Additional copies are available from your local ministry office. Also available are all forms mentioned earlier in this chapter.
4. Claim Card Submission Manual — available to all providers' offices. This manual assists administrative assistants in completing claims.
5. *Computer User Information* — this booklet is available on request for providers who are interested in learning more about billing by computer.
6. *Technical Specifications Manual* — this contains the detailed specifications required for claim input using diskettes.
7. Medical administrative assistant seminars — the ministry periodically conducts seminars in various cities. You will be invited to attend whenever one is to be held in your vicinity. These seminars have proved to be very popular and informative.

## How the MOH Communicates with Medical Administrative Assistants

All of the preceding information will prove helpful once you begin your work as a medical administrative assistant. However, it is intended as a basic outline only. As in all professions, additional on-the-job training must be gained before you are proficient in your field.

Remember that your local Ministry of Health office will be available for assistance whenever possible.

## Conclusion

Your instructor will provide you with the material required to complete the assignment.

## Assignment 6.1

Using the personal data information provided in Chapter 3, complete health claim cards (Working Papers, pp. 24–32) for the following procedures performed by Dr. Plunkett (0000-123456-00):

Mr. Mel Thompson, minor assessment on February 28, 19__ (diagnosis: influenza).

Mr. Jean Belliveau, two minor assessments on February 24 and 27, 19__ (diagnosis: (1) URI; (2) tension headache).

Mr. Thomas Bell, annual health exam, February 24, 19__.

Erik Shultz, special trip to hospital (no. 1100) during office hours on February 25, 19__ (sutured 4.5 cm laceration on head).

Peter John Scott, entered Ottawa General Hospital (no. 1179) on February 18, 19__ (Dr. Plunkett performed an emergency appendectomy, which involved complications such as gross perforation and peritonitis).

## Assignment 6.2

Amelia Jackson, intermediate assessment and Pap smear, February 20, 19__ (diagnosis: vaginitis).

Dr. Plunkett (0000-123456-00) has referred patients in the situations below. Complete health claim cards for each service. (It is not necessary to complete the consulting physicians' data.)

Mr. Thomas Bell was seen by an internal medicine specialist (first visit) on admission to Ottawa General Hospital (no. 1220) on February 16, 19__. The specialist made four subsequent visits on February 17, 18, 19, and 20 (diagnosis: cirrhosis).

Mrs. Hazel Davis delivered a baby by caesarean section in hospital no. 1220 on February 18, 19__. She was attended by an obstetrician.

Lisa Basciano was attended by a urologist on February 20, 19__, in Ottawa City Hospital (no. 2463). Three consecutive visits were made (diagnosis: urethritis).

Erik Shultz's wife, Mary (born June 6, 19__), had individual psychotherapy with a psychiatrist on February 23, 19__ for one hour (diagnosis: alcoholism).

After your work has been evaluated, insert cards for Peter John Scott, Thomas Bell, Hazel Davis, Lisa Basciano, and Mary Shultz in your portfolio.

## Workers' Compensation

The Workers' Compensation Board (WCB) is a statutory corporation created by an act of the Ontario Legislature in 1914. It is responsible for administering the Workers' Compensation Act and Regulations of Ontario. The board raises funds from the province's employers in order to provide compensation to workers who are injured on the job or who contract an industrial disease.

Compensation includes payment for loss of wages that may result from the injury or disease; future economic loss and/or noneconomic loss awards for permanent/partial disability; payment of health care expenses; a wide range of vocational and medical rehabilitation services; retraining programs; and survivor benefits in the case of a fatality.

If an injured worker is not satisfied with the decision rendered by any of the operating divisions at the Workers' Compensation Board, the injured worker may appeal the decision to the Appeals Branch, which is the final level within the board.

If the worker wishes to pursue a denial, he or she can appeal to the Workers' Compensation Appeals Tribunal, a body external to the board.

## Making a Claim

### Employee's Responsibilities

1. Get first aid immediately. (By law, the employer must have a first-aid station available and a person trained in first aid on duty at all times.)
2. Report the details of the accident to the employer, even if no further medical treatment is required.

**Illustration 6.19   Treatment Memorandum**

| Workers' Compensation Board | Commission des accidents du travail | 2 Bloor Street East<br>Toronto, Ontario<br>M4W 3C3 | 2, rue Bloor Est<br>Toronto (Ontario)<br>M4W 3C3 | Treatment Memorandum<br>*Avis de traitement* |
|---|---|---|---|---|

Practitioner/Hospital:   The worker claims to have been injured in our employ and requests treatment.  We , the employer, are sending a report to the Workers' Compensation Board.

*Praticien/ hôpital :   Le travailleur affirme avoir subi une lésion alors qu'il était à notre emploi et demande des traitemente.  En tant qu'employeur, nous ferons parvenir un rapport à la Commission des accidents du travail.*

| | | | | | |
|---|---|---|---|---|---|
| Worker Identification<br>*Identification du travailleur* | Last Name/ *Nom de famille* | | First Name/ *Prénom* | Initials/ *Initiale* | S.I.N./ *N° d'assurance sociale* |
| | Address (no.,street,apt. no.)/ *Adresse (n°, rue,app.)* | City,Town/*Ville* | Province | Postal Code<br>*Code postal* | |

| | | | |
|---|---|---|---|
| Employer Identification<br>*Identification de l'employeur* | Firm Name/ *Nom de l'entreprise* | | W.C.B. Firm No./ *N° d'entreprise à la CAT* |
| | Address/ *Adresse* | City,Town/*Ville* | Province | Postal Code<br>*Code postal* |

| | | | |
|---|---|---|---|
| Accident Information<br>*Renseignements sur l'accident* | Date  and hour of accidental injury<br>*Date et heure de l'accident*<br>dd/jj   mm/mm  yy/aa     time/ heure | Date and hour accident reported<br>*Date et heure où fut signalé l'accid.*<br>dd/jj   mm/mm  yy/aa   time/ heure | Nature of Injury/*Nature de la lésion* |
| | m | m | |

Important:   Please retain and file this document for future reference and submission to the Board if requested.

*Veuillez conserver ce document aux fins de références futures et de soumission à la Commission, sur demande.*

| Name of Company Officer/ *Nom du dirigeant de l'entreprise* | Date |
|---|---|

Please see other side/  *Voir au verso.*

Please submit your account to the Board/  *Veuillez envoyer votre facture à la Commission.*
0156C (07/86)

3. Ask the employer for a Treatment Memorandum, and take it to the doctor or hospital if medical attention is required (see Illustration 6.19). (Note: Read the Treatment Memorandum form for your information.)

4. Choose the physician or other qualified health care provider you want to administer treatment. (Note: Once you have made your choice, you must receive permission from WCB before changing to another doctor. It may be necessary to change doctors because you are moving, for instance; or you may be dissatisfied with the treatment you are receiving. If you find it necessary to change doctors for whatever reason, remember to get permission from WCB *before* making a change.)

5. Complete and return quickly any forms received from WCB. Be sure all forms are legible and in black ink, that all information is exact and complete (including postal code), and that you sign all forms. When an accident is reported to WCB, the injured worker is assigned a claim number. This number *must* appear on *every* form or letter that is sent to WCB.

## Employer's Responsibilities

1. Make sure first aid is administered immediately.
2. Complete and give a Treatment Memorandum to the employee if further medical treatment is required.

3. Record the details of the accident (date, time, place, type of injury, medical aid given).

4. If necessary, provide transportation to doctor's office, hospital, or home (within reasonable distance of workplace).

5. Complete an Employer's Report of Injury/Disease and send to WCB immediately if injury requires medical treatment (see Illustration 6.20). (Note: Read report details for your information.)

6. Supply any other information required by WCB.

## Physician's Responsibilities

In all cases where an injured worker has been treated for a work-related injury, complete and send to WCB a Physician's First Report (see Illustration 6.21) as soon as the injured patient has been examined.

## Administrative Assistant's Responsibilities

1. Secure the Treatment Memorandum on the arrival of the injured worker at the doctor's office. This has already been completed by the employer confirming the accident or injury.

2. Complete the Physician's First Report and send it to the WCB. This is done after the doctor has seen the patient, and has provided the necessary information. Complete the billing portion in the bottom right corner of the form to reimburse the physician for completing the report.

3. Keep a financial record of the charges for patients seen by the doctor on behalf of WCB. Payment for services rendered is received from the Ministry of Health. Complete and submit a Ministry of Health claim card using the same procedure as for regular health service claims. Enter "WCB" in the "Payment Program" block on the health claim card.

4. Keep a record of fees claimed for completing reports on behalf of WCB.

5. Complete a Health Care Accounts Inquiry Form and send it to WCB (see Illustration 6.22).

6. Obtain a WCB Medical Records Waiver Form, signed by the injured patient and witnessed by a second party (see Illustration 6.23), if WCB requires access to the patient's complete medical records. This form is completed *before* releasing the documents.

7. Forward a Physician's Progress Report (see Illustration 6.24). This will be done under certain circumstances only, and completed by the doctor. Be sure to complete the payment portion in the bottom right corner of the report form.

8. If a physician is required to submit to WCB a supporting document such as a consultation or operating report, a Form 0150 (see Illustration 6.25) should be completed and affixed to the bottom right corner of the report. Form 0150 is referred to as a "payment label" and can be ordered through the WCB office. You should ensure that all portions of the form contain the required information.

**Illustration 6.20   Employer's Report of Injury/Disease**

---

### Workers' Compensation Board — Commission des accidents du travail — Ontario

**Employer's Report of Injury/Disease**
**Form 7      (Page 1)**

Ce formulaire est disponible en français sur demande.

- Please read the instructions on the reverse of the Employer's Copy (yellow copy)
- Please type or print firmly in dark ink.
- Do not fold page 2 under page 1 when completing the form.

**WCB use only**
Claim Number

#### A. Worker Identification

| Last Name | First Name |
|---|---|

Address

City / Town

Province        Postal Code

Worker Reference Number        Miner's Certificate Number

Social Insurance Number

Occupation at Time of Injury/Awareness of Disease        Years Experience in Occupation

Date of Birth   day   month   year        Sex        Date of Hire   day   month   year

Worker's Preferred Language of Service
☐ English   ☐ French

Other language if worker speaks neither English/French

Fold                                                                                          Fold

Is the injured person a (sub) contractor, independent operator, owner, executive of the business or spouse or relative of the employer?   ☐ yes   ☐ no        Area Code   Telephone Number   (      )

#### B. Employer Identification

Employer Name        Firm Number        Rate Number

Address        City / Town        Province        Postal Code

Area Code   Telephone Number   (      )        Area Code   FAX Number   (      )        Description of Business Activity

Worksite Location, Branch, Plant, Department Where Worker Employed        Classification Unit Code See instructions

Do you have an early return to work, Co-operative Return To Work program or an accommodation program in your workplace?   ☐ no   ☐ yes        Is the injured worker represented by a trade union?   ☐ no   ☐ yes

#### C. Temporary Disability

Following the day that the injury/awareness of disease occurred, will the injured worker be absent from work because of the injury/disease?   ☐ unknown   ☐ yes   ☐ no

If you answered "no" to the above, will the injured worker as a result of the injury/disease:

- assume other work duties because the injury/disease prevents them from performing their regular duties?   ☐ yes   ☐ no
- earn less than their regular wages because of the injury/disease?   ☐ yes   ☐ no

**Note:** If your answer is "no" to all of these questions do not complete Section F, "Earnings Information".

#### D. Details of Injury/Disease

| Date and Hour of Injury/Awareness of Disease | | | Date and Hour Reported to Employer | | | Date and Hour Last Worked | | | Normal Working Hours on Last Day Worked |
|---|---|---|---|---|---|---|---|---|---|
| day | month | year   a.m. p.m. | day | month | year   a.m. p.m. | day | month | year   a.m. p.m. | from          to |

| Date and Hour Returned to Work | Actual Earnings for Last Day Worked | Normal Earnings for Last Day Worked | Do you have any information that the worker could have returned to work earlier? If so, provide details: |
|---|---|---|---|
| day   month   year   a.m. p.m. | $ | $ | |

1. What happened to cause the injury/disease?  If known, describe injury, part of body involved and specify left or right side.

2. Who was the injury/disease reported to?  If injury/disease was not reported immediately, provide reason for delay.

3. Describe the worker's activities at the time of the injury/disease.  Include details of equipment or materials used and the size and weights of objects being handled.

4. Where was the worker when the injury/awareness of disease occurred?  If the injury/disease occurred outside of Ontario, specify province, state or country.

5. Is there anyone else who may have witnessed or who may know about the injury/onset of disease?  If so, provide details below.
   Name(s)                          Address(es) and phone number(s) if available

0007A (11/94)          **WCB COPY - WHITE   WORKER COPY - PINK   EMPLOYER COPY - YELLOW**          **Please read and complete page 2**

**Illustration 6.20    Employer's Report of Injury/Disease (continued)**

| Workers' Compensation Board | Commission des accidents du travail | Employer's Report of Injury/Disease Form 7 (Page 2) |
|---|---|---|

Ontario

| | | **WCB use only** |
|---|---|---|
| Worker's Name | Social Insurance Number | Claim Number |

## E. Health Care

Did the worker receive health care?    ☐ yes  ☐ no  ☐ don't know

Initial or emergency health care: if known, provide the name and address of practitioner/facility.

Current or continuing health care: if known, provide the name, address and telephone number of practitioner/facility, if different than above.

## F. Earnings Information - Do not complete this section if you answered "No" to all questions in Section C on page 1.

**Rate of Pay** (before tax)    ☐ hourly  ☐ daily    $

Total Weekly Pay Hours

If weekly pay hours are irregular, please state average weekly hours.

Does the worker's work schedule change from week to week?    ☐ yes  ☐ no

From Revenue Canada TD1 provide:    Net Claim for Exemption

Net Claim Code

Enter Worker's Usual Work Days (F = full day, H = half day)    | S | M | T | W | T | F | S |

Are Benefit Plan (Health Care, Life Insurance, Pension) contributions continuing?    ☐ yes  ☐ no  ☐ not applicable

If "no", is the benefit plan a multi-employer benefit plan?    ☐ yes  ☐ no

The worker also receives the following earnings in addition to the Rate of Pay as reported above.    (Check all that apply.)

Will this benefit continue while the worker is absent from work due to this injury/disease?

If "no", please state value if known

| | | | |
|---|---|---|---|
| ☐ Vacation Pay | ☐ yes  ☐ no | $ | ☐ daily  ☐ weekly |
| ☐ Production Bonuses | ☐ yes  ☐ no | $ | ☐ daily  ☐ weekly |
| ☐ Profit Sharing | ☐ yes  ☐ no | $ | ☐ daily  ☐ weekly |
| ☐ Room and board and/or benefit from the worker's personal use of an employer's vehicle | ☐ yes  ☐ no | $ | ☐ daily  ☐ weekly |
| ☐ Cost of living allowance, shift differential, lead hand premium | ☐ yes  ☐ no | $ | ☐ daily  ☐ weekly |
| ☐ Tips and Gratuities | ☐ yes  ☐ no | $ | ☐ daily  ☐ weekly |
| ☐ Unemployment insurance benefits paid in a job creation or work-sharing program | ☐ yes  ☐ no | $ | ☐ daily  ☐ weekly |

Identify Type of Employment  (Check all that apply.)

☐ Full Time  ☐ Part Time  ☐ Casual  ☐ Seasonal  ☐ Apprentice  ☐ Student  ☐ Learner  ☐ Other _____

If the worker worked after the first absence, please enter dates.

| From | | | | To | | | |
|---|---|---|---|---|---|---|---|
| day | month | year | a.m. p.m. | day | month | year | a.m. p.m. |

**G. Advances**    If you have advanced or will be advancing anything to cover period of disability, give particulars including dates covered.

If advances are to be mailed to another address, please provide.

## H. Claim Information

To your knowledge has the worker had a previous similar injury/disease?    ☐ no  ☐ yes

If yes, provide details.  If the previous similar injury/disease was work-related, include prior WCB claim number if known.

Was any individual who does not work for you totally or partially responsible for the injury/disease?    ☐ no  ☐ yes    If yes, please explain.

If machinery, equipment or a motor vehicle was totally or partially responsible for the injury/disease, refer to the instructions on the reverse of the Employer's Copy and provide particulars.

Do you have any reason to doubt that the injury/disease is work-related?    ☐ no  ☐ yes    If yes, please explain.

Letter of explanation attached?    ☐ no  ☐ yes

Who is responsible for arranging the worker's return to work?  (Name and telephone number)

**I.**    It is an offence to deliberately make false statements to the WCB.  I declare that all of the information provided on pages 1 and 2 of this report is true.

| Name of Person Completing this Report | Official Title |
|---|---|

| Signature | Area Code ( ) | Telephone Number | Date |
|---|---|---|---|

| **WCB Use Only** | | | | | | |
|---|---|---|---|---|---|---|
| Allowed | Final | Pending | Lost Time | No Lost Time | Third Party | Out of Province |
| Signature | | | Date | Paid From | | Paid To |

0007A (11/94)    **WCB COPY - WHITE    WORKER COPY - PINK    EMPLOYER COPY - YELLOW**

**Illustration 6.21 Physician's First Report**

---

**Workers' Compensation Board** **Commission des accidents du travail** 2 Bloor Street East Toronto, Ontario M4W 3C3

**For WCB use only** >

**Physician's First Report Form 8**

| Firm No. | Rate No. | Claim No. |
|---|---|---|

**Message to Physician:**

- **Please complete in full and mail to the WCB within 48 hours if the patient's injury/disease is work related.**

- Section 51 (R.S.O. 1990) of the Workers' Compensation Act authorizes you to release this information to the WCB.

- To ensure prompt processing of the claim, please remind the patient to report the accident to the employer.

- Supplies of Physician's First Report, Form 8, are available on request from your local WCB office.

**Please complete in black ink or type and submit the original.**

| Patient's Last Name | First Name |
|---|---|

Full Address (No., Street, Apt.)

| City/Town | Province | Postal Code |
|---|---|---|

| Area Code | Phone No. | Social Insurance No. | Date of Birth day month year |
|---|---|---|---|

Employer's Name

Full Address

| City/Town | Province | Postal Code |
|---|---|---|

| Area Code | Phone No. | Date of Accident day month year |
|---|---|---|

---

**1** Date you first treated injured worker

**For WCB use only** >

| Status | Injury | Claims Adjudicator |
|---|---|---|

**2** Who rendered first treatment? | Date

**3** Patient's history of injury/disease

**4** Prior history of similar medical condition

**5** Symptoms and specify physical findings

**6** Diagnosis

**7** Will the worker be absent from work because of the workplace injury/disease on the day after it occurred? ☐ no ☐ yes

**8** Investigations ordered/Results

**9** Describe current or proposed treatment/program including physiotherapy/chiropractic/medications, etc.

Referral to a community clinic ☐ no ☐ yes

**10** Referral to specialist: Name of specialist(s) (please print) | Date(s) of appointment

**11** Complete recovery expected? ☐ no ☐ yes If yes, approximate time?

**12** List any medical restrictions that should be observed when the patient returns to work activities now

**13** Are there medical restrictions which prevent this patient from operating a motor vehicle? ☐ no ☐ yes

**14** Can the patient use public transport? ☐ no ☐ yes

| Health No. | Version Code |
|---|---|

Physician's name - please print.

WCB Agency Billing No.

Address | City/Town

Province | Postal code | Area code | Phone No.

Physician's signature | Date

| Your own invoice No. | Service date d d m m y y | Fee code M 6 4 0 |
|---|---|---|

0008C (06/94)

(Français au verso)

**Illustration 6.22 Health Care Accounts Inquiry Form**

Workers' Compensation Board / Commission des accidents du travail

Health Care Benefits Branch / *Direction de l'aide médicale*

**Accounts Enquiry/*Demande de renseignements***

**Return parts 1 and 2 to WCB/*Retournez les parties 1 et 2 à la CAT***

Claim No./*Dossier n^o^*

| Patient's Surname/*Nom de famille du patient* | Given Name(s)/*Prénom* | SIN/*N^o^ d'assurance sociale* | Accident Date/*Date de l'accident* |
|---|---|---|---|
| | | | |

Patient's Full Address/*Adresse du patient*

Nature of Injury/*Nature de la lésion*

Employer's Name & Address/*Nom et adresse de l'employeur*

| Acct. Ref. No./*N^o^ de réf. du compte* | Date of Service/*Date du service* | Details of Service/*Service rendu* | Desc. Code Billed *Code desc. facturé* | Amt. Billed/*Montant facturé* | Amt. Allowed/*Montant autorisé* | Agy. Reg't. No./*N^o^ enr. organisme* |
|---|---|---|---|---|---|---|
| | | | | | | |

Agency's Name & Full Mailing Address/*Nom et adresse postale de l'organisme*

**Nature of Service**
***Nature du service***

**Reason For Follow-up/*Raison du rappel***

☐ Account filed payment not received / *Paiement du compte non reçu*
☐ Balance still owing *Solde dû* $
☐ Other (specify) *Autre (précisez)*

Prepared by/*Préparé par*

Agency Telephone No. *N^o^ téléphone organisme* | Area Code/*Indicatif* | Date

0178C (07/85)

The medical administrative assistant is not required to have considerable knowledge concerning workers' compensation because reporting work-related injuries is the responsibility of the employer and employee. The doctor is responsible for diagnosing the injuries, and WCB makes the decision on compensation to the injured worker. The medical administrative assistant should, however, have a general knowledge of the system and be capable of completing all forms related to the doctor's involvement with WCB.

If you have questions or need clarification of information, call the Workers' Compensation Board's head office. The number is in the telephone directory in both the white pages and the blue pages "government services" section.

## Assignment 6.3

Dr. Plunkett provides you with the necessary information, and you are responsible for the completion of all reports, the doctor's account forms, and the submission of this information to WCB.

Using the following information, complete the Physician's First Report (Working Papers, pp. 33–34) and the Ministry of Health health claim card (Working Papers, pp. 24–32).

On February 16, 19__, Tim Peters was involved in an industrial accident. Dr. Plunkett was doing rounds at the hospital (no. 1220) and Tim was transported to the hospital for examination. On examination, it was discovered that he had a severe sprain in his left ankle. The doctor recommended bed rest for one week, after which time he felt Tim would be able to return to work. Dr. Plunkett feels that three weeks of physiotherapy (twice weekly) will be required to restore the muscles in the ankle.

Tim Peters's social insurance number is 416 274 963. He is employed at Smith and Smith Limited, 372 Parkview Drive, Ottawa. The claim number has not yet been issued. Dr. Plunkett first saw Tim at 1535.

**Illustration 6.23   Medical Records Waiver Form**

| Workers' Compensation Board | Commission des accidents du travail | 2 Bloor Street East Toronto, Ontario M4W 3C3 | Telephone: (416) 927-7222 For toll free calling, check your local telephone directory. |

**Medical Records Waiver**

*Autorisation d'accès au dossier médical*

| Claim number/Dossier n° | Desk/ Bureau | Alloc. no. N° D'Attrib. |
|---|---|---|
| Worker's name/ Nom du travailleur | | |

This will be your authority to allow a representative of the Workers' Compensation Board of Ontario to have access to my medical records and to receive copies thereof at:

*Par la présente, j'autorise un représentant de la Commission des accidents du travail de l'Ontario à consulter mon dossier médical et à en demander des copies à :*

| Name of Hospital (please print) Nom de l'hôpital (en lettres moulées S.V.P.) | Hospital ID Number Matricule de l'hôpital | Address/Adresse |
|---|---|---|
| | | Postal Code/ Code postal |

| Dates of treatment/ Dates des traitements | | | | Type of injury/Type de lésion |
|---|---|---|---|---|
| Admission/Admission | Emergency/ Urgence | Outpatient/Patient externe | Physiotherapy Physiothérapie | |

| Doctor's name/ Nom du médecin | Address/ Adresse |
|---|---|
| | Postal Code/ Code postal |

| Worker's name (please print)/ Nom du travailleur (en lettre moulées s.v.p.) | Worker's date of birth Date de naissance | S.I.N./ N.A.S. |
|---|---|---|

| Address (when receiving treatments)/Adresse (au moment des traitements) | Postal Code/Code postal | Worker's signature/ Signature du travailleur |
|---|---|---|

| Witness's signature/ Signature du témoin | Date/ Date | Next of Kin's signature Signature du plus proche parent | Relationship/ Lien de parente |
|---|---|---|---|

| Desk no. (for WCB use only) Bureau no (réserve à la CAT) |
|---|

**Section 53 of the Workers' Compensation Act States:**

Every physician, surgeon, hospital official or other person attending, consulted respecting, or having the care of, any worker shall furnish to the Board from time to time, without additional charge, such reports as may be required by the Board in respect of such worker. R.S.O. 1980, c.539, s.53.

*L'article 53 de la Loi sur les accidents du travail stipule que:*

*Le médecin, le chirurgien, le responsable d'hôpital ou une autre personne qui donne des soins, consultés au sujet d'un travailleur, ou chargés de le soigner, fournissent a l'occasion à la Commission, sans frais supplémentaires, les rapports demandes, le cas échéant, par la Commission au sujet de ce travailleur L.R.O. 1980, chap. 539, art. 53.*

0285C (03/88)

**WAIVER**

**Illustration 6.24    Physician's Progress Report**

**Workers' Compensation Board**    **Commission des accidents du travail**    2 Bloor Street East
Toronto, Ontario
M4W 3C3

**Physician's Progress Report Form 26**

**Section 51 (R.S.O. 1990) of the Workers' Compensation Act authorizes you to release this information to the WCB. Please <u>respond to all questions</u> in black ink or type and return the <u>original</u> to the WCB.**

Patient's name

Claim No.

Date of examination on which report is based

When will patient be seen again?

1. Current symptoms and physical findings

2. Diagnosis

3. Investigations ordered/results since last report

4. Describe current or proposed treatment program including physiotherapy/chiropractic/medications, etc.

Referral to a community clinic
☐ yes    ☐ no

5. Referral to specialist: Name of specialist(s) (please print)

Date(s) of appointment

6. Referral to a regional evaluation centre for a multi-disciplinary assessment?    ☐ no    ☐ yes    If yes, date of appointment

7. Any significant factors delaying recovery?    ☐ no    ☐ yes    If yes, please describe

8. Improvement expected?    ☐ no    ☐ yes    If yes, please describe and give approximate date

9. Complete recovery expected?    ☐ no    ☐ yes    If yes, approximate date

10. List any medical restrictions that should be observed should the patient return to work activities now

11. If you anticipate permanent restrictions, specify:

12. Are there medical restrictions which prevent the patient from operating a motor vehicle?    ☐ yes    ☐ no

13. Can the patient use public transport?    ☐ yes    ☐ no

Health No.

Version Code

WCB Agency Billing No.

Physician's name  (please print)

Signature

Address

Telephone

Date

Your own invoice No.

Service date
d    d    m    m    y    y

Fee code

**M | 6 | 4 | 3**

0896A (04/94)

(Français au verso)    26

**Illustration 6.25    Payment Label — Form 0150**

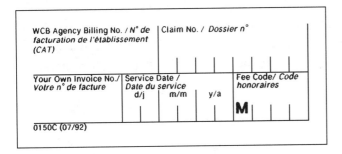

In addition to health care plans and workers' compensation, the public may wish to carry additional health care insurance to cover expenses not reimbursed by their respective plans.

Many private insurance companies issue group and individual policies to cover these additional expenses. London Life Mutual, Metropolitan Life, Prudential Insurance, and The Protectors Group are examples of third-party private insurance companies.

**Third-Party Insurance**

## Some Benefits Available through Third-Party Insurance

1. Semi-private hospital accommodation (available on an individual pay-direct or a group basis).
2. Extended health care plans (available on an individual pay-direct or a group basis) provide protection against the costs of health services not covered by basic government health plans. The plan can be tailored to the needs of any group.
3. Prescription drug plan (available on a group basis), to help protect group subscribers and their families against the costs of prescribed drugs and injectibles.
4. Vision care plan (available on a group basis), to provide payment toward the purchase of eye glasses and contact lenses.
5. Dental plan (available on a group basis).
6. Nursing home plan (available on a group basis).
7. Health plan for visitors (on an individual or a family basis), designed to provide visitors to Canada with protection against unexpected costs of hospital care.
8. Health plan for Canadians while travelling outside Canada (on an individual or a family basis), designed to protect people from unexpected costs of medical bills incurred while on business or vacationing anywhere outside Canada.

A general knowledge of what is available through third-party insurance companies is an asset. Although each private company offers its own plan, most benefits offered are very similar.

## Assignment 6.4

If your class is interested in more detailed information about third-party insurance, appoint a group to arrange for representatives of private insurance companies to visit your class to expand on the benefits offered by their particular organizations.

**Illustration 6.26   Examples of Provincial Health Cards**

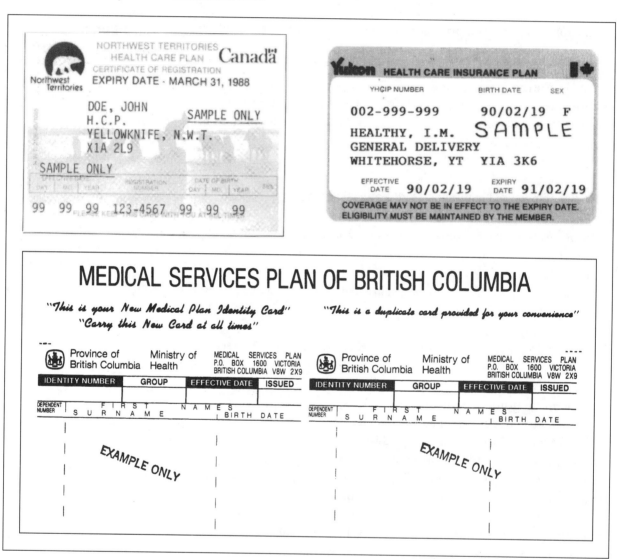

**Illustration 6.26   Examples of Provincial Health Cards (continued)**

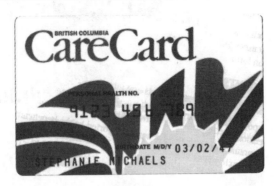

| | NAME AND MAILING ADDRESS | FIRST NAME & INITIAL | HEALTH IDENTITY NO. | DATE OF BIRTH | DATE ELIGIBLE |
|---|---|---|---|---|---|
| | DOE | John A. | 111 111 1111 | 12 Dec 12 | 01 01 83 |
| | John | Jane B. | 111 111111 | 12 Dec 12 | 01 01 83 |
| | Any Street | | | | |
| | Any Town, P.E.I. | | | | |
| | **HOUSEHOLD NUMBER** COA 1GO | | | | |

PRESENT THIS CARD FOR HOSPITAL/MEDICAL SERVICES

**Health and Community
Services Agency**
PO Box 3000
Montague
Prince Edward Island
C0A 1R0

*Telephone*
**902 838 4064**
*Charlottetown*
**902 368 5858**

Prince Edward Island
Health and Community
Services System

A claim must contain name of
Patient and Health Identity No.

# Chapter 7

# Financial

# Records

## Chapter Outline

## Learning Objectives

To learn
- how to record cash disbursements, cash receipts, and patient charges in journals
- how to prepare ledgers and post information from journals
- how to prepare patient statements of account
- how to control petty cash
- how to prepare cheques and cash for deposit
- how to reconcile bank statements
- how to interpret payroll deduction tables and prepare payroll sheets
- how to complete Revenue Canada payroll remittance forms

It is essential for any business to keep accurate and complete financial records. Large organizations such as hospitals, clinics, and health service organizations employ graduate accountants and have a separate finance department because their accounting systems are very complex. Generally, a small service organization maintains an adequate set of accounting records to enable a chartered accountant to complete the financial statements and process the proprietor's income tax returns.

A medical administrative assistant in a single-proprietorship practice should be knowledgeable about single-entry bookkeeping, writing cheques, bank deposits, petty cash records, completing patients' accounts and statements, and bank reconciliations. Most medical administrative assistants take care of these accounting functions at a time when the doctor is not seeing patients or other times when the office is not busy.

**Illustration 7.1   Cash Disbursements Journal**

| | | | | | | | U.I.C.<br>C.P.P. | Heat,<br>Hydro, | Auto<br>Maint. | Office<br>Rent & | | Travel<br>& | |
|---|---|---|---|---|---|---|---|---|---|---|---|---|---|
| | | | CASH DISBURSEMENTS JOURNAL | | | | | | | | | PAGE  1 | |
| Date | Explanation | Ch.<br># | Amount | Office<br>Supplies | Med.<br>Supplies | Wages | In. Tax | Tele. | & Gas | Maint. | Draw'ng | Enter. | Misc. |
| 19-<br>JAN. 2 | AFAXEL Co (needles) | 123 | 49 90 | | 49 90 | | | | | | | | |
| | | | | | | | | | | | | | |
| | | | | | | | | | | | | | |
| | | | | | | | | | | | | | |
| | | | | | | | | | | | | | |
| | | | | | | | | | | | | | |
| | | | | | | | | | | | | | |
| | | | | | | | | | | | | | |
| | | | | | | | | | | | | | |
| | | | | | | | | | | | | | |
| | | | | | | | | | | | | | |
| | | | | | | | | | | | | | |
| | | | | | | | | | | | | | |
| | | | | | | | | | | | | | |
| | | | | | | | | | | | | | |

Since billing methods vary among the provinces, this chapter will follow Ontario procedures.

In a single-entry bookkeeping system, a multicolumn journal is used to record all daily receipts and expenditures. Look at Illustration 7.1. This is a cash disbursements journal. You must record where the money is spent. Therefore, the payment entry is extended into a column that groups similar payouts. The accountant who sets up your doctor's accounting records will suggest basic column headings for disbursements. In many medical offices, all accounting procedures will be computerized, including medical plan billing, remittance advice reconciliation, cash receipts and disbursements, cheque writing, and so on. In order to fully understand the material necessary for computer input, it is first necessary to work with material using manual procedures.

## Recording in the Cash Disbursements Journal

On a typical day in the doctor's office, you might record the following transaction in your cash disbursements journal.

January 2, 19__, purchased 2 gross (1 gross = 12 dozen) needles from AFAXEL Co. at $24.95 per gross. This transaction has been recorded in Illustration 7.1 using the following procedures:

At the top of the date column, the year is entered. On line one, the month and day are entered. Do not repeat the month again until it changes. The year appears only at the top of the date column on each page. Following along horizontally, enter the reason for payment — company name and 2 gross needles — in the "Explanation" column; the number of the cheque used to make payment in the "Ch.#" column — 123; the amount of the purchase in the "Amount" column and also in the "Medical Supplies" column — $49.90.

## Exercise 7.1

(For the exercises in this chapter, record the transactions on the text illustrations or use the blank forms in the Working Papers [pp. 35–66].)

Following the same procedure described above, record these additional transactions (use consecutive cheque numbers from no. 123):

| | | |
|---|---|---|
| January | 2 | Establish petty cash fund for $50 |
| | 2 | The doctor entertained at a dinner party and spent $50 (Romeo's Cafe) |
| | 2 | Paid Purolator $7.62 for delivery of laboratory reports |
| | 3 | Purchased letterhead and envelopes $48.29 (ABC Supplies) |
| | 3 | Paid January rent $400 (Medical Services Inc.) |
| | 4 | Paid automobile credit card charges for gas and oil $71.65 (Jay's Gas Bar) |
| | 5 | Paid your wages $450, and janitor's wages $280 (Don James) |
| | 5 | The doctor withdrew $350 for personal use |
| | 8 | Sent cheque to Ontario Hydro for $147 |
| | 8 | Made $100 contribution to the United Way |
| | 9 | Paid telephone bill of $56.50 (Bell Canada) |
| | 11 | Paid Campbell's Florist $25 for roses sent to the doctor's wife for anniversary |
| | 12 | Paid your wages $450, and janitor's wages $280 (Don James) |
| | 12 | The doctor withdrew $350 |
| | 13 | Submitted cheque to the Receiver General of Canada for income tax $290; unemployment insurance, $15.18; Canada Pension $12.92 |
| | 13 | Reimbursed petty cash $47.41 |

Examine your entry on January 2 for the dinner party. If a businessperson entertains for the purpose of promoting the business, the expense is tax deductible. However, a businessperson must not charge personal expenses against the business. You may have entered the $50 dinner expense under "Travel and Entertainment," assuming it was a business engagement. Or you may have assumed it was a personal engagement, in which case the entry would be made under "Drawings."

**Illustration 7.2   Business Cheques**

| | | |
|---|---|---|
| BAL. | 3,912.10 | THE BANK OF NOVA SCOTIA · Scotiabank |
| DEP. | 1,069.00 | 126   JAN 2, 19-- |
| TOTAL | 4,981.10 | NO.   DATE |
| CHEQUE | 7.62 | |
| BAL. | 4,973.48 | |

PAY TO *Purolator*
*FOR LAB REPORTS*
SUM OF 7.62
DATE *JAN. 2/--* NO. 126

PAY TO THE ORDER OF — *Purolator*   $ 7.62
SUM OF — *SEVEN* — 62/100 DOLLARS
ACCOUNT NO. 00000

*J.C. Pentlett*

(second blank cheque — THE BANK OF NOVA SCOTIA · Scotiabank)

## Writing Cheques

A safe and convenient way to handle the payment of accounts is to write cheques. Since you will not have large amounts of cash on hand, you can eliminate the possibility of theft and loss. Also, mailing a cheque rather than going to someone to pay cash is a more efficient business practice. Never put cash in the mail. Cheques used by business are similar to those shown in Illustration 7.2 (The January 2 payment is recorded on the first cheque.)

A running balance is kept on the cheque stub. This allows a double check of your accounting accuracy. The cheque number, amount, name of person to whom the cheque is issued, and purpose of the cheque also appear on the stub. On the actual cheque, the amount of the cheque in figures, as well as in words, and the payer's signature must be recorded.

Write cheques for the first four entries in your cash disbursements journal. The beginning balance on cheque no. 123 is $4062. Assume that on January 2 you deposited $1069. (Extra cheque forms can be found in the Working Papers [pp. 37–38].)

**Exercise 7.2**

**Illustration 7.3    Patients' Charges and Payments Journal**

| | | | | | | | |
|---|---|---|---|---|---|---|---|
| PATIENTS' CHARGES AND PAYMENT JOURNAL | | | | | | PAGE  1 | |
| Date | Health Card No. | Patient's Name | Explanation | FO | Cash Payment Received | Amount Charged | |
| | | | | | | | |
| | | | | | | | |
| | | | | | | | |
| | | | | | | | |
| | | | | | | | |
| | | | | | | | |
| | | | | | | | |
| | | | | | | | |
| | | | | | | | |
| | | | | | | | |
| | | | | | | | |
| | | | | | | | |
| | | | | | | | |
| | | | | | | | |
| | | | | | | | |

## Patients' Charges and Payments Journal

The majority of providers are opted in; however, because some opt out of their provincial health plan, it is important to know how to bill for their services.

NP: Billing for most services is done on magnetic media; however, it is important to understand a manual billing process before applying it to a computerized system. The following is an explanation of manual billing.

### For Opted-Out Physicians

An opted-out physician submits a fee to the provincial health care plan on behalf of the patient and directly bills the patient. Full responsibility for payment rests with the patient.

The doctor's main source of revenue is the fee charged to the patient. The charge is taken from the billing card and recorded in a journal of patients' charges and payments (see Illustration 7.3).

**Exercise 7.3**

On January 2, 19__, the doctor examined the following patients, and their billing cards were returned to you to record the charges in your journal (Working Papers, pp. 39–40).

1. Lisa Basciano, annual health exam
2. Bob Baxter, counselling (40 minutes)
3. William Harris, sore throat and temperature (intermediate assessment)

Be sure the year is at the beginning of the date column. For patient (1), record the date January 2. Following along horizontally, record the health card number, the patient's name, reason for visit, and the charges in the "Amount Charged" column (look up charges in the Schedule of Benefits).

Following the same procedure described above, record patients (2) and (3).

## Ledger Cards

In addition to the patients' charges and payments journal, a separate card, called a ledger card, is kept for each patient. You must keep a record of all charges and payments for all patients. You may choose to record charges on a family or individual basis (see Illustration 7.4). At the end of the day, the entries made in the patients' charges and payments journal would be recorded on the patients' individual ledger cards as outlined in Exercise 7.4.

**Illustration 7.4  Patient Ledger Card**

PATIENT LEDGER CARD

NAME_____  HEALTH #_____ BIRTH DATE_____

ADDRESS_____  TELEPHONE #_____

_____  EMPLOYER_____

POSTAL CODE_____  CHILDREN_____ BIRTH DATE_____

SPOUSE_____ BIRTH DATE_____  _____  _____

| Date | Service Rendered | First Name | Ref | Charges | | Payments | | Balance | |
|------|------------------|------------|-----|---------|---|----------|---|---------|---|
|  |  |  |  |  |  |  |  |  |  |
|  |  |  |  |  |  |  |  |  |  |
|  |  |  |  |  |  |  |  |  |  |
|  |  |  |  |  |  |  |  |  |  |
|  |  |  |  |  |  |  |  |  |  |
|  |  |  |  |  |  |  |  |  |  |
|  |  |  |  |  |  |  |  |  |  |
|  |  |  |  |  |  |  |  |  |  |
|  |  |  |  |  |  |  |  |  |  |

## Exercise 7.4

Set up ledger cards (Working Papers, pp. 41–56) for Lisa Basciano, Bob Baxter, and William Harris. The header information can be found on the patient information forms in Chapter 3. Transfer the information from the charges and payments journal to Lisa Basciano's ledger card by recording the date of examination, purpose of visit, patient's first name, amount charged, and balance owing. As you transfer from the journal to the ledger card, place a check mark (✓) in the folio column on the journal page; on the ledger card, record the journal page (J1) in the reference column.

Complete the ledger cards for Baxter and Harris (enter a balance owing of $29.60 on the Harris card).

Now let us examine the procedure to follow when payment is made. You have submitted your charges to the Ministry of Health. When acting on behalf of the patient, the ministry does not submit payment directly to the doctor. The cheque is sent to the patient for the amount of the physician's service. The patient is then responsible for making payment to the doctor.

Let us assume that MOH sent a cheque to Lisa Basciano to pay for her examination. Mrs. Basciano could either deposit the cheque in the bank and write a cheque for the full amount of the charges, or she could endorse the cheque and turn it over to the doctor. In either case, the entry in the charges and payments journal would be: date (use January 15), patient's name, received payment under "Explanation," and the amount of the fee entered in "Payment Received" column; follow the same procedure to record patient (2).

What procedure do we follow if total payment is not received? Mr. Harris has a balance of $29.60 owing on his account. He has received his Ministry of Health cheque to pay for baby Harris's January 2 appointment. However, instead of signing the cheque to Dr. Plunkett, he cashed it and then came in and paid $25 on account. Follow the same procedure as for patients (1) and (2); however, this time the amount received will not pay the account in full. What is the balance owing? ($29.60 bal. + intermediate assessment charge − $25 payment).

After all three entries have been completed, transfer the transactions to the ledger cards.

You will note that the balance on the Basciano and Baxter cards is nil. However, there is a remaining balance on the Harris card.

### An Opted-In Physician

An opted-in physician submits a fee for each patient to the Ministry of Health and is reimbursed for these charges when his or her monthly medical insurance payment is received.

What procedures are followed when payment is made to an opted-in provider? You have submitted your charges to the Ministry of Health and they have made payment with the accompanying Remittance Advice that we examined in Chapter 6. The total amount of the cheque or direct bank deposit would be recorded in the charges and payments journal as follows:

Date, explanation (MOH payment received), and amount entered in "Cash Payment Received" column. We will assume that the cheque received covered payment for Lisa Basciano, Bob Baxter, and William Harris.

When you are employed by an opted-in provider, it is not necessary to make journal entries and keep ledgers for your patients. The only time a ledger would be required would be if the patient requested a service that was not covered by the provincial medical plan (for example, to have an insurance form completed). You would then be required to record the appropriate fee in the journal and transfer to a ledger.

Rather than enter each service in a journal and transfer it to a ledger, the administrative assistant should keep the source document for backup of the billing information. Such a source document may be the flimsy copy of the billing card or billing sheet produced by the physician. When the Remittance Advice is received with the physician's cheque for services rendered, the entries on the Remittance Advice are cross-checked with the applicable source documents on file. If the payment on the Remittance Advice agrees with the fees submitted, the billing source document can be discarded. If there is a discrepancy between the payment and charge, place a red check mark beside the entry on the Remittance Advice. After all entries have been examined, take action to rectify the discrepancies (complete and submit a Remittance Advice Inquiry form, for example).

## Patient's Statement of Account

At the end of each month, the administrative assistant must go through the patients' ledger cards and send a statement of account to those who show a balance owing. Of course, this procedure would be necessary only for those administrative assistants employed by an opted-out physician. The exception would be if an opted-in physician performed a service that was not covered by the provincial health care plan, for example, filling out an insurance claim form or writing a legal letter. Examine the statement of account in Illustration 7.5. A statement of account form may vary in its format, but the information required is generally the same:

1. Name of statement
2. Originator's name, address, and telephone number
3. The date the statement is issued
4. Name and address of the debtor
5. Date of each service
6. Explanation of the service
7. Amount of the charges
8. Amount of any payment received
9. Balance owing
10. Notification of service charge for overdue accounts

**Illustration 7.5   Statement of Account**

```
┌─────────────────────────────────────────────────────────────────────┐
│                        STATEMENT OF ACCOUNT                           │
│                                                                       │
│                       JOHN E. PLUNKETT                                │
│               PHM.B., M.D., C.M., F.R.C.P., F.A.C.P.                 │
│                      INTERNAL MEDICINE                                │
│                278 O'CONNOR ST., OTTAWA, ONT.                        │
│                                                                       │
│   To:                                       Date:                     │
│                                                                       │
│                                             Amount   $_____        │
│                                                                       │
│                                             Enclosed $_____        │
│                                                                       │
│   Please return this stub with your cheque                           │
│                                                                       │
└─────────────────────────────────────────────────────────────────────┘
```

| Date | | Explanation | Payments | | Charges | | Balance | |
|------|---|------------|----------|---|---------|---|---------|---|
| | | Balance Forward | | | | | | |
| | | | | | | | | |
| | | | | | | | | |
| | | | | | | | | |
| | | | | | | | | |
| | | Accounts due when rendered 1 1/2% per month charged on overdue accounts | | | | | | |

---

## Exercise 7.5

Using the form in Illustration 7.5 or one from the Working Papers (pp. 57–59), complete a statement of account for Brad Harris.

---

Sometimes a doctor is faced with unpaid accounts. After several unsuccessful attempts to collect the overdue account, a decision must be made whether to put the account in the hands of a collection agency or write off the account as a bad debt. The doctor's accountant generally makes this decision and takes the necessary action.

**Illustration 7.6   Petty Cash Record**

| PETTY CASH RECORD | | | | | | | | |
|---|---|---|---|---|---|---|---|---|
| Date | | Explanation | Receipts | | Payments | | Balance | |
| 19–<br>Jan | 2 | ESTABLISH PETTY CASH | 50 | – | | | 50 | – |
| | | | | | | | | |
| | | | | | | | | |
| | | | | | | | | |
| | | | | | | | | |
| | | | | | | | | |
| | | | | | | | | |
| | | | | | | | | |
| | | | | | | | | |
| | | | | | | | | |
| | | | | | | | | |
| | | | | | | | | |
| | | | | | | | | |

## Petty Cash

Most doctors' offices maintain a small petty cash fund to purchase stamps, coffee supplies, and so on. It is essential that an accurate record be maintained for the petty cash. This record does not have to be elaborate, but simply a record of the amount received to replenish the fund and a record of what payments were made from the fund (see Illustration 7.6).

Let us assume that on January 2, 19___, a cheque for $50 was issued to establish a petty cash fund. The entry would be: year at the top of the "Date" column; date, January 2; explanation — cheque no. 124 to establish petty cash; received, $50; balance, $50.

Using the form in Illustration 7.6 or p. 60 of the Working Papers, record the following transactions for January:

**Exercise 7.6**

January 2   Bought paper clips, $1.29
4   Paid for collect telegram, $1.35
8   Purchased sugar, cream, and coffee, $11.27
10   Bought stamps, $30
13   Doctor's lunch, $3.50

When the cash in your petty cash box gets low, it is time to replenish the fund. You should have $2.59 in your cash box to agree with the balance column in your petty cash record. In order to bring your petty cash up to $50, you would write a cheque made out to cash in the amount of $47.41, have the doctor sign it, and then cash it when you go to the bank.

The petty cash box is generally a small metal box approximately 20 cm × 15 cm × 8 cm (8 inches × 6 inches × 3 inches) and is kept in the administrative assistant's desk or a file cabinet. You should be able to lock the drawer containing the petty cash box. You should always ask for receipts when making payment from the petty cash box to verify the amount of cash paid out. Occasionally, fellow workers may ask to borrow money from the cash box. If you are responsible for petty cash, it is advisable to refrain from making such personal loans.

## Banking

The three main banking duties required of the administrative assistant follow:

1. Making deposits
2. Writing cheques
3. Reconciling the monthly bank statement

We discussed cheque writing earlier in this chapter. We will now examine depositing and reconciling the bank statement.

**Making deposits** — The doctor's main source of revenue is the fee paid by the patient for the doctor's services.

As explained previously, an opted-in doctor submits a service fee for each patient to the Ministry of Health. The ministry issues a cheque, or makes a direct deposit to the provider's bank, every month for the amount of fee submissions during the period covered by the cheque. If you receive the cheque, it is a good safety measure to use a "For Deposit Only" stamp on the back of the cheque (see Illustration 7.7). This is a form of endorsement.

**Illustration 7.7   "For Deposit Only" Stamp**

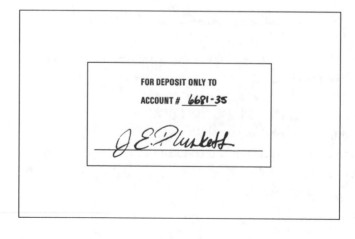

**Illustration 7.8    Deposit Slip**

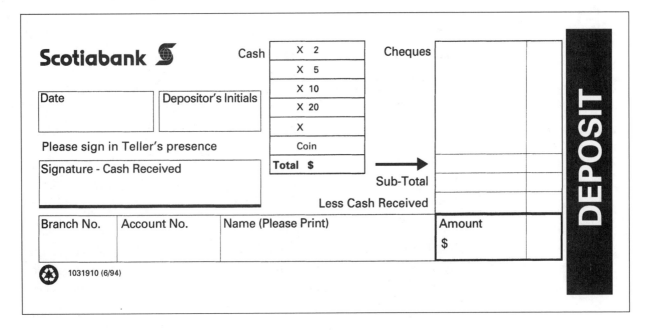

Patients often pay the opted-out physician with the cheque received from the Ministry of Health. Before stamping the cheque "For Deposit Only," ensure that the patient endorses the cheque.

If the cheque is lost or stolen but has this stamp, it cannot be cashed. Each time you receive a cheque, you deposit it in the doctor's business account. A deposit slip, similar to that in Illustration 7.8, must be completed before presenting the deposit to the bank teller.

It is never wise to accept a postdated cheque. You cannot deposit a post-dated cheque until it is due, and collection on a postdated cheque returned "not sufficient funds" (NSF) can sometimes cause problems.

Enter the following information on a deposit slip (Working Papers, p. 61) for Dr. Plunkett: date, January 13, 19__; cash $152.57 consisting of 9 ones, 4 twos, 3 fives, 6 tens, 3 twenties, and 57 cents in coin; cheques for $13.42 from E.C. Westran, $35 from C.S.A. Insurance Co. (for writing a patient history), $116.28 from W.C. Post, and $52.50 from R.A. James; account no. 6681-35; name of account, Dr. J.E. Plunkett (you made the deposit).

**Exercise 7.7**

Your instructor will provide you with the information required to complete this assignment.

**Assignment 7.1a and b**

**Illustration 7.9   Bank Reconciliation**

```
┌──────────────────────────────────────────────────────────────────────────┐
│  January 13, 19___                                                         │
│                                                                            │
│  Bank Balance              $2,769.20   Chequebook Balance      $1,326.50   │
│                                                                            │
│  Outstanding Cheques                    1) Service Charge          −3.50    │
│    (a) S.O.S.        $   732.60                                  1,323.00   │
│    (b) Jones           1,072.91         2) Interest earned       +127.50    │
│    (c) R.G. of                                                  1,450.50    │
│        Canada            427.50    2,233.01   3) Loan interest paid −200.00 │
│                                      536.19                     1,250.50    │
│    (d) Jan. 11                          4) Safety deposit box       −5.70   │
│        Deposit                     +543.21                      1,244.80    │
│                                         5) NSF Cheque Thomas Bell  −165.40  │
│        BANK BALANCE                $1,079.40   CHEQUEBOOK BALANCE  1,079.40  │
└──────────────────────────────────────────────────────────────────────────┘
```

**Bank Reconciliation** — Each month, the bank sends a statement of account and all cancelled cheques to its current account customers. (A business bank account is called a current account.) The administrative assistant must check his or her figures with the bank's balance to make sure the two accounts agree.

The cancelled cheques received from the bank are checked off the chequebook and a small check mark (✔) is placed beside the corresponding amount on the statement. After completing this procedure, you are ready to reconcile your statement. Divide a sheet of paper in two and write "Bank Balance" on one side and "Chequebook Balance" on the other (see Illustration 7.9).

On your statement, you see five items that are not checked off. Item (1) is a service charge for $3.50; item (2) is a credit memo for $127.50 for interest you received on your term deposit; item (3) is a debit memo for $200 interest charged on a loan; item (4) is a $5.70 charge for safety deposit box rental; and item (5) is a debit memo for an NSF cheque from Thomas Bell for $165.40.

The procedure to record these items is as follows:

No. 1   The bank has charged you for service, but you have not recorded the charge on your books. Subtract $3.50 from the chequebook side.

No. 2   A savings deposit at the bank has earned $127.50 interest. The bank has recorded it in your account; now you have to enter the amount in your records. Add to the chequebook side.

No. 3   The bank has made a loan to the business. Two hundred dollars for interest on the loan is deducted from your bank account. You must make an equal deduction from your chequebook record.

No. 4   The bank charges $5.70 yearly for rental of a safety deposit box. The bank has charged your account; you must charge your records with the same amount.

No. 5   A patient, Thomas Bell, gave you a cheque for $165.40. You deposited the cheque in the bank and added the amount to your records. When you received your bank statements, you discovered that Mr. Bell did not have sufficient funds in his account to cover the cheque. It was, therefore, returned to you. The bank did not add $165.40 to its records. You must therefore subtract the amount from your records.

Items (1), (3), and (4) would be entered in your cash disbursements journal after your statement is reconciled. Although you would not write cheques for these items, you would have to subtract the amounts from your chequebook stubs in order to keep your running balance accurate. For item (2) you would record it on your chequebook stub in the deposit space and label it "interested earned." Item (5) would require a notation in the patients' charges and payments journal beside the entry that recorded the receipt of Mr. Bell's payment, indicating that the cheque was returned NSF. The amount of the cheque would have to be deducted from the chequebook stub, and an adjustment to Mr. Bell's ledger card would have to be made.

When you examine your chequebook stubs, you discover that three cheques you have written have not been cashed. The cheques are to Smith Office Supplies, $732.60; Jones Medical Service, $1072.91; and the Receiver General of Canada, $427.50.

You have deducted all these cheques from your chequebook. But since they have not been cashed, the amounts have not been deducted from your bank account. See items (a), (b), and (c) in Illustration 7.9.

Your bank statement was mailed on January 12, and on January 11 you made a deposit of $543.21. You notice that the amount does not appear on your statement. You have added this deposit to your chequebook; you must now add it to your bank statement (d).

Your bank statement and your chequebook balance are now in agreement.

Many offices do not require the completion of a formal printed reconciliation statement. However, you should be aware of the correct format. Based on the information used in Illustration 7.9, a formal keyed bank reconciliation statement would resemble that shown in Illustration 7.10.

### Illustration 7.10   Bank Reconciliation Statement

**J.E. PLUNKETT M.D.**
**Bank Reconciliation Statement**
**January 13, 19___**

| | | |
|---|---|---|
| Balance as per bank statement, January 13 | | $2,769.20 |
| Add:  Deposit of January 11 not recorded by bank | | 543.21 |
| | | $3,312.41 |
| Deduct Outstanding Cheques: | | |
| #236  S.O.S. | $   732.60 | |
| #239  Jones Medical Services | 1,072.91 | |
| #244  Receiver General of Canada | 427.50 | 2,233.01 |
| Adjusted Bank Balance | | $1,079.40 |
| Balance as per Chequebook, January 13 | | $1,326.50 |
| Add:  Interest on term deposit | | 127.50 |
| | | $1,454.00 |
| Deduct:  Debit memo for safety deposit box rental | $     5.70 | |
| Bank interest on demand loan | 200.00 | |
| Monthly service charge | 3.50 | |
| NSF Cheque of J.D. Smith | 165.40 | 374.60 |
| Adjusted Chequebook balance | | $1,079.40 |

## Exercise 7.8

Using the following information, prepare rough draft bank reconciliation statements for Dr. Plunkett.

a.  The bank reported the balance of $2751.16. Your records show a balance of $2823.70. A cheque issued to us from J.P. Sands for $50.75 was returned NSF. Cheque no. 42 is still outstanding. The bank charged $2 for service. Cheque nos. 46 and 53 are outstanding. The account was debited $10 for interest on the demand loan. Cheque no. 55 for $127.50 is outstanding. Cheque stub no. 40 revealed an error: the cheque was recorded as $36 when it should have been $72. The amounts of cheque nos. 42, 46, and 53 are $19.75, $75.80, and $68.30 respectively. Bank deposit made but not recorded on bank statement $295.14. Bond interest paid by bank $37.50. Safety deposit charges $7.50. Date the statement November 30, 19___.

b.  Final bank balance as shown on bank statement $3241.82. Cash account balance (agreeing with chequebook balance on February 29) $3544.22. Outstanding cheques: no. 140, $31.40; no. 144, $40.00; no. 147, $7.15. Deposit in night depository on last day of February, outstanding on bank statement, $234. Dishonoured cheque from W.J. Krestel, $144. Bank service charge $2.75. A cheque issued to Kraus Novelty Company (no. 141) was issued for $14.40, but incorrectly recorded in the cash journal and on the cheque stub as $14.20. Date the statement March 31, 19___.

## Assignment 7.2

Prepared a bank reconciliation statement for Dr. Plunkett using the following information. Date the statement April 1, 19___. Students may use a computer software package or a typewriter.

Cash account $2140 and March 31 bank statement $2012. Deposit entered in books on March 30 was not taken to the bank until March 31 (amount $530). The bank sent a credit memo for $215 for interest earned on Canada Savings Bonds. The amount is shown on the account. However, the memo has not yet been received. Bank service charges $6. A patient's cheque for $50, included in the March 27 deposit, has been charged back by the bank on the statement as NSF. The patient is J. Wren. Cheque no. 502 was made out to cash for $35 to reimburse the petty cash; this cheque is recorded in the cash payments journal as $53. The following cheques were not returned by the bank with the March statement: no. 521 to R. Smith for $10; no. 523 to J. Jones Ltd. for $50; no. 524 to Metrics Limited for $100 (certified on March 27); no. 525 to P. Brown for $75; and no. 526 to J. Smith and Company for $90.

## Payroll

In order to follow this section of the chapter, each student must have a copy of the Canada Pension Plan (CPP), Unemployment Insurance (UI), and Income Tax Deduction tables.

Before beginning the instructions for payroll, please read the preambles at the beginning of the CPP/UI and income tax tables. It is essential that anyone working with payroll be familiar with the instructions given in these two manuals. Because you require the tables to compute any payroll, reprinting the guidelines in this text is unnecessary.

In a large organization, payroll is fairly complicated and requires several employees to process the employee paycheques each pay period. However, in a small organization, of say ten or less, the payroll procedure is fairly simple. You can purchase a payroll book from an office supply store to cover 52 pay periods (or one year). Each employee has a separate sheet similar to that in Illustration 7.11. Many offices use a computerized payroll system. However, in order for you to understand a payroll process, we are providing information on the manual procedure.

Let us assume that in your office you are the only salaried employee. The doctor does not have a registered nurse. A part-time janitor looks after cleaning and maintenance duties and is paid on an hourly basis. The doctor is not on the payroll; he or she is the proprietor of the business. A proprietor cannot draw wages from his or her company. The money the doctor extracts for personal use is called "drawings," which you learned about earlier in the chapter.

The first step is to complete the personal data portion on the payroll page. In order to read the Income Tax Deduction table, you must establish the employee's code. This is done by completing a TD1 form, which lists your total exemptions and places you in one of fourteen categories in the Income Tax Deduction table.

**Exercise 7.9**

Let us assume that you are single with no dependents; your deductions would be read from column 1. The janitor's deductions are read from column 4. Using blank payroll forms from the Working Papers (pp. 62–65), we will complete the payroll for the week of January 15, 19__.

You are paid $450 weekly and work 40 hours. The janitor, Mr. Don James, earns $8 an hour. Mr. James lives at 321 Jane Street, Manotick, K2E 7Z3. His phone number is 626-9731. He was formerly employed as a toolmaker at Tool and Die Co. Ltd. He was born September 25, 1939, and is a widower. He looks after his elderly mother and two teenage children. He began working in Dr. Plunkett's office two years ago on June 12 at a salary of $7 an hour. He receives a 50-cent-an-hour increase every year on the anniversary of his employment. His vacation period is negotiable. He is paid every two weeks. Complete Mr. James's data portion of the payroll sheet. Mr. James's social insurance number is 472 237 942.

Complete your portion of the personal data sheet on the payroll. You are paid every week, were not previously employed, were hired on the first day of June this year, and have not received an increase in your salary. Your vacation is negotiable. Use your regular street address and Ottawa as the city in which you live.

## Illustration 7.11 Payroll Journal

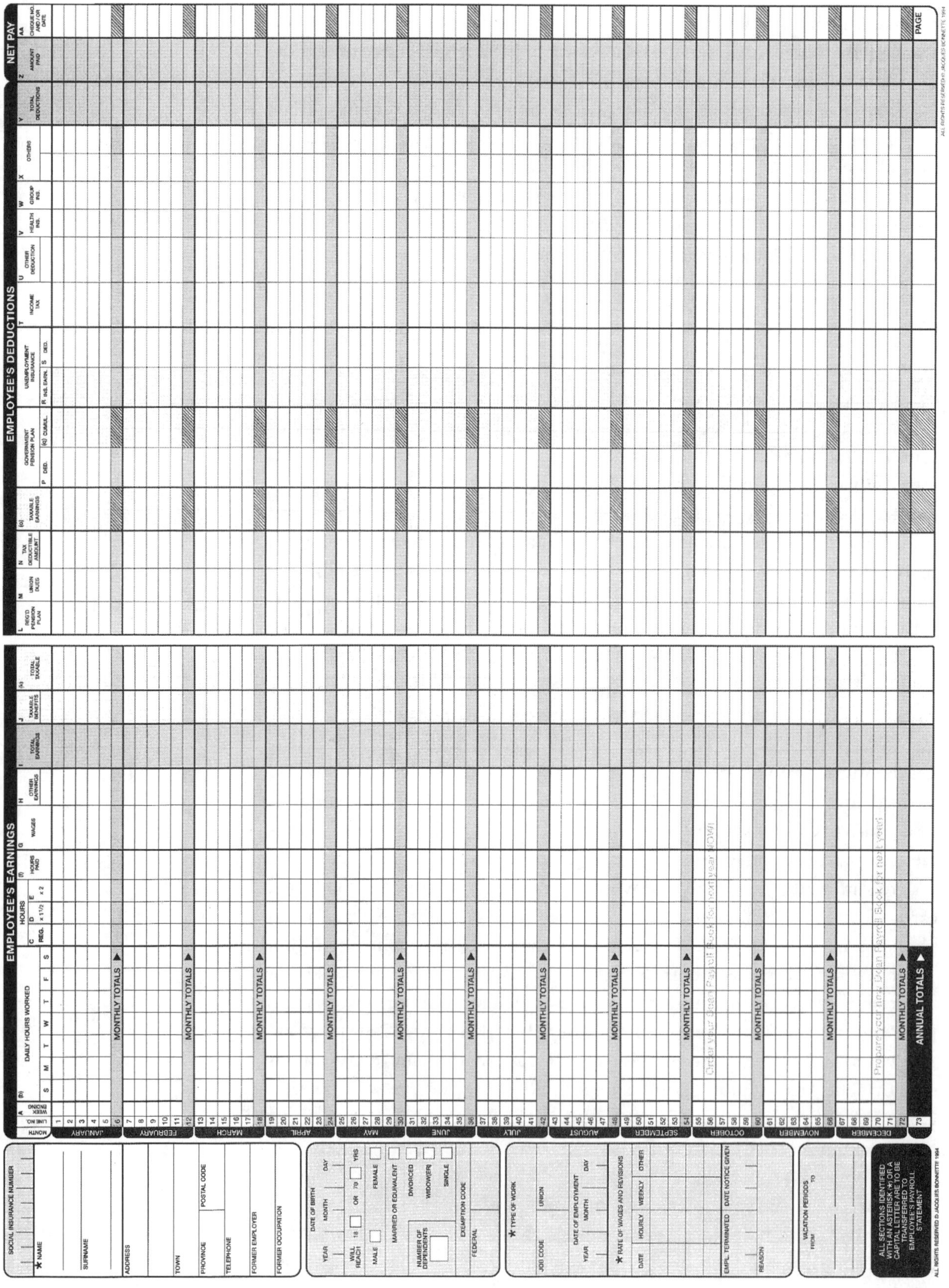
SOCIAL INSURANCE NUMBER
★ NAME
SURNAME
ADDRESS
TOWN
PROVINCE
POSTAL CODE
TELEPHONE
FORMER EMPLOYER
FORMER OCCUPATION
DATE OF BIRTH
YEAR MONTH DAY
WILL REACH 18 OR 70 YRS
MALE FEMALE
MARRIED OR EQUIVALENT
DIVORCED
WIDOW(ER)
SINGLE
NUMBER OF DEPENDENTS
EXEMPTION CODE
FEDERAL
★ TYPE OF WORK
JOB CODE
UNION
DATE OF EMPLOYMENT
YEAR MONTH DAY
★ RATE OF WAGES AND REVISIONS
DATE HOURLY WEEKLY OTHER
EMPL. TERMINATED
DATE NOTICE GIVEN
REASON
VACATION PERIODS
FROM TO
ALL SECTIONS IDENTIFIED WITH AN ASTERISK ★ OR A CAPITAL LETTER ARE TO BE TRANSFERRED TO EMPLOYEE'S PAYROLL STATEMENT
ALL RIGHTS RESERVED © JACQUES BONNETTE 1984
EMPLOYEE'S EARNINGS
MONTH
LINE NO.
A WEEK ENDING
(b) DAILY HOURS WORKED
S M T W T F S
HOURS
C REG.
D x 1 1/2
E x 2
(f) HOURS PAID
G WAGES
H OTHER EARNINGS
I TOTAL EARNINGS
J TAXABLE BENEFITS
(k) TOTAL TAXABLE
JANUARY
FEBRUARY
MARCH
APRIL
MAY
JUNE
JULY
AUGUST
SEPTEMBER
OCTOBER
NOVEMBER
DECEMBER
MONTHLY TOTALS ▶
ANNUAL TOTALS ▶
EMPLOYEE'S DEDUCTIONS
L REG'D PENSION PLAN
M UNION DUES
N TAX DEDUCTIBLE AMOUNT
(o) TAXABLE EARNINGS
GOVERNMENT PENSION PLAN
P DED.
(q) CUMUL.
UNEMPLOYMENT INSURANCE
R INS. EARN.
S DED.
T INCOME TAX
U OTHER DEDUCTION
V HEALTH INS.
W GROUP INS.
X OTHERS
Y TOTAL DEDUCTIONS
NET PAY
Z AMOUNT PAID
AA CHEQUE NO. AND/OR DATE
PAGE
ALL RIGHTS RESERVED © JACQUES BONNETTE 1984

Now complete the earnings and deductions portion of the payroll. Mr. James has worked the following hours over the past two weeks. Week ending January 8: Sunday 4½ hours, Tuesday 5 hours, Thursday 6 hours, Friday 4 hours. Week ending January 15: Sunday 8 hours, Monday 8 hours, Tuesday 10 hours, Wednesday 8 hours, Thursday 10 hours, Friday 8 hours. Mr. James is paid time-and-a-half for hours worked from 41 to 49 inclusive, and double time for hours above 49. In addition to deductions for CPP/UI and income tax, Mr. James pays $28.35 each pay period for OHIP and $5 each pay period for group insurance. Mr. James also contributes $10 each week to his registered pension plan and $1 each pay period to the United Way.

Your $450 salary is paid every week. In addition to CPP/UI and income tax, you pay $5 each week to a registered pension, $6.50 for OHIP, $2 for group insurance, and $1 to the United Way.

(Keep this payroll assignment for use in Assignment 7.4 at the end of the chapter.)

## Employee Payroll Statement

An important part of any payroll system is the employee payroll statement. The statement may be attached to the employee's cheque, or it may be included as a separate statement in the employee's pay envelope. Illustration 7.12 is an example of an employee payroll statement.

You will note that it gives a complete account of hours worked, earnings, each deduction, and the net amount of the paycheque. For practice, after you have completed Mr. James's payroll sheet for the two-week period ending January 15, fill in his employee payroll statement on Illustration 7.12 or use a statement form from the Working Papers (p. 66).

### Illustration 7.12   Payroll Statement

## Payment of UI, CPP, and Income Tax Deductions

On the fifteenth day of each month, an employer must submit to the Receiver General of Canada the amount of money deducted from employees' cheques, combined with the employer's contribution to CPP and UI. A Statement of Account for Source Deductions form (Illustration 7.13) must be completed to accompany the payment. The top half of the form is retained by the employer as a record of payment. The administrative assistant should calculate the total amount required for CPP, UI, and income tax and insert the figures in the proper areas of the form. If payment is made at the bank, the teller will stamp the receipt and return part 1. If you remit by mail, send part 3 in with your cheque and keep part 2 for your records. Let us assume that for the month of March, $47.52 has been deducted from your employees for UI, $57.64 for CPP, and $237.98 for income taxes. The calculations for your payment would be as follows:

| | | |
|---|---|---|
| UI | Employee contribution | $  47.52 |
| | Employer contribution | |
| | (47.52 × 1.4) = | 66.53 |
| | Total UI submission | $114.05 |
| | | |
| CPP | Employee contribution | $  57.64 |
| | Employer contribution | $  57.64 |
| | Total CPP submission | $115.28 |
| | | |
| Income Tax (amount deducted according to tax schedule) | | $237.98 |

You should write a cheque for the Receiver General of Canada in the amount of $114.05 + 115.28 + 237.98 = $467.31. The Statement of Account for Source Deductions form is completed as follows (see Illustration 7.13):

Part 1:  Write amounts for CPP and UI premium contributions, tax deductions, current payment, gross monthly payroll, and number of employees in the appropriate boxes.

The current payment is the sum of UI premiums, CPP, and income tax. Part 1 is kept by employers for their records.

Part 2:  This section is retained for communiqués from Revenue Canada.

Part 3:  Write proper amounts in the corresponding boxes.

After the first submission, the government will send a blank form for you to complete for the next remittance. The form will have the following information preprinted on it:

Part 1:  Date of last remittance, amount of remittance, any balance owing, and taxation centre contact

Part 2:  Employer account number and name, and address of business

Part 3:  Employer account number

**Illustration 7.13   Statement of Account for Source Deductions**

---

**1** | Revenue Canada / Revenu Canada

Account number  72734

**STATEMENT OF ACCOUNT FOR SOURCE DEDUCTIONS**

PD7A(E) Rev.95

Employer name  J.E. PLUNKETT

| Statement of account as of | Amount paid for | Assessed amount owing | You can make your payment where you bank or to: |
|---|---|---|---|
| **APRIL 15, 19___** Transactions processed after this date will appear on the next statement | For enquiries contact: | | Taxation Centre |

• IMPORTANT - SEE REVERSE •

**EXPLANATION OF CHANGES**

| Date | Description | Amount |
|---|---|---|
| | | |

Indicate remittance information in this area for your records

| CPP contributions | UI premiums | Tax deductions | Current payment | Gross monthly payroll | No. of empl. - last period |
|---|---|---|---|---|---|
| 115.28 | 114.05 | 237.98 | 467.31 | 2169.60 | 2 |

**2**

PD7A(E) Rev.95

Account number  72734

Employer name  Dr. J.E. Plunkett
278 O'Connor
Ottawa, ON J5Z 2X8

PIERRE GRAVELLE, QC
DEPUTY MINISTER OF NATIONAL REVENUE

---

**3** | Revenue Canada / Revenu Canada

**CURRENT SOURCE DEDUCTIONS REMITTANCE**

**PD7A(E)** Rev.95

**6**

| Account number | For Taxation use only |
|---|---|
| 72734 | |

**Amount of payment** ▷  | 4 | 6 | 7 | 3 | 1 |

**Month for which deductions were withheld** ▷   Year | _ | _ |   Month | 0 | 3 |

**Gross monthly payroll (dollars only)** ▷  | 2 | 1 | 7 | 0 | 0 | 0 |

**Number of employees in last pay period** ▷  | 2 |

⑈0 2000⑈⑈⑈ 96

## Assignment 7.3

In Chapter 2, you were instructed to book appointments for several patients. Complete health claim cards for each patient and transfer the information to the appropriate accounting documents (Working Papers, pp. 39–59). (Note: The diagnosis for the Harris baby was strep throat and an infected ear.) Personal data information is on the patient information sheets. Use February 28, 19__, as the date for these cards. Use the health claim cards provided in the Working Papers (pp. 24–32), or a computer billing system if one is available.

For the purpose of this assignment only, assume that Amelia Jackson and Hazel Davis have balances from January on their accounts in the amount of $33.50 and $14.25, respectively. Complete statements of account for these two patients.

Dr. Plunkett has asked you to write a letter to Thomas Bell informing him that his cheque for $32.50 was returned NSF and asking him to make arrangements to rectify the situation. (Use your imagination.)

Mr. Harris has not yet paid his account in full. It is now four months overdue. Dr. Plunkett sends a statement of account the first month, a reminder notice the second month, an inquiry the third month, and an appeal the fourth month. You have completed the statement of account. Compose the correspondence for the remainder of the collection series. (Use an appropriate reference book from the library and your imagination to assist you in completing the letters — *do not copy* letters from a textbook.) The balance outstanding on Mr. Harris's account is $37.50.

The cost of living has been increasing rapidly over the past year, and you and Mr. James have negotiated a 10 percent cost of living increase in your salary schedule. Complete the payroll book for the weeks of January 22 and January 29. Mr. James worked 8 hours each day Monday to Friday the week of January 22. For the week of January 29 he worked 12 hours Monday, 14 hours Tuesday, 10 hours Wednesday, he was off work Thursday, and he worked 8 hours Friday. During the week of January 22, you were granted two days off work to participate in a curling bonspiel. Of course, you were not paid for those two days. The salary increase became effective the week of January 22.

Calculate the CPP, UI, and income tax deduction figures for January to be submitted to the Receiver General of Canada, and insert them in the appropriate areas on the remittance form. (Include the figures from Exercise 7.9 for salaries paid January 8 and 15.)

## Assignment 7.4

Complete an employee payroll statement for Mr. James's two-week pay period, January 22 and 29, and one for yourself for the week of January 29. Use the payroll sheets from Assignment 7.3.

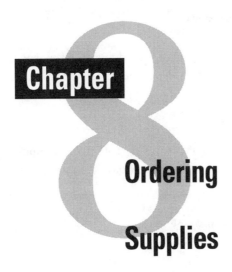

# Chapter 8

# Ordering

# Supplies

## Chapter Outline

- Ordering Procedures
- Purchasing and Inventory Control
- Cash Discounts
- Sales Taxes
- Assignments 8.1a, b, c, and d
- Assignment 8.2

## Learning Objectives

To become familiar with
- proper ordering procedures for billing supplies, medical supplies, drugs, cleaning products, and office supplies
- purchasing and inventory records
- cash discounts
- sales taxes

An important responsibility of the medical administrative assistant is to ensure that adequate supplies for all facets of the practice are readily available.

It is the administrative assistant's duty to check through the stock of supplies in the cupboard to see how much is being used daily or weekly. You should ensure that you always have supplies available and that reordering of stock is done before supplies are exhausted. It is advisable to produce a list of supplies contained in a specific area and post it in a readily visible place. This serves as a good reminder to check for depleted stock.

It is an easy task, when carefully monitored, to see how quickly supplies are used and to maintain a sufficient balance of stock.

## Billing Supplies

As you learned in Chapter 6, in order for providers to make a claim for their services, they must submit billing information for each patient seen. A busy doctor may see as many as 200 patients each week. The majority of physicians submit their fee for service to the Ministry of Health via electronic media.

It is essential that you maintain an adequate supply of tapes or diskettes to ensure that billing information can be submitted in a timely fashion.

## Medical Supplies

Doctors use a large quantity of different medical supplies in their practice. Dressings, disposable needles, surgical gloves, sutures, adhesive, tongue depressors, and thermometers are just a few of the necessities. Salespersons usually contact the physician, who, in turn, will inform you of the companies with which to place medical supply orders.

## Drugs

If you are responsible for ordering drugs, remember that drugs deteriorate. Do not make quantity purchases without consulting your employer. Drugs that are kept in the office include vaccines for influenza and other common diseases, adrenalin, various ointments and creams, antibiotics, aspirin, morphine, novocaine, penicillin, and so on. *All painkillers, sleeping pills, and tranquilizers should be kept securely locked and carefully controlled.*

In the past, when a drug's shelf life expired, it was usually flushed down the toilet. It is no longer acceptable to dispose of drugs in this manner because of the harm it may cause to the environment. Outdated drugs must be incinerated. Many drug companies will collect outdated drugs and have a disposal company incinerate them. If you cannot arrange for this service, contact a local company or the pharmacy at your community hospital, to ensure that disposal is carried out in an environmentally safe manner.

Drug manufacturers have salespersons who call on doctors to keep them informed of new drugs. Most doctors are aware of the services provided by these people and will give them a few minutes if possible.

## Toiletries and Cleaning Products

Items such as soap, paper towels, toilet paper, disinfectants, cleansers, and cleaning cloths are necessary to maintain a clean and sanitary environment. A local cleaning and maintenance supplier can provide you with these items.

## Office Supplies

The medical administrative assistant requires many items to perform the daily office duties. The physician generally has stationery preprinted such as letterhead, envelopes, statements, and prescription forms. In addition, a supply of pens, pencils, paper clips, staples, notepads, photocopier paper and toner, erasers, plain bond paper, file folders, and requisition and business forms should always be available. It may be helpful to flag supplies at a point where reordering should take place.

Arrangements should be made with equipment suppliers to have all equipment (computers, printers, fax machines, photocopiers, scales) serviced on a regular basis. In order to have an efficient office, equipment must be in good working order.

Prescription pad forms are often obtainable free of charge through drug suppliers.

Contact your local hospital to secure their requisition forms.

The administrative assistant should have an order book in which to keep a record of supplies ordered, the name and address of the supplier, the cost of the item, and the date the order was placed. This information can be used for reference when reordering and for cost comparisons. It will also give you a general idea of how long a quantity of a certain item lasts and when it is necessary to reorder. You should make routine reference to your order book to ensure your supply room is always adequately stocked.

## Purchasing and Inventory Control

**Illustration 8.1   Purchase Order**

**PURCHASE ORDER**

JOHN E. PLUNKETT
PHM.B., M.D., C.M., F.R.C.P., F.A.C.P.
INTERNAL MEDICINE
278 O'CONNOR ST.   OTTAWA, ONT.

TO:  Readymade Office Equipment
     225 Rideau Crescent
     Ottawa, Ontario
     J3X 7X6

DATE:        Sept. 25, 19____
ORDER NO.: 3754
REQ'D BY:   A.S.A.P.
SHIP VIA:   Paxy Transport
TERMS:      2/10/n/30

| ITEM NO. | QUANTITY | DESCRIPTION | UNIT | UNIT PRICE | | TOTAL | |
|---|---|---|---|---|---|---|---|
| 1 | 1 | Pedestal Desk | 1 | $525 | 00 | $525 | 00 |
| 2 | 500 | Hanger Files | 100 | 25 | 00 | 125 | 00 |
| | | Total | | | | $650 | 00 |
| | | Add G.S.T. 7% | | | | 45 | 50 |
| | | Add P.S.T. 8% | | | | 52 | 00 |
| | | Total Invoice | | | | $747 | 50 |

## The Purchase Order

In some office environments, ordering will be done by telephone or fax machine. A copy of the order will serve as a record. In some large organizations, it may be necessary to complete a purchase order (see Illustration 8.1).

A copy of the purchase order should be kept in a pending file until the material is received. If quoted prices have been received prior to the order, the amount should appear on the purchase order.

## The Packing Slip

A packing slip (Illustration 8.2) will be enclosed with your supplies shipment. The items and quantities listed on the packing slip should be compared with

**Illustration 8.2   Packing Slip**

PACKING SLIP

**READYMADE OFFICE EQUIPMENT**
225 Rideau Crescent
Ottawa, ON J3X 7X6
Telephone: (613) 387-5567
Fax: (613) 387-5568
Toll Free: 1-800-772-8893

INVOICE NO.  337815-33

DATE: ___/09/29

SOLD TO:
Dr. John E. Plunkett
278 O'Connor St.
Ottawa, ON J5Z 2X8

SHIP TO:
Dr. John E. Plunkett
278 O'Connor St.
Ottawa, ON J5Z 2X8

CUSTOMER ORDER NO.  3754

| ITEM NO. | QUANTITY ORDER | QUANTITY SHIP | DESCRIPTION |
|---|---|---|---|
| 1 | 1 | | 1 Pedestal Desk |
| 2 | 500 | | 400 Hanger Files |
| | | | 100 Hanger Files on Backorder |

Customer Signature

the contents of the package. After it has been confirmed that there are no discrepancies in the shipment received, the packing slip should be compared with the order record to ensure that your supplies requirements have been met.

## The Invoice

The invoice (Illustration 8.3) is a statement of the amount owing for goods shipped by the supplier. The quantities on the invoice should match those documented on the packing slip. If you were quoted prices prior to shipment, the prices on the invoice should match your order record.

If there are any discrepancies in price and/or quantity, the supplier should be contacted.

**Illustration 8.3   Invoice**

INVOICE

READYMADE OFFICE EQUIPMENT
225 Rideau Crescent
Ottawa, ON J3X 7X6

INVOICE NO. 337815-33                                    DATE: ___/09/29

SOLD TO:                                                 SHIP TO:
Dr. John E. Plunkett                                     Dr. John E. Plunkett
278 O'Connor Street                                      278 O'Connor Street
Ottawa, ON J5Z 2X8                                       Ottawa, ON J5Z 2X8

CUSTOMER ORDER NO. 3754

| ITEM NO. | QUANT. ORDER | QUANT. SHIP | DESCRIPTION | UNIT | UNIT PRICE | | TOTAL | |
|---|---|---|---|---|---|---|---|---|
| 1 | 1 | 1 | Pedestal Desk | 1 | $525 | 00 | $525 | 00 |
| 2 | 500 | 400 | Hanger Files | 100 | 25 | 00 | 100 | 00 |
| | | | Sub Total | | | | $625 | 00 |
| | | | Add G.S.T. 7% | | | | 43 | 75 |
| | | | Add P.S.T. 8% | | | | 50 | 00 |
| | | | Total Invoice | | | | $718 | 75 |

_____
Customer Signature

## Cash Discounts

Suppliers often allow a cash discount on purchases to encourage prompt payment; the cash discount is referred to as the "credit terms." The credit terms on a purchase may be "2 percent 10 days, net 30 days," meaning that if payment is received within 10 days after purchase, 2 percent can be deducted from the total cost; otherwise, payment is due within 30 days of the purchase. The terms are written "2/10/n/30" and expressed as "2, 10, net, 30."

## Sales Taxes

A 7 percent federal Goods and Services Tax is added to many items that you will purchase. In some provinces, a provincial sales tax is also added. The amount of the tax varies from province to province. For example, in Ontario, 8 percent is added to the invoice as a tax on the sale. There are also many variations in types of goods that are taxed. The medical administrative assistant is not expected to know the federal and provincial sales tax laws, but should be aware of the types of medical supplies that are not taxable. Information can be obtained by calling your provincial government sales tax branch (usually through a toll-free line). Most suppliers are aware of sales tax implications on the goods they supply and will add tax where applicable. However, if you know which items are taxable, you may wish to add the tax onto your purchase order.

## Assignment 8.1a

Prepare a purchase order (Working Papers, pp. 67–68) for 2 boxes of pencils, HB lead, at $2.50 a box; 2000 carbon packs at $10 per thousand; 4 ballpoint pens/blue at 59 cents each; 10 boxes of paper clips at $2.32 per box; 4 ballpoint pens/red at 69 cents each; and 250 ⅕ cut file folders at $10.35 per 100.

The purchase order no. 423 is dated February 16, 19__, and is required by February 19, 19__. Ship via Purolator. Supply company is Ottawa Valley Office Supplies, 213 Bank Street, Ottawa. Their terms are 2 percent 10 days and net 30 days.

## Assignment 8.1b

Your instructor will provide you with a copy of the packing slip that accompanied your order from Assignment 8.1a. Compare the slip and note discrepancies, if any.

## Assignment 8.1c

Your instructor will provide you with the invoice for goods ordered in Assignment 8.1a. Compare the invoice with the order record and packing slip and note discrepancies, if any.

## Assignment 8.1d

When you compared the order record, packing slip, and invoice, you noted some discrepancies. Document the discrepancies and the follow-up action you would take. Select a classmate and role play your conversation with the supplier. Remember that it is important to maintain a good relationship with your suppliers. Diplomacy and tact should be used when dealing with this and every situation.

**Assignment 8.2**

Before completing this assignment, select two students in your class to contact your provincial sales tax branch (if sales tax is collected in your province) and inquire if sales tax is applicable to the items to be included in the following purchase order.

Medical supplies are ordered from Merke & Parker Medical Suppliers, 337 Main Street, Ottawa. Their terms on all purchases are 2 percent if paid in 20 days and net due in 60 days; they have their own delivery service. You require 200 disposable needles at $50 per 100; 500 disposable thermometers at $72.50 per 100; 12 dozen pairs surgical gloves at $14.25 per pair; 20 dozen 5 cm × 10 cm gauze dressings at $8.75 per dozen; and 10 adhesive rolls (245 cm × 5 cm) at $7.50 per roll. A purchase order form can be found in the Working Papers (pp. 67–68).

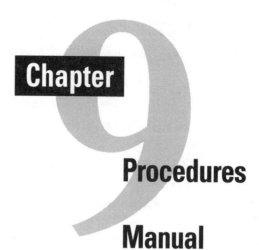

# Chapter 9

## Procedures Manual

**Chapter Outline**

- Assignment 9.1
- Assignment 9.2
- Assignment 9.3

**Learning Objectives**

To identify
- components of a procedures manual
- set-up and style of a procedures manual
- uses of a procedures manual

All businesses, whether they are manufacturers, wholesalers, retailers, or services, should have a procedures manual for easy reference by all employees.

## Components and Style

A procedures manual describes the necessary steps involved in completing any and all jobs relating to the business. If you are the only person dealing with the administration, it is a simple task to describe in detail how you go about completing individual duties in specific areas. If you are one of many employees and you are responsible for producing a procedures manual, you will have to ask each employee to describe the procedures involved in completing his or her particular job.

The manual should be printed on looseleaf sheets, alphabetized by job description, and organized in a reference manual. Tabbed dividers can be used to identify each section. Illustration 9.1 is a sample of how a page in a procedures manual might be formatted.

If you are employed in an office that does not have a procedures manual or that has a manual that needs updating, some topics you might consider covering are the following:

**Illustration 9.1 Procedures Manual**

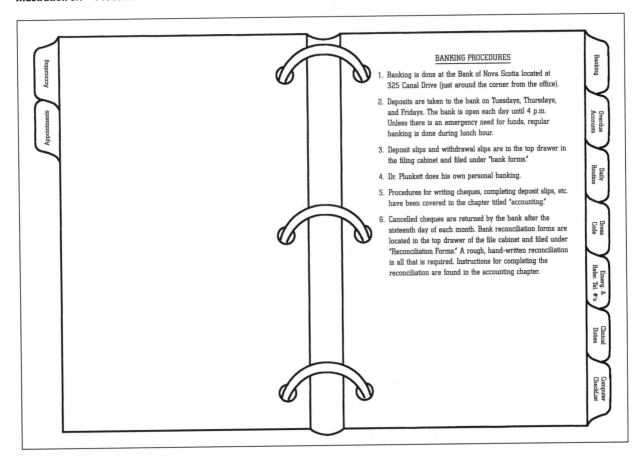

The following pages are indexed in the binder shown. The tabs on the left read (top to bottom): Accounting, Appointments. The tabs on the right read (top to bottom): Banking, Overdue Accounts, Daily Routine, Dress Code, Emerg. & Refer. Tel. #'s, Clinical Duties, Computer Checklist.

**BANKING PROCEDURES**

1. Banking is done at the Bank of Nova Scotia located at 325 Canal Drive (just around the corner from the office).

2. Deposits are taken to the bank on Tuesdays, Thursdays, and Fridays. The bank is open each day until 4 p.m. Unless there is an emergency need for funds, regular banking is done during lunch hour.

3. Deposit slips and withdrawal slips are in the top drawer in the filing cabinet and filed under 'bank forms.'

4. Dr. Plunkett does his own personal banking.

5. Procedures for writing cheques, completing deposit slips, etc. have been covered in the chapter titled 'accounting.'

6. Cancelled cheques are returned by the bank after the sixteenth day of each month. Bank reconciliation forms are located in the top drawer of the file cabinet and filed under 'Reconciliation Forms.' A rough, hand-written reconciliation is all that is required. Instructions for completing the reconciliation are found in the accounting chapter.

Accounting Procedures

Appointments

Banking

Bill Collections (overdue)

Daily Activity Routine

Dress Code

Emergency and Referral Telephone Numbers

Employee Benefits

Equipment

Health Card Billing

Hospital Forms

Insurance — Claim Forms and Policies Carried

Insurance Forms — Completion for Patients

Inventory

Job Description

Letter, Memo, Report, Manuscript Set-Up

Office Overload Agencies (for emergency and holiday staff replacement)

Office Policies

Ordering Supplies

Patient Ledgers
Personnel
Petty Cash
Reprographics
Salary Schedules
Telephone
Travel Arrangements
Work Schedule

Specific procedures are unique to each organization. You would add to or delete from the above list as required.

The chronological order or time sequence (daily, weekly, or monthly) in which jobs should be completed should also be recorded in the manual so that no job is left undone. Looking through the manual, the new administrative assistant can check if any vital duties have been overlooked.

## Uses

When explicit instructions are documented for all jobs, a substitute employee can effectively handle any emergency tasks. A procedures manual is also helpful for new employees. After reading the manual, the new employee has a general overview of the job requirements of the organization.

Of course, to be effective, the manual must have explicit information, such as the exact location of the petty cash box, where the list of medical supply companies and their addresses can be found, what time the mail is collected, and where important phone numbers are listed.

Preparing a procedures manual can sometimes reveal poor time management in a particular job. Because you are involved in writing a comprehensive description of how to handle a job, it is possible that you may discover you are duplicating a process or performing a facet of the job that is unnecessary. From time to time, you should review your manual so that any changes can be incorporated.

Cost savings and time management are important to the success of any business. As a responsible medical administrative assistant, you should take a personal interest in minimizing waste of both time and material. If you see others being inefficient, and you feel you can diplomatically bring it to their attention, you should do so. If the organization does not make a profit, you will soon find yourself out of a job.

---

## Assignment 9.1

When you begin your duties for Drs. Plunkett and Pelham, assume that the office does not have a procedures manual. Using your imagination, prepare a section for the manual describing the handling of petty cash. The description should include such things as appearance of petty cash box, where it is stored, proper procedures for reimbursements and withdrawals, and so on.

Following is an excerpt from an actual medical procedures manual. Key the instructions, improving on format and information provided.

**Assignment 9.2**

PATIENT DISCHARGE

Therapist sends note of discharge to the office.

Patient's Rolodex index card is removed and a large filing card is printed with the same information. The small card is stapled to the back of the large filing card and filed in the discharge file cardex.

Date of discharge appears in red on the large filing card.

Patient's file is removed from the file shelf and all papers, letters, and reports are placed in a manila folder.

Insert patient's name, birthdate, address, phone number on the folder.

Admittance information sheet is attached to the inside left of the manila folder and all other reports and correspondence are attached to the right side.

Place the manila folder in the discharge filing cabinet under the appropriate year.

Stroke out the patient's name on the master sheet and write the discharge date on the sheet.

Leave the coloured disc on the master sheet until statistics are recorded at the end of the month and then remove.

Record discharge date in the admittance book at the back.

Remember, the important thing to decide before completing this assignment is whether you would be able to perform the patient discharge procedures from the above information. If not, you must improve the instructions so that *anyone* who may be involved in following the procedure would be able to do so without having to ask questions.

Assume this is an office where there is only one administrative assistant, and he is ill. You have been called to substitute during his illness. You have never been in the office before. A patient is being discharged from the centre and you must complete the patient discharge procedures. The only instructions available for undertaking the task are found in the procedures manual as above.

It will be necessary to use your imagination to fill in missing information and clarify the information provided.

**Assignment 9.3**

Prepare a page for a medical office procedures manual entitled "Daily Activity Routine." You will have to imagine what duties you would perform and the order in which they would be done. Also, decide whether the doctor has office hours all day or just in the morning or afternoon. Choose the type of medical office (private practice, hospital admitting, clinic reception, or other) in which you hope to find employment when you graduate. Insert this assignment in your portfolio.

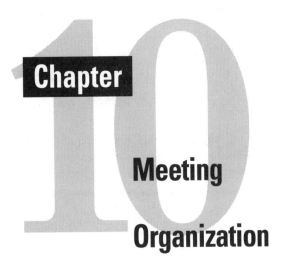

# Chapter 10

# Meeting

# Organization

## Chapter Outline

- Assignment 10.1
- Assignment 10.2
- Assignment 10.3

## Learning Objectives

To review
- the preparation of a notice of meeting
- agenda
- minutes

A medical administrative assistant may be responsible for arranging meetings as well as recording and producing minutes. A meeting can be very informal with a committee of three or four persons, or a convention of several hundred participants.

The administrative assistant may also be responsible for sending out notices of the meeting, reserving an appropriate meeting place, deciding on and supervising the arranging of suitable table placement, having beverages (coffee, tea, water, juice) available for participants, compiling an agenda, recording the minutes, and producing and distributing printed copies of the minutes. For large convention-type meetings, public address systems and meals may also have to be considered.

## Notice of Meeting

When the date and time of the meeting have been established, the first responsibility of the administrative assistant is to find an appropriate physical space in which to hold the meeting. The number of participants will determine the size of the room; if participants will be taking notes, tables, notebooks, and pencils should be available; if a number of people will be participating, a public address system may be necessary. These requirements, and

**Illustration 10.1   Notice of Meeting**

NOTICE OF MEETING

A meeting of the Medical Aid Association will be held at 5 p.m. on December 15, 19__ in the Blue Room at the Holiday Inn, 215 Front Street, Ottawa, Ontario. All committee heads are required to have their annual reports completed for presentation.

(handwritten signature)

any others necessary for a well-organized meeting, must be taken into consideration. Once an appropriate area has been reserved, the administrative assistant must inform the participants of the details. This would be done with a notice of meeting (see Illustration 10.1).

This notice should be distributed approximately ten days before the meeting. Timing of notices is crucial: if sent too early, they may be forgotten; if sent too late, members may have made other commitments for the date you have arranged.

## Meeting Agenda

Discuss with the chairperson of the meeting the topics to be covered. A planned order for the meeting will avoid confusion, wasted time, and missed items.

Some groups have an agenda committee as part of their executive. In this case, the administrative assistant would attend an agenda meeting approximately two weeks prior to the meeting; an appropriate agenda would be discussed and the administrative assistant would print and distribute the details. Illustration 10.2 is an example of an agenda.

## Assignment 10.1

Assume that your doctor/employer has just informed you that the meeting outlined in Illustration 10.2 will be held. You are responsible for making all physical arrangements for this meeting. The doctor is also secretary of this society, and has asked you to take care of all the secretarial duties.

With your instructor's help, prepare a checklist of all items that you will have to attend to, including phone calls, paper work, and so on. After you have completed your first list, determine the approximate date on which each task should be completed, and then prepare a chronological list of these tasks.

**Illustration 10.2    Agenda**

---

MEETING

MEDICAL AID ASSOCIATION

December 15, 19___

I.  a) Meeting called to order
    b) Roll call
    c) Minutes of meeting, November 14, 19___

II.  Correspondence

III.  Financial Report

IV.  Business Arising from the Minutes

    a) Purchase of Resuscitating Equipment    G. Farley
    b) Revision of Constitution    D. Moore

V.  New Business

    a) Charity Project for 19___    Nominating
    b) Election of Officers    Committee

VI.  Guest Speaker    "Crib Death"    J.A. Coons,
    M.D.

VII.  Adjournment

---

## Convention Agenda

Preparation for a convention begins several months in advance. A planning committee is responsible for all facets of the event including engaging speakers, setting the agenda, and publicity. Once details are finalized, the administrative assistant produces the agenda (Illustration 10.3) and ensures that all those registered to attend the convention receive a copy. The agenda may be sent out prior to the convention, or used as a handout the day of the event.

**Assignment 10.2**

Assume you are employed as the administrative assistant of the doctor responsible for organizing a convention. Prepare a printed copy of the convention schedule outlined below using an appropriate and attractive format (use your creativity). A copy of the schedule would be mailed to each convention delegate. Insert a copy of the completed schedule in your portfolio.

The schedule for the convention is the same each day except for the registration beginning at 10 A.M. on May 14 and the dinner on May 18 at 6 P.M.

On May 14, the convention meetings begin at 1 P.M. and conclude at 4 P.M. On May 15, 16, and 17, morning sessions begin at 9 A.M. and conclude at 11:30 A.M.; afternoon sessions are from 2 P.M. to 4 P.M. On May 18, sessions conclude at 11:30 A.M., and the afternoon is free.

The afternoon sessions are lecture meetings and the morning sessions are workshops. The speakers are Dr. John McGilvray, anaesthetist, on "Advances in Administering Techniques"; Dr. Scott Hayes, pediatrician, on "Learning Disabilities"; Dr. Fraser McGee, heart specialist, on "The Killer Disease"; and Dr. Terry Fisher, neurologist, on "The Human Mind."

The workshops are discussions pertaining to the previous afternoon's lecture.

## Illustration 10.3   Convention Agenda

### AGENDA

**Friday, June 2, 19__**

|  |  |
|---|---|
| 2:00 - 6:00 | Registration |
| 6:30 | Barbecue |
| 8:30 | Travelling Theme Party |

**Saturday, June 3, 19__**

|  |  |
|---|---|
| 7:30 - 9:00 | Breakfast (8:00 President's Round Table) |
| 9:00 - 9:30 | Opening Ceremonies and Welcome |
| 9:30 - 10:00 | Annual Meeting |
| 10:00 - 10:15 | Coffee |
| 10:15 - 11:00 | "Rules My Grammar Never Taught Me" - Sylvia Smith |
| 11:00 - 12:00 | "M.O.R.E." (Multiple Organ and Retrieval Exchange) - L. Lars, Representative • Heart Transplant Recipient • Lung Transplant Recipient • Mother of a young donor |
| 12:00 - 1:00 | Lunch |

|  |  |
|---|---|
| 1:00 - 2:00 | "Emergency Medicine" - Dr. A. Vince Emergency Department Peterborough Civic Hospital |
| 2:00 - 2:45 | "What's Happening in Health Care ... What's Coming Up" - D. Jones Health Policies O.M.A. |
| 2:45 - 3:00 | Coffee |
| 3:00 - 4:00 | "Laughter is the Best Medicine" - Tom White, Humourist |
| 5:30 | President's and International Reception |
| 6:30 | Social Time (Cash Bar) |
| 7:00 - 9:00 | Banquet Awards/Presentations |
| 9:30 | Academy Awards |

**Sunday, June 4, 19__**

|  |  |
|---|---|
| 8:00 - 9:00 | Continental Breakfast (Delivered personally to your cottage) |
| 9:30 - 11:30 | Country Store & Craft Sale |
| 11:30 - 1:00 | Buffet Brunch Fashion Show |

Visit the displays
on Saturday
in the Whistle Stop Room

**Elmhirst Resort Total Convention Package is $242.94 per person**

Includes:  All Taxes and Gratuities
2 Nights Accommodation/
Fully Equipped Cottages
All Meals/Entertainment
Use of All Facilities/
Pool/Hot Tub/Sauna
Nature Trails

To reserve your accommodations or meal packages, please see enclosed flyer.

**Convention Registration**

Registration Fee:

| | |
|---|---|
| Members | $30.00 |
| Non-Members | $75.00 |
| Retirees | $30.00 |

Please complete the reverse side, tear off this portion and return to OMSA by April 27, 19__.

To be eligible for an **Early Bird Draw**, registrations must be received at Head Office by May 1, 19__.

## Minutes

You may be required to attend the meeting and record the minutes, or your employer may record the minutes and ask you to prepare them from hand-written notes; or a recording device may be used, and you would produce the minutes from the transcription tape. Regardless of the method used to record the minutes, they must be printed and distributed to the participants in an acceptable form. A general guideline for producing minutes follows:

1. Centre and capitalize the word "Minutes" on line 8 or 9, followed by a double space and the name of the organization.
2. Triple-space after the heading.
3. Minutes may be single- or double-spaced. Use a 15-cm (6-inch) line and standard 21.5 cm × 28 cm (8½ inch × 11 inch) paper.
4. Use the prepared agenda as a guideline for producing the minutes. It should be noted if deviation from the agenda order occurs.
5. Place subject captions in such a manner that they are easily located; for example, leave a wide margin with captions in capital letters within the margin as in Illustration 10.4.
6. Some minutes are produced with "Motion" captions formatted in the same manner as the subject captions.
7. The words "motion carried" or "motion defeated" should be in all capitals, underlined, and should follow each motion. The recording secretary might also wish to note the number "for," "against," and "abstaining."
8. Do not record personal comments or opinions such as, "John Smith thought it would be wise if . . ." Only business matters are recorded.
9. Try to summarize discussions; motions should be recorded exactly as presented.
10. If a thank-you letter is requested, or an expression of gratitude recommended, it should be in the form of a resolution.
11. Attach any pertinent reports to the minutes.
12. Errors in minutes should be corrected in red ink and noted in the margin, making reference to the minutes of the following meeting when the error was reported.
13. After the last line of the body of the minutes, leave five or six spaces followed by a line of underscores from the left margin for the president's or chairperson's signature, and a line of underscores to the right margin for the secretary's signature (see Illustration 10.4).
14. All motions must be seconded and voted on by the membership (a motion of adjournment is an exception). Be sure to include both the "mover" and "seconder" when producing the minutes.

**Illustration 10.4    Format Style for Minutes**

MINUTES

MEDICAL AID ASSOCIATION MEETING

A meeting of the Medical Aid Association was held on December 15, 19___ in the Blue Room of the Holiday Inn.

The meeting was called to order by President Joe Hayes at 5:15 p.m.

THOSE PRESENT     J. Hayes, R. Mastrianni, T. Intersoll, A. Mosia, C. Fortran, M. Zincovich, T. Cavanagh, D. Moore, G. Farley, T. Fergus, D. Dudey, J. Bluett, and Treasurer E. Chambers

MINUTES     T. Cavanagh noted that Paragraph 2, Section V of the November 14, 19___ minutes should read ". . . at a purchase price of $218.28."

Moved by D. Moore, seconded by T. Fergus that the minutes be accepted as amended.

MOTION CARRIED

CORRESPONDENCE     Letters were received from the Homecare Workers requesting a donation of baked goods for their Christmas Tea and Bazaar to be held on Wednesday, December 3, 19___; and from the Heavenly Home for the Aged inviting our association to attend their Christmas Party on December 10, 19___; tickets are $8.

FINANCIAL REPORT     Treasurer Eleanor Chambers reviewed the financial statement (copy attached).

Moved by C. Fortran and seconded by M. Zincovich that the financial report be adopted as read and that all accounts be paid when properly vouched.

MOTION CARRIED

BUSINESS ARISING
FROM THE MINUTES     a) G. Farley reported on his investigation into the cost of purchasing resuscitating equipment for use by the fire department. The TX60 equipment discussed at the November meeting can be acquired for $4,926.50. Mr. Farley has discussed the purchase with the fire chief and he feels the TX60 would improve their efficiency 100 percent when dealing with cardiac and drowning victims. A. Mosia moved that we purchase the TX60 package at a cost of $4,926.50. D. Dudey seconded the motion.

MOTION CARRIED

b) D. Moore reported that the Constitution Committee is still meeting twice a month and they will be ready to present a draft revision at the January meeting.

NEW BUSINESS     a) T. Intersoll recommended that our charity project for 19___ be directed toward providing tables, chairs, cards, and trays for the Senior Citizens' Bridge Club. A brief discussion ensued. No other suggestions were brought forward.

J. Bluett moved that we defer this topic to the next meeting and hopefully more suggestions will be made at that time. R. Mastrianni seconded the motion.

MOTION CARRIED

**Illustration 10.4   Format Style for Minutes (continued)**

Minutes
Medical Aid Association Meeting
December 15, 19__
Page Two

      b) The nominating committee presented a slate of officers for 19__ and an election was held. The new executive is:

| | |
|---|---|
| President | -- R. Mastrianni |
| Vice-President | -- J. Bluett |
| Secretary | -- T. Intersoll |
| Treasurer | -- E. Chambers |

GUEST SPEAKER    Dr. J.A. Coons was introduced by A. Mosia. His presentation on crib deaths was both interesting and informative. G. Farley thanked Dr. Coons on behalf of the membership.

ADJOURNMENT    D. Moore moved that the meeting adjourn at 7:15 p.m.

_____        _____
      PRESIDENT                    SECRETARY

---

## Assignment 10.3

You are the administrative assistant to Dr. John Lawson, chairperson of the medical records committee. Using the following minutes as a guide,

1. Produce a notice of the meeting and the agenda that would be sent to the committee members prior to the meeting.
2. Reproduce the minutes using the format shown in Illustration 10.4. Place major headings in the margin and use run-in style for other headings.

### MINUTES

Minutes of a meeting of the Medical Records Committee held on May 20, 19__, at 1215 hours in Conference Room A, Peterborough Civic Hospital.

PRESENT:  Dr. J. Lawson, Dr. T. Chromie, R. Smith, Dr. Trims, S. Adams, R. Sevich, L. Bazio, N. Taylor, A. Rawlins, P. Clark, Z. Copping, T. Kezia, R. Jacobs, Dr. Roberts, T. Dawson.

MINUTES:  The minutes of the previous meeting were approved on a motion by Dr. M. Roberts, seconded by Mrs. S. Adams.

BUSINESS ARISING FROM THE MINUTES

1.  New Medical Records Policy for Incomplete Charts

Dr. Chromie noted that the policy recommended by this committee has now been passed by the Medical Advisory Committee and the Board of Governors. It is now up to the Medical Records Committee to decide when and how the new policy should be implemented. It was agreed that a notice should be sent to all medical staff members explaining the policy and including a copy of the policy. Mrs. R. Smith noted that the next count would be taken on Friday, May 21. It was agreed that overdue charts would be ignored for this one week. The notice to physicians would be sent out as quickly as possible and implementation of the new policy would begin the week of May 25.

2.   Patient Profile Form

There is nothing to report on this form at the present time. Dr. Chromie noted that he suggested to Miss Dawson that she obtain suggestions for the Patient Profile Form from all medical departments. Committee members agreed that medical staff input is necessary.

3.   Obstetrical Form

Mrs. Adams noted that the Obstetrical Form, which includes intrapartum risk factors, was used on a trial basis for several months. At the end of this time, its use was reviewed by the department of obstetrics, which has recommended to discontinue use of the form.

Dr. Trims drew the attention of committee members to the vast amount of duplication from physicians completing medical records. He asked that the committee be aware of this when new forms are being considered, and that all possible attempts be made to avoid duplication wherever possible.

4.   Diet Order Form

Mrs. Sevich reported that the new Diet Order Forms have been printed and are now in use throughout the hospital.

5.   Dictating Line in Special Procedures Room

It was noted that this line has now been installed in the special procedures room and is in use.

6.   Unit Number System

Mrs. Bazio reported that the conversion to a unit number system is complete and all admitted patients' and surgical outpatients' charts are now being handled in this fashion. It was noted that the unit numbering system is not used for emergency patients. She noted that during the initial use of the new system, it was taking more time; however, once staff become more familiar with the system, it will be a time saver.

NEW BUSINESS

1.  Letter from Wellesley Hospital re Transfer of Information

    A letter was received from Wellesley Hospital asking precisely what information is sent with a patient being transferred from Civic Hospital to another hospital. Wellesley Hospital is gathering this information from a number of hospitals in an effort to determine what is actually required when patients are transferred.

    Mrs. Rawlins noted that what is sent with the patient depends on where the patient is being sent and what procedures are going to be done. She noted that it is one thing for a patient being transferred to Princess Margaret, and that it is quite a different situation if a patient is being transferred to Sunnybrook Medical Centre. Dr. Chromie noted that when a patient comes back from Toronto, we receive copies of almost the total chart, and he finds this very useful. He noted that it is difficult for one hospital to know what will be useful in another hospital and, therefore, sending the whole chart is often helpful. He stated that for patients being sent to Toronto for a CT scan, the whole chart (not copies) is sent with the patient and then returned when the patient comes back to Peterborough.

    Mrs. Smith noted that nursing staff find it very helpful to receive the nursing notes with the patient and not at a later date. Dr. Trims noted that it can take up to six months for final notes to be received on patients being sent back to Peterborough from another facility.

    Mrs. Sevich will respond to the Wellesley Hospital request, noting that it is very helpful to receive as much information as possible at the time of patient transfer.

2.  Preop Histories

    This item was included on the agenda because of an incident where one physician insisted on having a medical transcriptionist called back to the hospital at night to transcribe a preop history. This is an ongoing problem. On the day of surgery, transcriptionists frequently spend a great deal of time hunting for the preop history dictation. Mrs. N. Taylor noted that there are two outside priority lines that are cleared very early every morning. If preop histories are dictated on these lines, there should be no problem with histories being available for surgery that day.

    Mr. Clark made the suggestion that for all elective surgery, preop histories be required before the patient is admitted; if no history is available, the patient is not admitted to the hospital.

    Committee members agreed that the whole preop package should be reviewed once again, not just in light of difficulties in obtaining histories but also in light of laboratory work, and so on.

As an interim measure, Mr. Clark suggested that a cutoff time, after which preop histories will not be transcribed in the hospital, be set and if this deadline is not met, it then becomes the physician's responsibility to have the history transcribed elsewhere.

It was further suggested that doctors should be educated to dictate preop histories when they see the patient in their offices. If this were done, problems would be minimized.

Mr. Copping suggested that Mr. Jacobs and Mrs. Kezia be delegated to look at the whole problem and bring back suggestions to this committee. In the meantime, he noted, no transcriptionist should be called back after hours to transcribe preoperative histories.

3.  Availability of Old Charts

Mrs. Kezia noted that the physicians like to have old charts added to their patients' current charts. The anaesthetists in particular find this most desirable, and it has been recommended that the old chart be added to the current chart in the ward. Mrs. Bazio outlined the procedure used for surgical patients. She is attempting to organize the logistical problems in order to reach the goal of having all old charts attached to current charts in the ward.

Mrs. Smith noted that she has received some complaints about physicians having to use microfilm charts. She noted, however, that space is an ongoing problem and in her department, there is little alternative to microfilming.

Mrs. Sevich noted that she is looking at ways in which to increase the storage potential in her department; however, she noted that those charts that have been microfilmed in the past cannot be restored to their previous form.

4.  Chart Review

This item was tabled because of lack of time to deal with it adequately.

5.  Problem Charts

Ms. Dawson noted that there were two charts for which she was unable to determine which physician should complete the record. Committee members looked at these charts and assigned them to physicians for completion.

ADJOURNMENT

Dr. Chromie moved the meeting be adjourned at 1530.

John Lawson, M.D., Chairman
Medical Records Committee

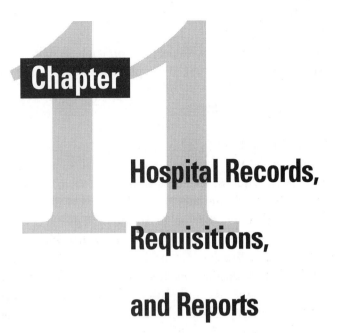

# Chapter 11

# Hospital Records, Requisitions, and Reports

## Chapter Outline

- Assignment 11.1a, b, and c
- History and Physical Report
- Assignment 11.2
- Assignment 11.3
- Assignment 11.4
- Discharge Summary/Final Note
- Consultation/Admission Note
- Assignment 11.5
- Operative Record
- Assignment 11.6
- Delivery Report

- Assignment 11.7
- Assignment 11.8
- Assignment 11.9
- Completion of Requisition Forms
- Assignment 11.10
- Assignment 11.11
- Appendix A — Common Abbreviations Used in the Health Care Field
- Appendix B — Laboratory Medicine
- Appendix C — Pharmacology
- Appendix D — Reference Sources

## Learning Objectives

To learn
- how to initiate hospital records
- proper procedures for completing hospital requisitions
- the processing of discharge records
- recognized filing systems for health records departments
- how to complete requisitions in a physician's office

To identify appropriate formats for
- history and physical reports
- discharge summaries/final notes
- consultation notes
- operative records
- delivery reports
- patient admission forms
- patient consent forms
- request for accommodation forms

To review
- the various types of investigative reports generated in a medical environment
- proper procedures for preparing investigative reports

In addition to learning how to process hospital records, you will learn how to complete hospital requisitions in the physician's office.

## Initiation of Hospital Records

The hospital record begins in the admitting department of the hospital with the admission of the patient. There, essential sociological information is obtained: name, address, telephone number, and so on. This information is very important for future reference, billing, and statistical purposes. The reason for admission is recorded on an Admission/Discharge Record (Illustration 11.1), which helps the attending physician know what initial investigations might be required. When a patient is being admitted on a prearranged basis, such as for surgery, this information will have already been recorded on the Admission/Discharge Record, based on information received from the patient's physician. A plastic hospital card, or addressograph (Illustration 11.2), is also prepared at time of admission and used during the patient's stay to imprint his or her identification onto all records. In some hospitals, the addressograph card is given to the patient on discharge to be used for future visits. The Admission/Discharge Record is the first of several documents that will make up the patient's chart.

The chart is then sent to the nursing unit, where the patient will be treated, and various nursing forms are added, such as Nurse's Record (Illustration 11.3), Temperature Chart (Illustration 11.4), Nursing History Chart, often referred to as Kardex (Illustration 11.5), and the Nursing Care Plan (Illustration 11.6). In some hospitals this process is computerized.

The attending physician adds the patient's complaints regarding the onset and course of the illness, the patient's personal and family history, and a complete report of the physical examination. This information is recorded on a History and Physical Examination Report (Illustration 11.7). The physician may choose to dictate a History and Physical Examination Report. The content of a History and Physical Report is covered on page 184.

The doctor then fills out a Physician's Orders Form (Illustration 11.8) with the appropriate medication and treatment ordered according to the patient's diagnosis. A consultant may be requested to see the patient, and findings will be recorded either by dictating or writing a Consultation Report (Illustrations 11.9 and 11.10). The consultant may give additional orders.

If surgery is required, other records are completed and appended to the chart. The information is recorded on appropriate preprinted forms, such as Consent for Surgical Operation (Illustration 11.11), Anaesthetic Record (Illustration 11.12), Physician's Operative Report (Illustration 11.13), Nurse's Operative Record (Illustration 11.14), and Postanaesthetic Record (Illustration 11.15).

Changes that occur in the patient's condition are recorded on Progress Notes (Illustration 11.16), and additional orders are written as necessary.

**Illustration 11.1   Admission/Discharge Record**

## ST. JOSEPH'S HOSPITAL & HEALTH CENTRE
384 ROGERS STREET
PETERBOROUGH, ONT.  K9H 7B6

### ADMISSION / DISCHARGE RECORD

HOSPITAL #1772

| Patient's Surname | Patient's First Name | Patient ID Number |
|---|---|---|
| Register Number | Admission Date DD MM YY / Time Hr. | Health Card # |

| Amb. | Lang | RTS | RFP | Birthdate DD MM YY | Sex | Language | Mar. Stat. | Prev. Pat. | Alternate or Previous Name | Certificate Holder's Initials |

| Age Group | Residence Code | Type | Address (Include Township, County, District, If Necessary) |

Postal Code        Phone        Religion

In Emergency Notify - Name, (Relation), Address, Phone

OHIP Group - Name & Address

Responsibility For Payment & Other Insurance Data

☐ OHIP

| Accom. | Requested | Assigned | Room No. | Rate | Transferred From |

Family Physician        Referring Physician        Attending Physician

Admitting Diagnosis        Expected Date of Disc.

Allergies

I agree to assume responsibility for charges not paid by any other agency.

Signature of Patient or Guarantor

Discharged ☐ Date
Signed Out ☐ and
Death ☐ Time:        Day  Month  Years / hours

Autopsy: Yes ☐ No ☐     Coroner: Yes ☐ No ☐   name

Transferred to:        Days Stay

**Diagnosis Most Responsible For Length of Stay    Do Not Use Abbreviations**

**Complications (conditions arising during the hospital stay)    Do Not Use Abbreviations**

**Other Diagnoses    Do Not Use Abbreviations**        Did it influence L.O.S.?

Yes ☐ No ☐
Yes ☐ No ☐
Yes ☐ No ☐
Yes ☐ No ☐

**Operations and procedures:**

**Discharge Summary**        Note Dictated:  Yes ☐  No ☐

I.C.U. Days
Physio ☐ O.T. ☐
Speech ☐ Resp. ☐
Other ☐ Other ☐
Social Serv. ☐ Disch. Planning ☐

The undersigned confirms all orders for treatment contained in the herein doctors' order sheets, whether signed or not and the discharge of the patient on the date shown above.

D  M  Y

#6520 REVISED 11/92

Signature of the most Responsible Physician        Date

**SUMMARY SHEET**

Abst. by:
Date:

**Illustration 11.2   Addressograph**

EXAMPLE A

| | |
|---|---|
| Patient's Unit # | 40442 |
| Patient's Sex/Name | M       Shultz, Erik |
| Patient's Address | 17 Bond St., Ottawa, ON |
| Health Card # | 7819749313 |

EXAMPLE B

| | |
|---|---|
| Patient's Unit #/Visit Specific # | 40442          95-03751 |
| Patient's Sex/Age/Name | M55 yrs        Shultz, Erik |
| Patient's Visit Date/Birth Date | 16 Oct 95 BD26 May 19__ |
| Patient's Address | 17 Bond St., Ottawa, ON |
| Health Card #/Doctor's Name | 7819749313   Dr. Plunkett |

Example A depicts a card that would be given to a patient to be used for each and every visit to the health care facility.

Example B depicts a card that would be specific to each visit made to the health care facility. In this case the card would not be given to the patient but would be destroyed by the facility when the patient is discharged.

**Illustration 11.3   Nurse's Record**

Erik Shultz
17 Bond Street
Ottawa, Ontario   May 26, 19___
7819749313

**NURSE'S RECORD**

| DATE TIME | DIET – MEDICATION – TREATMENTS | Ur-ine | St-ool | OBSERVATIONS – PROGRESS |
|---|---|---|---|---|
| | | | | |
| | | | | |
| | | | | |
| | | | | |
| | | | | |
| | | | | |
| | | | | |
| | | | | |
| | | | | |
| | | | | |
| | | | | |
| | | | | |
| | | | | |
| | | | | |
| | | | | |
| | | | | |
| | | | | |
| | | | | |
| | | | | |
| | | | | |
| | | | | |
| | | | | |
| | | | | |
| | | | | |
| | | | | |
| | | | | |
| | | | | |
| | | | | |
| | | | | |
| | | | | |
| | | | | |
| | | | | |
| | | | | |

**Illustration 11.4    Temperature Chart**

PETERBOROUGH HOSPITALS
MINDEN HOSPITAL
HALIBURTON HOSPITAL

NURSING DEPARTMENT
VITAL SIGNS RECORD

| DATE | | |
|---|---|---|
| TIME | | |

| TEMP (BLACK) | 41 | | | 41 |
|---|---|---|---|---|
| | 40 | | | 40 |
| | 39 | | | 39 |
| | 38 | | | 38 |
| | 37 | | | 37 |
| | 36 | | | 36 |
| | 35 | | | 35 |

| BP (BLACK) | 240 | | | 240 |
|---|---|---|---|---|
| | 230 | | | 230 |
| | 220 | | | 220 |
| | 210 | | | 210 |
| | 200 | | | 200 |
| PULSE (BLACK) | 190 | | | 190 |
| | 180 | | | 180 |
| | 170 | | | 170 |
| | 160 | | | 160 |
| | 150 | | | 150 |
| APICAL x (BLACK) | 140 | | | 140 |
| | 130 | | | 130 |
| | 120 | | | 120 |
| | 110 | | | 110 |
| | 100 | | | 100 |
| | 90 | | | 90 |
| | 80 | | | 80 |
| | 70 | | | 70 |
| | 60 | | | 60 |
| | 50 | | | 50 |
| | 40 | | | 40 |
| | 30 | | | 30 |
| | 20 | | | 20 |
| | 10 | | | 10 |

| RESP (BLACK) | 40 | | | 40 |
|---|---|---|---|---|
| | 35 | | | 35 |
| | 30 | | | 30 |
| | 25 | | | 25 |
| | 20 | | | 20 |
| | 15 | | | 15 |
| | 10 | | | 10 |
| | 5 | | | 5 |

| WEIGHT (kg) | | |
|---|---|---|

FORM #1519 JF: JANUARY, 1992

## Illustration 11.5   Nursing History Chart

**NURSING HISTORY**

Erik Shultz
17 Bond Street
Ottawa, Ontario    May 26, 19___
7819749313

**ADMISSION:**   Date: _____ Time: _____ From: _____ How: _____ Age: 55

Dr. Notified:  YES  NO _____ Admission  Bld. Work Drawn:  YES  NO

**DIAGNOSIS:** _____ Pt's Expected Length of Stay _____

Pt's Own Words re Reason Admitted: _____

Other Health Problems: _____

**MEDICATIONS:**   Taking At Home: _____   Taken Today: _____   Brought to Hospital: (list) _____

_____   _____   _____
_____   _____   _____
_____   _____   _____
_____   _____   _____
_____   _____   _____
_____   _____   _____

**OBSERVATIONS:**   T_____ p.o./rectal  P_____ reg/irreg  R_____ easy/difficult  B/P_____ Wt._____ Ht._____ Denture:  Upper  Lower

Prosthesis (explain) _____ Glasses _____ Hearing Aid _____ False Fingernails _____     Partial

_____ Contacts _____ Hospital I.D. Band _____ Ostomy:  YES  NO  Selfcare/with help

General Appearance, Skin Condition & Physical Limitations: _____

_____

Emotional & Mental Status: _____

Other Comments: _____

Allergies: _____ Bladder Habits: _____

Diet: _____ Bowel Habits: _____ Sleep Habits: _____

Valuables Record Understood & Signed by Pt. and/or Family?  YES  NO   Has Pt. ever had a Blood Transfusion?  YES  NO

**SOCIAL PROFILE:**  Marital Status:  M  S  W  D  R     Religion: _____ Anointed: _____ Smoker - Nonsmoker: _____

Ethnic Origins: _____ Languages Spoken: _____ Previous Hospitalization: _____

Occupation (or retired from) _____ Employed/Unemployed: _____ _____

Hobbies & Normal Activities: _____

Social Problems: _____

Discharge Plans: _____

Significant Others: _____

Persons to Notify in Case of Emergency:  (1) _____ Phone Number _____

(2) _____ Phone Number _____

Signature of Nurse _____

## Illustration 11.5   Nursing History Chart (continued)

| OBSERVATION & SUPERVISION | | AGE: 55    DATE OF ADMISSION | | |
|---|---|---|---|---|
| ☐ Isolation | ☐ Urine S & A | Family Physician: | | Erik Shultz |
| | | Diagnosis: | | 17 Bond Street |
| ☐ Vital Signs | ☐ Weight | | | Ottawa, Ontario    May 26, 19__ |
| B/P | Due: | Surgery: | | 7819749313 |
| TPR | ☐ Measurements: | | | |
| ☐ Pedal Pulses | ☐ Head Injury Routine | Surgeon: | | Other Health Problems: |
| R/L | | Consultant(s): | | |
| | ☐ Other Supervision | | | |
| ☐ CVP | | Allergy: | | Transfers: |
| Swan Ganz | | | | |
| Art Lines | | PC Level: | | Revised: |

| Hygiene | Comfort/Activity | Nutrition | Elimination | Respiration |
|---|---|---|---|---|
| Bath | Up ad Lib. | Diet: | Self Care | ☐ O$_2$ |
| ☐ Self | ☐ Up in Chair | | ☐ Bathroom with Help | LPM |
| ☐ Partial | ☐ Walking | | | ☐ Humidifier |
| ☐ Complete | Devices | ☐ Self | Urinal | |
| | | ☐ With Help | ☐ Bedpan | ☐ Cough & Deep Breath |
| ☐ Tub/Shower | Total Bedrest | ☐ Complete Feed | Commode | |
| | BRP | ☐ Fluids | ☐ Incontinence | ☐ Trach Care |
| S M T W T F S | ☐ Skin Care & Position | | Condom | ☐ Aerosol |
| | | ☐ Bottle Fdg/Baby Food | ☐ Diapers | |
| ☐ Oral Hygiene | | | ☐ Catheter | ☐ Suction |
| ☐ Beard Shave | ☐ Active/Passive Exercises | ☐ Gavage (eg. Barron's) | ☐ Change: | OTHER |
| | | | | ☐ Teach |
| ☐ Hair Wash | Restraints Siderails | | | ☐ Communication |
| S M T W T F S | ☐ Traction, Stockings | | ☐ Ostomy | |
| | Bandage, Prosthesis | ☐ Intake – Output | | |

**Illustration 11.5   Nursing History Chart (continued)**

| Date | MEDICATIONS ☐ | ERIK SHULTZ | 0700 | 1500 | 2300 | Renew | INTRAVENOUS ☐ THERAPY | I.V. TUBING ☐ CHANGE DATE: |
|------|---------------|-------------|------|------|------|-------|------------------------|----------------------------|
|      |               |             |      |      |      |       |                        |                            |

| | | | ☐ REMINDERS | | ☐ Diagnostic Workup |
|--|--|--|--|--|--|
| | | | | Date | |

| Date | PRN MEDICATIONS | Renew |
|------|-----------------|-------|
|      |                 |       |

| Other Disciplines | ☐ Treatments |
|-------------------|--------------|
|                   |              |

PATIENT'S NAME:                              ROOM:

## Illustration 11.6    Nursing Care Plan

| | NURSING CARE PLAN | | | |
|---|---|---|---|---|
| NAME:  ERIK SHULTZ | | | | |
| Date | PATIENT PROBLEMS | NURSING APPROACH | Date | Evaluation |
| | | | | |

**Illustration 11.7 History and Physical Examination Report**

## History & Physical Examination

Name_____ Age_____

Address_____

**HISTORY**

Chief Complaint:_____

Present Illness:_____

_____

_____

| Functional Enquiry: | Normal | Abnormal | Comments | ALLERGIES |
|---|---|---|---|---|
| Metabolic/Endocrine | | | | |
| Respiratory | | | | |
| Cardiovascular | | | | MEDICATIONS |
| Gastrointestinal | | | | |
| Neurological | | | | 1. |
| Genitourinary | | | | 2. |
| Development | | | | 3. |

Past History:_____ 4.

_____ IMMUNIZATIONS

_____ (   ) Up-to-date **or**

Family History:_____

_____ G.    P.    T.    A.    L.

Personal/Social History:_____

**PHYSICAL EXAM** Temp._____ B.P. _____/_____ Pulse:_____ Weight:_____ Height:_____

| | Normal | Abnormal | If Abnormal, specify*** |
|---|---|---|---|
| General | | | |
| Head & Neck | | | |
| Chest | | | |
| Cardiovascular | | | |
| Abdomen | | | |
| Genitourinary | | | |
| Back & Extremeties | | | |
| Skin & Breast | | | |
| Neurological | | | |

***Further Details:_____

_____

**DIAGNOSIS** 1._____ **TREATMENT** 1._____

2._____ **PLANS** 2._____

3._____ 3._____

Copy to: Dr._____ _____M.D. _____ _____
Signature                        date        time

3507 JF   Oct 89

**Illustration 11.8    Physician's Orders Form**

| DATE/TIME | ORDERS | | EXECUTED |
|---|---|---|---|

Erik Shultz
17 Bond Street
Ottawa, Ontario    May 26, 19___
7819749313

# PHYSICIAN'S ORDERS

START NEW SECTION FOR EACH NEW ORDER. MORE THAN ONE SECTION MAY BE USED FOR A LONG ORDER. DO NOT USE SECTION IF COPY IS MISSING.

ALLERGIES:

1

2

3

4

PHYSICIAN'S ORDERS                WRITE FIRMLY!

**Illustration 11.9    Consultation Report**

---

Page 1 of 2

| | |
|---|---|
| **PATIENT:**   Shultz, Erik | **TYPE OR REPORT:**   Consultation |
| **ADDRESS:**   17 Bond Street, Ottawa | **COPIES TO:**   Dr. Hart |
| | Dr. Plunkett |
| **D.O.B.:**   May 26, 19___ | |

**DATE OF ADMISSION:**   July 1, 19___

**DATE OF REPORT:**   July 1, 19___

**DATE OF DISCHARGE:**                    **CHART #:**   66686                    **ROOM #:**   ICU

---

Erik Shultz is a _____-year-old man, who is a resident of Ottawa. He presented to the Emergency Room on the morning of July 1, 1986 with chest discomfort, was assessed and admitted to the Intensive Care Unit by Dr. Plunkett. He requested a cardiology consultation to assist with the management of his probable myocardial infarction.

**Previous Surgery**
Cholecystectomy, Orthopaedic surgery to the foot, repair of incisional hernia.

**Pre-Admission Medications**
A.S.A. p.r.n.

**Medication Allergies**
None known

**Myocardial Infarction**
This man noted the onset of soreness in his central chest about ten minutes after arising this morning. It was associated with left arm discomfort, nausea and profuse sweating. He took food hoping that this would pass. This made no difference to the discomfort and shortly thereafter he vomited and noticed accelerating chest discomfort. He came to the Emergency Room by ambulance and was admitted to the Intensive Care Unit.

This man had a similar episode approximately three years ago and was hospitalized for several days only. He is unaware that his cardiac status was clarified at this point in time.

In retrospect, this man has had exertion-related central chest discomfort identical in character but less intensive than the current complaint over the past few days only.

Prior to admission today, this man has not had shortness of breath on exertion.

**Cardiac Risk Factors**
The patient is somewhat overweight, an ongoing cigarette smoker, but has no personal history of hypertension, diabetes, stroke or claudication. The family history is negative for coronary artery disease. The patient's cholesterol status is unknown to him.

**Systems Review**
There is no established upper gut pathology or symptoms to suggest that this has been overlooked previously.

**6514**
**APR ___**

**Illustration 11.9    Consultation Report (continued)**

Mr. Erik Shultz (Continued - Consultation Note)

### Physical Examination

The approximate systolic blood pressure present is 120-130. The rhythm is sinus with a heart rate of approximately 115-120. The jugular venous pressure appears to be normal, but is difficult to assess because of the patient's body habitus. The apical impulse is palpable. Cardiac auscultation identifies first and second heart sounds. I believe there is a 4th sound and I suspect that there is an intermittent 3rd sound, but this is uncertain. There is no abdominal tenderness. Examination of the periphery identifies full pulses.

### E.K.G.

Three electrocardiograms have been done here today. All of them are compatible with an acute anteroseptal myocardial infarction. The E.K.G. changes are widespread and extend across to lead 1 and AVL as well as through all the precordial areas.

Several runs of wide complex tachycardia have been documented with a fairly slow ventricular response rate.

### ASSESSMENT

This man has a risk factor profile compatible with the development of atherosclerosis. It is my understanding there has been no previous overt expression of coronary disease in his case. Today his electrocardiogram and clinical presentation are perfectly compatible with myocardial infarction. The E.K.G. suggests this might be extensive. Because of the patient's body habitus it is difficut to be sure that the infarct has not been complicated by failure and there is some indirect evidence that this may be the case (i.e. sinus tachycardia).

Further, the myocardial infarction has been complicated by ventricular irritablility refractory to Xylocaine.

I believe that the management of this case would be assisted greatly by the use of Swan-Ganz catheter to assess left ventricular filling pressures. This should clarify for us whether his tachycardia is secondary to congestive failure.

If he is indeed in failure with such an apparent widespread myocardial infarction, his prognosis remains guarded at this point in time. Antiarrhythmic drugs will be switched from Xylocaine to Procainamide because of the clear failure of Xylocaine to control his rhythm disturbances.

A.Hart, M.D., F.R.C.P.(C), Cardiologist

AH:11

D.-July 1/___
T.-July 1/___

**Illustration 11.10 Consultation Request/Report**

Erik Shultz
17 Bond Street
Ottawa, Ontario    May 26, 19___
7819749313

**CONSULTATION REQUEST/REPORT**

Patient's Name: _____ Erik Shultz _____

To Dr.: _____

From Dr.: _____ Date: _____

Reason for request: _____

_____

An order should also be written on
the Doctor's Order Sheet indicating the
consultant's care status:

_____

☐ consultation      ☐ consultation with concurrent care      ☐ total transfer of responsibility

REPORT:

Date: _____ Hour: _____ Signature: _____ M.D.

6505
Oct 84       GOLD – Patient's chart       WHITE – Consultant's copy

**Illustration 11.11    Consent for Surgical Operation, Treatment, Diagnostic Test, or Anaesthetic**

**PATIENT'S CONSENT**

1. I hereby authorize Dr. _____ , and/or such surgeons or assistants as may be selected by him or her, to perform the following procedure(s): _____

_____

_____

(STATE NATURE OF PROCEDURE(S) TO BE PERFORMED)

with the administration of such anaesthetics as he or she may deem advisable, on _____

NAME OF PATIENT OR "MYSELF"

2. I certify that the nature and purpose of this operation and/or treatment have been explained to me by Dr. _____ . I acknowledge that no guarantee has been made as to the results that may be obtained.

3. If, during the course of the procedure(s) noted above, the surgeon in charge should discover any condition not now realized, I authorize him or her to make any immediate surgical correction, as a logical extension of the original procedure(s).

4. Any tissues or parts surgically removed may be disposed of by the Hospital in accordance with its usual practice.

DATE: _____ , 19_____

TIME: _____ HOURS

I CERTIFY THAT I HAVE READ, OR HAD READ TO ME, AND FULLY UNDERSTAND THIS CONSENT; AND THAT ALL BLANKS WERE FILLED IN, AND ANY DELETIONS OR ALTERATIONS WERE MADE AND INITIALLED BEFORE I SIGNED.

_____
SIGNATURE OF WITNESS

_____
SIGNATURE OF PATIENT OR PERSON LEGALLY AUTHORIZED
TO CONSENT ON PATIENT'S BEHALF

_____
SIGNATURE OF WITNESS

_____
SIGNATURE OF PATIENT'S SPOUSE – WHERE REQUIRED
BY HOSPITAL BY-LAWS OR RULES

CONSENT SIGNATURE
VERIFIED BY: _____        DATE: _____

**SURGEON'S CERTIFICATION OF NECESSITY TO PROCEED**

I hereby certify that I believe delay caused by attempting to obtain consent and/or consultation, as ordinarily required by the laws of the Province or by-laws and rules of the Hospital, would endanger the life of the patient.

_____
DATE AND TIME

_____
SURGEON'S SIGNATURE

**Illustration 11.12   Anaesthetic Record**

# ANAESTHETIC RECORD
## PRE ANAESTHETIC EVALUATION

Page 1

Erik Shultz
17 Bond Street
Ottawa, Ontario   May 26, 19___
7819749313

| PRE MEDICATION |
| PROCEDURE |
| SIGNED CONSENT ☐ |

| HISTORY | PHYSICAL | LAB |
|---|---|---|
| — GENERAL | — GENERAL | — HGB        — URINE |
| — CVS | — CVS | — OTHER |
| — RESPIRATORY | — RESPIRATORY |  |
| — CNS | — AIRWAY ASSESSMENT | ECG |
| — RENAL/HEPATIC | — CNS | X-RAY |
| — ALLERGIES | — DENTITION |  |
| — ANAESTHETIC HX | — OTHER | MEDICATIONS |
| — FAMILY Hx | — WEIGHT |  |

| POTENTIAL PROBLEMS AND COMMENTS | BLOOD CXT |
|---|---|
|  | NPO from: |
|  | FLUIDS |
|  | SOLIDS |

| ASA CLASS | 1 | 2 | 3 | 4 | 5 | E |
|---|---|---|---|---|---|---|

_____   _____
EVALUATING PHYSICIAN           DATE

### IMMEDIATE POST-OP ANAESTHETIC EVALUATION

COMMENTS

POST-OPERATIVE CONDITION

_____
SIGNATURE OF ATTENDING ANAESTHETIST

3505
Medical Staff
Jan 85

**Illustration 11.12 Anaesthetic Record (continued)**

Page 2

| NAME: | SURGEON (PRINT) | ANAESTHETIC RECORD |
| | | DATE |
| PROCEDURE: | ANAESTHETIST (PRINT) | ANAESTHETIC TIME |

TIME

| O2 | L/MIN |
| N2O | L/MIN |
| FIO2 | |
| VOLATILE AGENTS | % |

**SYMBOLS**

BP ✕ (angled)

PULSE ●

START ANAES ▣

START OPER'N ⊙

END ANAES. ⊗

RESP ◯

220
200
180
160
140
120
100
90
80
70
60
50
40
30
20
10

CVP
TEMP
URINE

IV AGENTS AND FLUIDS

| IV GAUGE | | MONITORS | | | GENERAL ANAESTHESIA | | REGIONAL |
|---|---|---|---|---|---|---|---|
| SITE | | STETH | OES ☐ PRECORD ☐ | | TECHNIQUE | | TYPE |
| | | BP | CUFF ☐ ART LINE ☐ | | AIRWAY ☐ | MASK ☐ | |
| FLUIDS | | SITE | # | | TUBE & TYPE | SIZE | LOCATION |
| IN— | | PULSE ☐ | ECG ☐ | | ORAL ☐ | NASAL R☐ L☐ | |
| | | CVP ☐ | TEMP ☐ | | CUFF ☐ | PACK ☐ | AGENT |
| | | LOW PRESS ☐ | O2 ☐ | | POSITION CHECK ☐ | | |
| | | OTHER | | | SYSTEM | | DOSE |
| TOTAL | | | | | CO-AXIAL ☐ | T PIECE ☐ | |
| OUT—BLOOD—SUCTION | | PRE-ANAESTHETIC CHECK LIST ☐ | | | CIRCLE ☐ | | REMARKS |
| —SPONGES | | | | | OTHER | | |
| —DRAPES | | POSITION | | | VENTILATION | | |
| —TOTAL | | | | | SPONT ☐ | ASSIST ☐ | |
| —URINE | | PROTECTION: | EYES ☐ | | CONTROL ☐ | VENTILATOR ☐ | |
| —OTHER | | ELBOWS ☐ | OTHER ☐ | | VT | RATE | |

**Illustration 11.13   Physician's Operative Report**

PATIENT:   Shultz, Erik

OPERATIVE REPORT:

ADDRESS:   17 Bond Street, Ottawa

COPIES TO:

D.O.B.:   May 26, 19___

DATE OF OPERATION:                    CHART #:                    ROOM #:

SURGEON:                    ASSISTANT:                    ANAESTHETIST:

PRE-OPERATIVE DIAGNOSIS:

POST-OPERATIVE DIAGNOSIS:

OPERATION:

PROCEDURE CARRIED OUT
AND FINDINGS AT OPERATION:

**Illustration 11.14   Nurse's Operative Record**

NURSE'S OPERATIVE RECORD     ☐ SJH & HC  ☐ PCH

Erik Shultz
17 Bond Street
Ottawa, Ontario   May 26, 19____
7819749313

Date_____ Theatre_____ Room Ready_____

Patient Entry_____

Anaesthetic Start_____ Total_____

Anaesthetic Stop_____

Surgeon Start_____

Surgeon Stop_____ Total_____

Patient Left_____ Overall Total_____

Wound Classification: ☐ Clean  ☐ Contaminated  ☐ Clean/Contaminated  ☐ Dirty
☐ Session  ☐ Non-Session  ☐ Elective  ☐ Non-Elective

Operation: _____

Surgeon: Dr. _____ Assistants: Dr. _____ Dr. _____

Anaesthetist: Dr. _____ Anaesthetic: ☐ General ☐ Local ☐ Neuro ☐ Spinal ☐ Epidural
☐ Other ☐ Bear Hugger ☐ Fluid Warmer   S.N. _____

Circ. Nurse 1. _____ R.N.  2. _____ R.N.   ESU Pad Position

Scrub Nurse 1. _____  2. _____   ESU S/N _____   Skin Condition Post-Op _____

Relief Circ. Nurse 1. _____ R.N.  2. _____ R.N.   Relief Scrub Nurse 1. _____  2. _____

POSITION:   LITHOTOMY   SUPINE   PRONE   KIDNEY   JACKNIFE   REV. TREND   TREND   RT./LT. SIDE

| Counts | Nil | Correct | Incorrect | If incorrect see action taken below |
|---|---|---|---|---|
| Sponge | | | | |
| Instruments | | | | |
| Needle | | | | |

**PROTECTION DEVICES**

| | | | |
|---|---|---|---|
| Safety Strap | ☐ | Padding: Elbow | L ☐ R ☐ |
| Induction Only | ☐ | Hand/Wrist | L ☐ R ☐ |
| Wrist Ties | L ☐ R ☐ | Knee | L ☐ R ☐ |
| Skids: Wrist | L ☐ R ☐ | Heel | L ☐ R ☐ |
| Elbow | L ☐ R ☐ | Other | L ☐ R ☐ |
| Bolsters | ☐ | | ☐ |
| Donut | ☐ | Armboard | L ☐ R ☐ |
| Head rest | ☐ | Stirrups | L ☐ R ☐ |
| Kidney rest | ☐ | Sandbags | _____ |
| Other | ☐ | Pillows | _____ |

In _____ R.N.   In _____
Out _____ R.N.   Out _____
Circ. Nurse Signature(s)         Scrub Nurse Signature(s)

Pathology_____ Cytology_____ Culture_____

**TOURNIQUET TIME**     S.N. _____

| Location | Pressure | Up | Down | Location | Pressure | Up | Down |
|---|---|---|---|---|---|---|---|
| R. Arm | | | | R. Leg | | | |
| L. Arm | | | | L. Leg | | | |

**CODES**

| PRIORITY CODE | DELAY | COMPLICATION | CANCELLATION |
|---|---|---|---|
| | | | |

| Penrose | Catheter | Other | Packing | Hyster. Drain | Hemovac |
|---|---|---|---|---|---|
| | | | | | |

**REMARKS**



GRASP _____     _____ R.N.
Circulating Nurse Signature

PATIENT TO PACU_____   I.C.U._____   DISCHARGE PACU_____   FLOOR_____
Time                  Time                        Time

1566JF 11/93

**Illustration 11.15   Postanaesthetic Record**

Erik Shultz
17 Bond Street
Ottawa, Ontario   May 26, 19____
7819749313

**POST-ANAESTHETIC RECORD**

DATE: _____

| PROCEDURE: | POST-ANAESTHETIC RECORD SCORE | ADM. | 15 min. | 30 min. | D/C |
|---|---|---|---|---|---|
| | RESPIR-ATIONS:  BREATHING DEEPLY) <br> ADEQUATE COUGH  )  2 <br> AIRWAY REQ.ATTENT- 1 <br> APNEA - 0 | | | | |

PROCEDURE:

ADMISSION TIME: _____

**AIRWAY**     NIL     ORAL     NASAL     E.N.T.
AIRWAY REMOVED @
ANAESTHETIC _____
**OXYGEN**     NIL     MASK     CATHETER
T-PIECE       AEROSOL       RESPIRATOR

POSITION ON ARRIVAL _____
_____

DRAINS _____

PACKING _____

CATHETER _____

DRESSING DRAINAGE _____
NAUSEA AND/OR VOMITING

MONITOR _____

BLOOD WORK _____

& RESULTS _____

X-RAY _____
OUTPUT:
    URINE _____
    OTHER _____

POST-ANAESTHETIC RECORD SCORE

| | ADM. | 15 min. | 30 min. | D/C |
|---|---|---|---|---|
| RESPIR-ATIONS:  BREATHING DEEPLY)<br>ADEQUATE COUGH  )  2<br>AIRWAY REQ.ATTENT- 1<br>APNEA - 0 | | | | |
| MOVE-MENTS:  PURPOSEFUL - 2<br>SOME PURPOSEFUL - 1<br>ATHETOID - NONE - 0 | | | | |
| COLOUR:  NORMAL - 2<br>PALE, DUSKY - 1<br>CYANOTIC  - 0 | | | | |
| CONSCIOUS-NESS:  FULLY AWARE - 2<br>AROUSABLE ON CALL)<br>DROWSY       )  1<br>NOT RESPONDING - 0 | | | | |
| CIRCU-LATION:  B/P P- $\pm$ 10 of PRE-OP-2<br>B/P P- $\pm$ 20 of PRE-OP-1<br>B/P P- $\pm$ 30 of PRE-OP-0 | | | | |

PRE-OP
B/P _____  P. _____

CODE FOR D/C          POOR    6
GOOD 8-10          FAIR 6 - 8

COMMENTS:

I.V. THERAPY

| I.V. SOLUTION | ABS. IN OR | ABS. IN RR | TOTAL |
|---|---|---|---|
| 3.3% D.-0.3% SAL. | | | |
| 5% GL/.2% SAL. | | | |
| Ringers Lact. | | | |
| 5% D/Plas. 56 | | | |
| Normal saline | | | |
| | | | |
| | | | |

M  15  30  45     15  30  45     15  30  45     15  30  45
240
220
200
180
160
140
120
100
 80
 60
 40
 20
  0
Resp.
Temp.

MEDICATIONS

| TIME | DRUG | ROUTE | REASON GIVEN & EFFECT | SIGNATURE |
|---|---|---|---|---|
| | | | | |
| | | | | |
| | | | | |
| | | | | |

DISCHARGE TIME: _____     CONDITION     GOOD     FAIR     POOR

SIGNATURE _____ R.N.

Revised 6/86

Form #142

REPORT GIVEN TO _____ R.N.

**Illustration 11.15   Postanaesthetic Record (continued)**

| TIME | FEET TEMP. COLOUR | DSG. | C.V.P. | PEDAL R. | L. | POST TIB. R. | L. | HAND GRIPS R. | L. | MEASUREMENTS | | PUPIL R. | L. | URINE | BLOOD PARAMETERS | TIME | RESULT |
|---|---|---|---|---|---|---|---|---|---|---|---|---|---|---|---|---|---|
| | | | | | | | | | | | | | | | Hgb. | | |
| | | | | | | | | | | | | | | | Hct. | | |
| | | | | | | | | | | | | | | | Cl. | | |
| | | | | | | | | | | | | | | | Na. | | |
| | | | | | | | | | | | | | | | K. | | |
| | | | | | | | | | | | | | | | B.U.N. | | |
| | | | | | | | | | | | | | | | P.H. | | |
| | | | | | | | | | | | | | | | CO2con | | |
| | | | | | | | | | | | | | | | PCO2 | | |
| | | | | | | | | | | | | | | | H2CO3 | | |
| | | | | | | | | | | | | | | | HCO3 | | |
| | | | | | | | | | | | | | | | PO2 | | |
| | | | | | | | | | | | | | | | H-HRat | | |
| | | | | | | | | | | | | | | | B.Exc. | | |
| | | | | | | | | | | | | | | | % Sat. | | |

CODE   D. & I.  – Dry & Intact        R.B.  –  React Briskly
       C.O.     – Cold                R.S.  –  React Slowly
       C.       – Cool                F.    –  Fixed
       M.       – Mottled

NURSE'S COMMENTS

_____

_____

_____

_____

_____

_____

_____

_____

_____

_____

_____

_____

_____

_____

_____

**Illustration 11.16    Progress Notes**

Peterborough Hospitals

Peterborough Civic Hospital
St. Joseph's General Hospital
Haliburton Hospital
Minden Hospital

Name of Patient: _____

| DATE | DISCIPLINE | TIME | MULTI-DISCIPLINARY NOTES | SIGNATURE |
|------|-----------|------|--------------------------|-----------|
|      |           |      |                          |           |
|      |           |      |                          |           |
|      |           |      |                          |           |
|      |           |      |                          |           |
|      |           |      |                          |           |
|      |           |      |                          |           |
|      |           |      |                          |           |
|      |           |      |                          |           |
|      |           |      |                          |           |
|      |           |      |                          |           |
|      |           |      |                          |           |
|      |           |      |                          |           |
|      |           |      |                          |           |
|      |           |      |                          |           |
|      |           |      |                          |           |
|      |           |      |                          |           |
|      |           |      |                          |           |
|      |           |      |                          |           |
|      |           |      |                          |           |
|      |           |      |                          |           |
|      |           |      |                          |           |

Form # JF 3514 Revised Dec./91

## Completion of Requisitions in Hospitals

The medical administrative assistant has the responsibility of completing requisitions from written orders. Accuracy in recording this information is essential to ensure appropriate care for the patient. Medical administrative assistants are important members of the health care team because they generally have responsibility for transferring information from the record to requisitions. Disastrous complications can result from inefficiency and carelessness.

The following example demonstrates the appropriate requisitioning to carry out the doctor's orders for Erik Shultz. (Refer to Illustration 11.17 for this example.) Mr. Shultz has been admitted to the hospital by Dr. Plunkett after complaining of severe thirst, headaches, and dizziness. The admitting clerk has completed the admission form. The diagnosis is diabetes mellitus/obesity as indicated at the top of the order sheet. Let's analyze the others:

1. CBC and ESR mean a complete blood count and sedimentation rate are required. On the Haematology Form (Illustration 11.18), the boxes beside "Hemogram" and "E.S.R." would be checked. Hemogram and "CBC" are interchangeable.
2. Weight please: the patient's weight would be recorded by the nurse on the Nursing History Chart (Illustration 11.5).
3. Dietician to see: the dietician would be telephoned, and an appointment time arranged.
4. 1200 Cal. DD, NAS means a diabetic diet of 1200 calories with no added salt. The information would be recorded on the Nursing History Chart (Illustration 11.5) under nutrition diet.
5. Urine bid ac & hs for sugar: the ward nurse is required to check the patient's urine twice a day, before breakfast and at night, to determine if there is sugar in the urine. This would be done by using keto sticks, and recording the results of the tests on the Nursing History Chart under the section reminders. The box beside "urine S & A" would also be checked.
6. Daily FBS means that a fasting blood sugar test is to be done daily. The request for this test would be recorded on the Biochemistry Requisition (Illustration 11.19) by placing a check mark beside "glucose" and circling "(F)."
7. 2 hours ac lunch BS means a blood sugar to be done two hours before lunch, requiring another Biochemistry Requisition to be completed, but this time circling the "(R)" for routine under "glucose."
8. Tylenol No. 2 tabs 1 q8h prn gives permission to administer one Tylenol No. 2 tablet every 8 hours as needed.

The information for prescribed drugs is recorded on the Nursing History Chart. Regardless of the medication administration system used by the hospital, it is imperative that an accurate record of all medication orders be kept for each patient. Illustration 11.20 is an example of a Medical Administration Record Sheet. This particular example is used for *prn* (as needed) medication orders.

**Illustration 11.17   Physician's Orders Form**

<table>
<tr><td colspan="3">

Erik Shultz
17 Bond Street
Ottawa, Ontario      May 26, 19___
7819749313

*D.M. Obese*

</td><td colspan="2">

**PHYSICIAN'S ORDERS**

START NEW SECTION FOR EACH NEW ORDER. MORE THAN ONE SECTION MAY BE USED FOR A LONG ORDER. DO NOT USE SECTION IF COPY IS MISSING.

ALLERGIES:

</td></tr>
<tr><td>DATE/TIME</td><td colspan="2">ORDERS</td><td>1</td><td>EXECUTED</td></tr>
<tr><td></td><td colspan="2">1) CBC & ESR</td><td></td><td></td></tr>
<tr><td></td><td colspan="2">2) Weigh please</td><td></td><td></td></tr>
<tr><td></td><td colspan="2">3) Dietician to see</td><td></td><td></td></tr>
<tr><td></td><td colspan="2">4) 1200 cal. D.D. NAS</td><td></td><td></td></tr>
<tr><td></td><td colspan="2">5) Urine bid ac & hs for sugar</td><td>2</td><td></td></tr>
<tr><td></td><td colspan="2">6) Daily FBS</td><td></td><td></td></tr>
<tr><td></td><td colspan="2">7) 2 hour pc lunch BS</td><td></td><td></td></tr>
<tr><td></td><td colspan="2">8) Tylenol #2 tabs i q 8h prn.</td><td></td><td></td></tr>
<tr><td></td><td colspan="2">9) Halcion 0.25 mgs. hs. prn.</td><td></td><td></td></tr>
<tr><td></td><td colspan="2">10) BRP</td><td></td><td></td></tr>
<tr><td></td><td colspan="2">11) LES prn</td><td></td><td></td></tr>
<tr><td></td><td colspan="2">12) CXR</td><td></td><td></td></tr>
<tr><td></td><td colspan="2">13) ECG</td><td></td><td></td></tr>
<tr><td></td><td colspan="2">14) BUN</td><td></td><td></td></tr>
<tr><td></td><td colspan="2">15) Lytes</td><td></td><td></td></tr>
<tr><td></td><td colspan="2">16) Proteins</td><td>3</td><td></td></tr>
<tr><td colspan="3">PHYSICIAN'S ORDERS</td><td colspan="2">WRITE FIRMLY!</td></tr>
</table>

**Illustration 11.18   Haematology Form**

# HAEMATOLOGY

184969

### CODE DEFINITIONS FOR RESULTS

| | | |
|---|---|---|
| + + + + + = | Results over printable range | L = Result is lower than lab action limit |
| − − − − − = | Results voted out | H = Result is higher than lab action limit |
| . . . . . = | Incomplete computation occurred | + = Result exceeds linearity |
| R = | Review results | X = Abnormal condition |
| * = | Abnormal condition caused other | S = Suspect |
| | parameters to flag | |

AFFIX
BAR CODE LABEL
HERE

CASS. NO.

TIME            INITIALS

I.D.

| SA | OP. CODES | NORMAL VALUES |
|---|---|---|
| | | Lkcs M 4.0-11.0 x 10⁹/L F 4.0-11.0 x 10⁹/L |
| | • | Ercs M 4.5-6.0 x 10¹²/L F 4.0-5.5 x 10¹²/L |
| | | Hb M 130-175 g/L F 120-155 g/L |
| | • | Hct M 0.40-0.54 F 0.37-0.47 |
| | • | MCV M 80-100 fL F 80-100 fL |
| | • | MCH M 27.0-32.0 pg F 27.0-32.0 pg |
| | • | MCHC M 320-360 g/L F 320-360 g/L |
| | • | RDW M 11.5-14.5 % F 11.5-14.5 % |
| | • | Plts M 150-450 x 10⁹/L F 150-450 x 10⁹/L |
| | | ESR M 0-10 mm/h F 0-20 mm/h |
| | | RETICS M 20-100 x 10⁹/L F 20-100 x 10⁹/L |
| | • | MPV M 8.9 ± 1.5 F 8.9 ± 1.5 |
| • | | LYMPHS M 0.20-0.45 F 0.20-0.45 |
| • | | MONO M 0.02-0.10 F 0.02-0.10 |
| • | | NEUT M 0.40-0.75 F 0.40-0.75 |
| • | | EOS M 0.01-0.06 F 0.01-0.06 |
| • | | BASOS M <0.02 F <0.02 |
| | • | LYMPH # M 1.5-3.5 x 10⁹/L F 1.5-3.5 x 10⁹/L |
| | • | MONO # M 0.2-0.8 x 10⁹/L F 0.2-0.8 x 10⁹/L |
| | • | NEUT # M 2.0-7.5 x 10⁹/L F 2.0-7.5 x 10⁹/L |
| | • | EOS # M 0.04-0.4 x 10⁹/L F 0.04-0.4 x 10⁹/L |
| | • | BASOS # M <0.1 x 10⁹/L F <0.1 x 10⁹/L |

### CHECK TEST REQUIRED

HEMOGRAM ✓
(INCLUDES Lkcs, (WBC),
Ercs (RBC) Hgb, Hct,
MCV, MCH, MCHC, RDW, MPV
Platelets)

DIFFERENTIAL ☐

CELL MORPHOLOGY ☐

E. S. R. ✓

RETICULOCYTES ☐

MORPH. REPORT

| W B C | | | | | |
|---|---|---|---|---|---|
| W | LYMPHO-PENIA | | | LYMPHO-CYTOSIS | |
| | NEUTRO-PENIA | | | NEUTRO-PHILIA | |
| B | ATYP LYMPHS | | | MONO-CYTOSIS | |
| C | BLASTS | | | EOSINO-PHILIA | |
| | IMMGRAN BANDS | | | BASO-PHILIA | |
| | NRBC | | | ANISO | |
| R | POIK | | | MICRO | |
| B | RBC FRAG | | | MACRO | |
| C | RBC AGG | | | HYPO | |
| P | PLT CLUMPS | | | LARGE PLTS | |
| L T | GIANT PLTS | | | SMALL PLTS | |

DATE/TIME REPORTED

TIME SPECIMEN RECEIVED

O.R.     DATE        TIME

RESULTS PHONED

BY:              TIME:

TO:

SPECIMEN TO BE TAKEN

M   D   YR.   TIME   INITIALS

ROUTINE   MEDICAL EMERGENCY

SPECIMEN COLLECTED     TIME:

BY:

CLINICAL INFORMATION

PATIENT'S LAST NAME (PRINT)

PATIENT'S FIRST NAME

ADDRESS

DOCTOR

**PETERBOROUGH HOSPITALS**
0505056 JF REV. 3/95          PCH ☐     SJH&HC ☐

**Illustration 11.19   Biochemistry Requisition**

## BIOCHEMISTRY REQUISITION

Name: Erik Schultz
Address: 17 Bond St.
City: Ottawa, Ontario
DOB: May 26, 19__
Diagnosis: Diabetes Mellitus
Room No.: 14
Hospital No.: 67572
Dr. Plunkett

S.I. UNITS

ROUTINE ☐
STAT ☐
PRE-OP ☐

(MARK IN RED)

DATE TO BE COLLECTED _____
TIME COLLECTED _____ BY: _____
ORDERING PHYSICIAN: _____
NURSE: _____

O.R. DATE:          O.R. TIME:

LAB NO.

CHECK DETERMINATION REQUIRED ✔

DATE/TIME SPECIMEN RECEIVED

DATE/TIME REPORT RELEASED

St. Joseph's Hospital & Health Centre
DEPARTMENT OF LABORATORY MEDICINE
PETERBOROUGH

| | | | | | |
|---|---|---|---|---|---|
| ✔ Glucose Ⓕ (R) | AST | Triglyceride | Ethyl Alcohol | B12 |
| Glucose (2h p.c.) | LD | Cholesterol (Total) | Barbiturates | Folate |
| ✔ Urea | CK | Osmolality | Salicylates | TSH |
| Creatinine | CK - 2 (MB) | | Acetaminophen | |
| Calcium | Alk. Phosphatase | | Theophylline | |
| Phosphate | Gamma Glutamyl Transpeptidase | | Phenytoin | Cholinesterase |
| | Acid Phosphatase-T | | Carbamazepine | |
| Bilirubin Total | Acid Phosphatase-P | | Phenobarbitol | Magnesium |
| Direct | Amylase | Iron | Digoxin | Ferritin |
| Urate | ✔ Sodium | TIBC | | |
| Total Protein | ✔ Potassium | Saturation | | Cortisol AM |
| Albumin | ✔ Chloride | | | Cortisol PM |

TESTS:          PHONED TO:          TIME:          BY:

Form FO 155 Reviewed March/95

9. Halcion 0.25 mg hs prn gives permission to administer 0.25 mg of Halcion at night as needed (see Illustration 11.20).

10. BRP means that the patient is allowed bathroom privileges and would be so recorded on the Nursing History Chart beside "BRP."

11. LES prn gives permission to administer, when necessary, a laxative, enema, or suppository (see Illustration 11.20). Laxatives and suppositories are treated as prn medications. The enema order would be recorded on the Nursing History Chart (Illustration 11.5) under treatments.

12. CXR is a request for a routine chest X-ray. This would include a P.A. (posterior/anterior) and lateral view. The information would be recorded on the Diagnostic Imaging Requisition (Illustration 11.21).

13. ECG means that an electrocardiogram is to be taken and the appropriate requisition (Illustration 11.22) would be completed.

14. BUN stands for blood, urea, and nitrogen, and a check mark would be placed beside "urea" on the Biochemistry Requisition (Illustration 11.19) to order the test.

### Illustration 11.20 Medication Administration Record Sheet

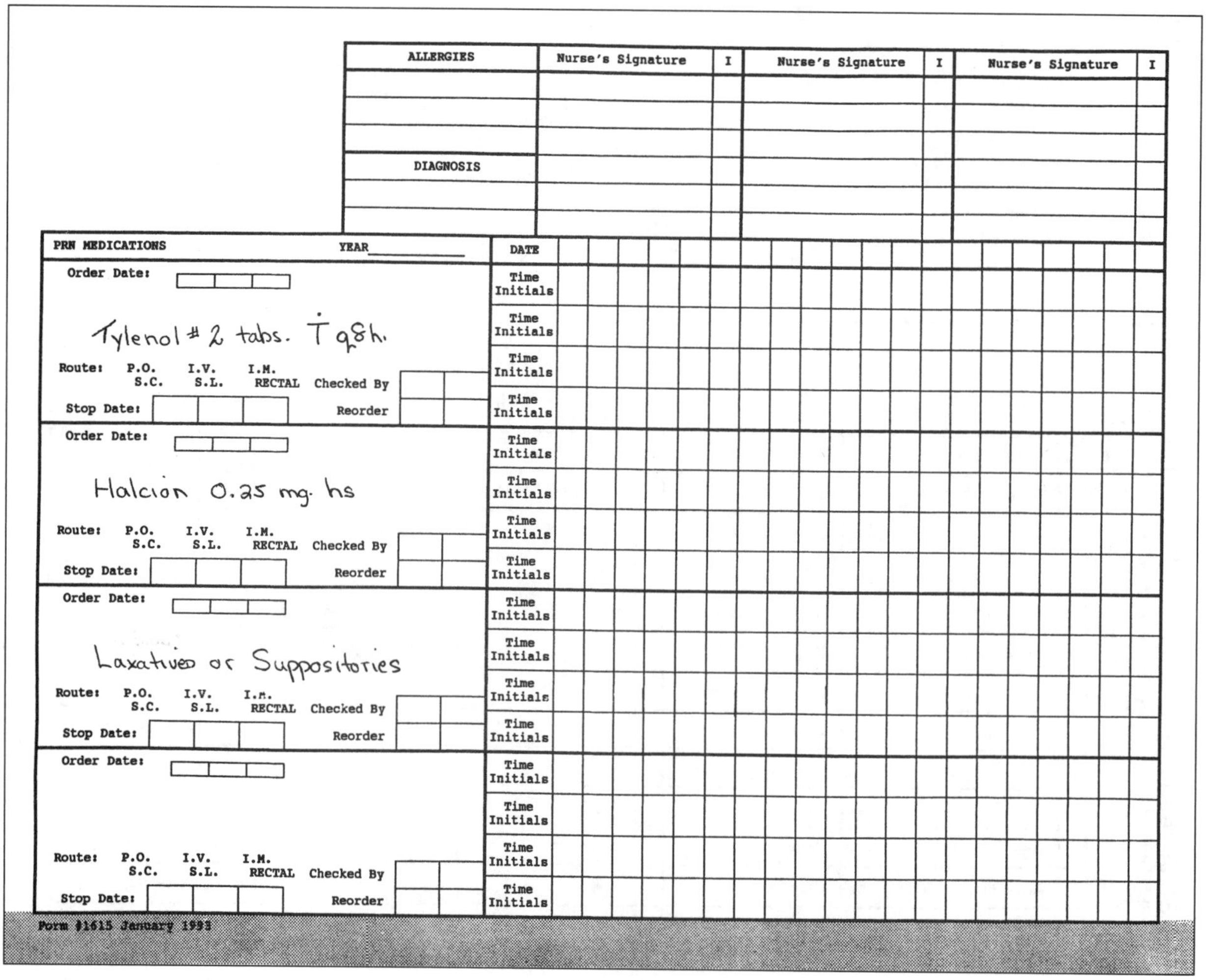

ALLERGIES | Nurse's Signature | I | Nurse's Signature | I | Nurse's Signature | I

DIAGNOSIS

PRN MEDICATIONS YEAR______ DATE

Order Date:

Tylenol # 2 tabs. i q8h.

Route: P.O. I.V. I.M. S.C. S.L. RECTAL Checked By

Stop Date: Reorder

Order Date:

Halcion 0.25 mg. hs

Route: P.O. I.V. I.M. S.C. S.L. RECTAL Checked By

Stop Date: Reorder

Order Date:

Laxatives or Suppositories

Route: P.O. I.V. I.M. S.C. S.L. RECTAL Checked By

Stop Date: Reorder

Order Date:

Route: P.O. I.V. I.M. S.C. S.L. RECTAL Checked By

Stop Date: Reorder

Time Initials

Form #1615 January 1993

15. Lytes means a testing of sodium, potassium, and chloride is requested. This test would also be ordered on the Biochemistry Requisition by placing a check mark beside "sodium, potassium, and chloride."
16. Proteins are checked through urinalysis, and the order would be processed by completing a Urinalysis Requisition (Illustration 11.23) and placing a check mark beside "protein."

**Illustration 11.21   Diagnostic Imaging Requisition**

Peterborough Hospitals

## *Diagnostic Imaging Requisition*

*Patient Data (print or place imprint upper left corner)*

Last Name _____

First Name _____

Address _____

City _____   Code _____

Phone _____   DOB [ ] [ ] [ ]
                              d    m    y

HC no.  [ ][ ][ ][ ]  [ ][ ][ ][ ]  [ ][ ][ ][ ]

WCB/Adm. no. _____

⇑ Place patient imprint in the above space only ⇑

### Transportation (circle)

P            portable
ambulatory
(wheelchair)
stretcher
isolation
ambulance

Radiography ☑        Ultrasound ☐        Nuclear Medicine ☐

Examination(s) Requested:

*CHEST (P.A. & LAT.)*

History

*Physician Data (print or imprint below)*

Name

Phone

Billing no.

Copies to:

Diabetes               yes ☐      no ☐

Kidney Disease         ☐          ☐

Previous IV contrast?   yes ☐     no ☐

Adverse Reaction?       ☐         ☐

If yes, describe

_____        _____
Date ordered            Physician's Signature

↖ All of the above must be completed in full and signed by the physician

### To the Out Patient

Appointment location: _____

time: _____   ☞ *You must bring this requisition with you!*

date: _____

If you think you might be pregnant, please inform the technologist
Please see over for instructions.  Your doctor will check the appropriate box.

Peterborough Civic Hospital

☎ 876-5039

Saint Joseph's Hospital
& Health Centre

☎ 740-8084

Form JF2209 Rev 2/95 Peterborough Civic Hospital (clipart by Corel)

**Illustration 11.22    Electrocardiogram Requisition**

```
                          ELECTROCARDIOGRAM REQUISITION

                          HOSP.NO. _67572_____  ROOM __14__
                          NAME _Erik Shultz_____
                          ADDRESS _17 Bond St._____
                          CITY _Ottawa_____
                          PHYSICIAN _Plunkett_____
                          D.O.B.Day_26_ Month__05__ Yr _19—_
                          HEALTH                     VERSION
                          CARE # _7819749313_____  #_____

  ↑↑ ADDRESSOGRAPH SPACE ↑↑   REQUISITION COPIED FOR BUSINESS OFFICE
                                    YES ☐        NO ☐
  _____
  DATE REQUESTED__Feb. 14,19—_____  MEDICATION:(HEART,FLUID,BLOOD PRESSURE)
  NURSE_____ ___       Please specify below
  DATE TO BE DONE__A.S.A.P._____  _____
  O.R. DATE_____  O.R. TIME_____  _____
  PATIENT: HEIGHT_6'_ WEIGHT___90 kg___  _____
  ADDITIONAL INFORMATION_____  _____
  _____
  PROCEDURE PERFORMED                        FORM # 2230
  DATE_____  TIME_____ SIGNATURE_____  REV. NOV/90
```

## Assignment 11.1a

Your instructor will provide you with a Physician's Orders Form for Erik Shultz. Mr. Shultz was admitted to the hospital last July 1. Requisitions were completed on July 2, 19__, hospital no. 56762, Room 2. You were the medical ward administrative assistant responsible for transferring the doctor's orders onto the appropriate requisitions. You will find the necessary forms in the Working Papers (pp. 70–74). After completing the requisitions, transcribe the orders on a sheet of plain white paper (for example, FBS would be fasting blood sugar; tid, three times in a day, and so on). Insert the completed assignment in your portfolio.

For the Assignments 11.1b and 11.1c (pp. 180–81), use plain paper or write directly on the form and translate the physician's orders; indicate the appropriate requisition that would be used to document the order. Some orders have not been covered in the text. These assignments are intended to assess your ability to determine what requisitions would be needed to initiate the necessary action. Use Appendix B as a reference source.

**Illustration 11.23    Urinalysis Requisition**

# URINALYSIS

ADDRESSOGRAPH

| DATE AND TIME RECEIVED IN LABORATORY | DATE AND TIME REPORT RELEASED | | |
|---|---|---|---|

☐ ROUTINE
☐ URGENT
☐ PRE-OP

O.R. DATE:
O.R. TIME:

| REFERENCE RANGE | | |
|---|---|---|
| | NEG. | GLUCOSE |
| | NEG. | BILIRUBIN |
| | NEG. | KETONES |
| | 1.010-1.030 | SPEC. GRAVITY |
| | NEG. | BLOOD |
| | 5 - 8 | pH |
| | ≤ 0.15 | PROTEIN |
| | ≤ 16 | UROBILINOGEN |
| | NEG. | NITRITE |
| | ≤ 15 | LEUKOCYTES |

☐ ROUTINE

**APPEARANCE**
☐ CLEAR
☐ CLOUDY
☐ TURBID

**COLOUR**
☐ STRAW/PALE
☐ YELLOW
☐ AMBER
☐ ATYPICAL

☐ MICROSCOPIC

☐ DIPSTICK SCREEN INDICATES MICROSCOPIC NOT WARRANTED

| | |
|---|---|
| LEUKOCYTES/hpf | |
| ERYTHROCYTES/hpf | |
| EPITHELIAL CELLS/hpf | |
| CASTS/hpf | |

COMMENTS:

| | |
|---|---|
| MUCOUS THREADS/hpf | |
| CRYSTALS/hpf | |
| AMORPH. PHOSPHATES | |
| AMORPH. URATES | |
| PHOSPHATE | |
| URATE | |
| OXALATE | |
| OTHER | |
| BACTERIA/hpf | |
| YEAST/hpf | |

**OTHER TESTS**

| | TEST | RESULT | REFERENCE RANGE |
|---|---|---|---|
| ☐ | PREGNANCY TEST | | Neg. |
| ☐ | OCCULT BLOOD | | Neg. |

| | | REF. RANGE |
|---|---|---|
| ☐ RANDOM URINE | | |
| ☐ 24 HOUR URINE | | |
| ☐ CREATININE mmol/d | | F  7-16  M  9-18 |
| ☐ CREAT. CLEARANCE mL/s | | 1.25-2.10 |
| ☑ PROTEIN (Quant.) g/d | | ≤ .15 |
| ☐ SODIUM mmol/d | | 25-285 |
| ☐ POTASSIUM mmol/d | | 25-125 |
| ☐ AMYLASE U/d | | 60-400 |
| ☐ PHOSPHATE mmol/d | | 13-42 |
| ☐ URATE mmol/d | | 1.5-4.5 |
| ☐ CALCIUM mmol/d | | 1.25-6.20 |
| ☐ OSMOLALITY mmol/kg. | | 50-1200 |

LAB USE    SPECIMEN VOLUME _____ mL

HT. _____ cm
WT. _____ kg    } FOR CREAT. CLEARANCE

LAB USE    S.A.

**PLEASE CHECK**
☑ IN PATIENT    ☐ OUT PATIENT    ☐ REFERRED IN
☐ HAL.    ☐ MIN.    OTHER

DATE / TIME COLLECTED

ORDERING PHYSICIAN:

NURSE:

DATE:                    PHONE:

TECH:                    BY:

**URINALYSIS**                    FORM 2214  REV. 5/94

**St. Joseph's Hospital & Health Centre**
PETERBOROUGH  •  HALIBURTON  •  MINDEN    **HEALTH RECORDS**

## Assignment 11.1b

**PHYSICIAN'S ORDERS**

START NEW SECTION FOR EACH NEW ORDER. MORE THAN ONE SECTION MAY BE USED FOR A LONG ORDER. DO NOT USE SECTION IF COPY IS MISSING.

EXPECTED DATE OF DISCHARGE

ALLERGIES: nil

| DATE/TIME | ORDERS | 1 | EXECUTED |
|---|---|---|---|
| | DAT | | |
| | AAT | | |
| | Must sign on + off floor | | |
| | Prozac 20 mg PO q prn | 2 | |
| | Psych consult | | |
| | Social work consult | | |
| | Tylenol E.S. ī-īī PO q4h prn. | | |

SEND TO PHARMACY

ADDRESSOGRAPH BACK - SEND TO PHARMACY

ADDRESSOGRAPH BACK - SEND TO PHARMACY

ADDRESSOGRAPH BACK - SEND TO PHARMACY

0505014 JF    **PHYSICIAN'S ORDERS**    **WRITE FIRMLY!**

## Assignment 11.1c

**PHYSICIAN'S ORDERS**

START NEW SECTION FOR EACH NEW ORDER. MORE THAN ONE SECTION MAY BE USED FOR A LONG ORDER. DO NOT USE SECTION IF COPY IS MISSING.

EXPECTED DATE OF DISCHARGE

ALLERGIES:

| DATE/TIME | ORDERS | 1 | EXECUTED |
|---|---|---|---|
| | Dx - acute (L) sciatica | | |
| | | | |
| | DAT | | |
| | bedrest c̄ BRP | | |
| | Vitals - routine | 2 | |
| | CT scan - Lumbar spine | | |
| | CBC, lytes, BUN, creatinine, B.S. | | |
| | Demerol 50 mg. ī q 4-6 h. prn | | |
| | Tyl. pl ī - īī q4h prn | | |
| | Sirax 15 mg qhs prn | | |

SEND TO PHARMACY   ADDRESSOGRAPH BACK - SEND TO PHARMACY   ADDRESSOGRAPH BACK - SEND TO PHARMACY   ADDRESSOGRAPH BACK - SEND TO PHARMACY

0505014 JF   **PHYSICIAN'S ORDERS**                    **WRITE FIRMLY!**

## Processing Hospital Records upon Discharge of Patient

Upon discharge of the patient, the complete chart is collected by the staff of health records and assembled into two sections: medical and nursing. The medical section is analyzed by health record technicians for missing information and signatures. Hospitals have bylaws, rules and regulations, accreditation standards, and legislation that govern the content as well as the completion of records. If physicians do not comply with the regulations, various penalties may result, including loss of admitting privileges and a request to appear before the Medical Advisory Committee (Administrative Committee of Medical Staff); sometimes a report on the infraction may be sent to the College of Physicians and Surgeons.

Upon completion of the chart by the physicians involved, the health records staff assigns diagnosis and procedure codes as recorded under the Admission/Discharge Record "code number" (Illustration 11.1). These are coded from the International Classification of Diagnoses and Procedures.

The chart is then filed according to a recognized filing system. The system generally used in health record departments is called *unit numbering*. In this method, the patient receives a number on the first admission to the hospital and keeps that number for all subsequent admissions. For instance, if John Smith comes in today and the next unused number is 35769, that number is assigned to him, and that number is used on each readmission.

The key to the filing system used is the central patient index. In a manual system, which is becoming obsolete, cards are filed alphabetically in a master filing cabinet, usually on 8 cm × 13 cm (3 inch × 5 inch) cards. On the patient's first admission, a card is started with the basic identifying information such as name, address, and date of birth; a number is then assigned from a number control book. These cards are updated with each admission. See Illustration 11.24 for an example of these cards.

Many hospitals have established a computerized central patient index so that in the case of a readmission, the patient's information can be readily accessed on the terminal and can easily be updated if necessary. In the case of a first admission, the data will be collected in the admitting department and

### Illustration 11.24    Unit Numbering Systems

| Sample B – Unit | | |
|---|---|---|
| Smith, George (Wife – Mary)<br>Anytown, Ontario | | NO. 66666<br>AGE 29/3/48 |
| **ADMITTED** | **DISCHARGED** | **PHYSICIAN** |
| June 3/73 | June 14/73 | Dr. Jones |
| July 8/79 | July 30/79 | Dr. Jones |
| Sept. 3/85 | Sept. 10/85 | Dr. Harrison |
| June 11/93 | June 15/96 | Dr. Harrison |

transmitted to health records for their use. This is a very beneficial system that provides close linkage between admitting and health records.

In the future, computerized records will be used throughout the hospital. These systems eliminate many manual steps; time is saved, communication between departments is improved, patient test results are returned faster, patient information is easier for the health care professionals to access, and statistical information is readily available.

When a local area network computer system is in place linking admitting, the nursing unit, and the laboratory, test requisitions can be sent electronically through the network to the laboratory. When tests are completed, the laboratory sends the test results back through the network to the nursing unit and they are printed at the unit. This is called order entry.

The position in the health records department that would most likely be of interest to the graduate medical administrative assistant would be that of medical transcriptionist. The medical transcriptionist transcribes all medical reports dictated by the physicians. Illustration 11.9, the Consultation Report, is a sample of one type of report.

Each patient file is kept for many years in the health records department. The length of time is governed by provincial legislation. Records may be kept in the original file order or placed on microfilm for compact storage. At present, most hospitals do not use computer storage for complete patient charts, although some hospitals are moving toward optical disk storage. The volumes of information produced in a hospital often necessitate off-site storage. This costly process has made optical disk storage much more attractive. If a patient is readmitted to the hospital, records are readily available for the attending physician's perusal.

## Processing Patient Records

Each hospital has formats for completion of its patient reports. These are either on a preprinted form or stored as a macro in a computer. The personal information, patient's hospital number, doctor(s) involved, dates, and so on are recorded in the appropriate spaces — usually at the beginning of the report. The originator of the report, the transcriptionist's initials, copy notations, and date of processing are included at the end of the report. The letters D and T appear as the last item on many reports, with D being date dictated and T date transcribed. All hospital reports require more than one copy, and the copy notations appear single-spaced below the transcriptionist's initials.

The above instructions are general. There is no best method, and each hospital has its own style preferences. Once the general format is understood, the administrative assistant will be able to adapt to the hospital's style.

When an individual first engages a physician (as a family doctor, a specialist for a specific problem, or in an emergency ward in a hospital), the physician must investigate such things as the reason for the visit (chief complaint).

## History and Physical Report

History of the present illness, past illnesses, family's health, and the patient's lifestyle must be reported because they may play a part in diagnosing the illness. The physician will then proceed with a physical examination, and subsequently prepare a report on his or her findings. The report is called a History and Physical Report (Illustrations 11.25 to 11.28).

The information contained in a History and Physical Report is generally documented in a specific order as follows:

**Sociological Information** — The patient's name, address, date of birth, and so on are recorded. If the patient is seen in the hospital, information such as date of admission, hospital records number, and room number is required.

**Chief Complaint** — This refers to the reason the patient has engaged the physician.

**Present Illness** — The patient is asked to give a detailed outline of the chief complaint, for example, when the discomfort first began and the severity of the discomfort. If the patient has been referred by another physician, the patient may be asked for details of previous tests and treatments. (The Present Illness section is sometimes referred to as History of Present Illness or History of Chief Complaint.)

**Past History** — The patient is asked about such things as previous surgery, illnesses, and diseases. This section may be broken into specific areas with appropriate subheadings such as Surgeries and Diseases.

**Family History** — The section comprises documentation of the medical history of the patient's parents, brothers and sisters, grandparents, and so on. Other details such as age and cause of death of any of the above may be significant.

**Personal History** — This includes such things as hobbies, alcohol or drug use or abuse, use of tobacco, socioeconomic and marital status, and type of employment. (This section may be included with Past History and entitled Past and Personal History.)

After the above details are recorded, the physician will undertake the physical examination. This section of the report may be entitled Physical Examination, or it may be referred to as a Systemic Review, Functional Inquiry, or Inventory of Systems.

The examination usually begins with the head area, and contains the following subheadings:

**Skin** — An examination of the appearance of the skin including rashes, discolouration, and so on.

**Hair** — Including thickness and texture.

**HEENT** — Pertains to the head, eyes, ears, nose, and throat and includes such things as use of glasses, blurred vision, loss of hearing, dizziness, pain, discharges, ability to smell, colds, condition of teeth, taste, dentures, gums, swallowing, neck movement, and so on.

**Cardiorespiratory (CR)** — Refers to the patient's heart and respiratory system.

**Gastrointestinal (GI)** — This is an examination of the digestive system and may include questions about appetite, indigestion, change in weight, and diet or bowel habits.

**Genitourinary (GU)** — Refers to the urinary organs and genitals and may include urgency, frequency, venereal disease, incontinence, hesitancy, and pain.

**Neuropsychiatric (NP)** — Refers to headaches, pains, paralysis, emotional state, convulsions, and so on.

**Musculoskeletal (MS)** — Discusses such things as pain, stiffness, movement ability, and fractures.

The physician does not necessarily cover all of the above details. If the patient's history or any other aspect of the examination has been covered previously, the report will state, for example, "Past Illness: as outlined on previous charts." A physician's personal preference of terms will also determine the subheading titles; for example, "Gastrointestinal" may be broken down into "Abdominal" and "Rectal."

If the examination of a system does not reveal any problems, the physician may record "unremarkable" or "nothing of note" beside the subheading. If an examination of a system is not performed, the record may state "deferred" or "not done."

Usually, the report will conclude with a diagnosis of the complaint. The subheading may be "Impression," "Admission Diagnosis," "Clinical Impression," or perhaps "Analysis and Plan."

There are four styles used for preparing History and Physical Reports:

1. Block style (Illustration 11.25)
2. Modified block style (Illustration 11.26)
3. Indented style (Illustration 11.27)
4. Word processing style (Illustration 11.28)

Make particular note of the capitalization, use of underscore, and varied spacing with each different style.

**Illustration 11.25    History and Physical Report — Block Style**

---

**NAME:**    Jackson, Amelia

**DOB:** _____   **SEX:** F

**ADDRESS:** _____

**DOCTOR:** B. Good

**ADMISSION DATE:** 31 08 ___

**PATIENT NO:** 57069

---

CHIEF COMPLAINT:
Shortness of breath.

HISTORY OF PRESENT ILLNESS:
This _____-year-old lady has a long history of chronic asthmatic bronchitis and emphysema. She has only been home from hospital for a couple of weeks, after a hospitalization for a month or so because of her chronic chest disease. She was reasonably well in hospital at the time of discharge and was able to walk about halls without undue dyspnea and was fine at rest.

She has been taking ventolin by aerosol and theo-dur orally 300 mg q.i.d. A theophylline level received the day prior to admission was 30 mg percent and therefore her dose will be decreased. She has been taking prednisone 15 mg and prednisone 5 mg on alternate days and was heading towards 15 mg every second day.

FUNCTIONAL INQUIRY, PAST ILLNESSES:
As outlined by her previous charts.

PHYSICAL EXAMINATIONS:
The patient was in moderate respiratory distress at rest on admission. She did have a dry cough, which increased her distress considerably.

Head and neck: She has had a fenestration operation on her ear and has had cataract surgery. Pharynx was normal with no inflammation and was somewhat dry. Neck showed no enlarged nodes and the thyroid was not enlarged.

Chest: She was using her accessory muscles of respiration. The AP diameter of her chest was increased. There was a slight audible wheeze. Her respirations were 30 per minute. They were faint expiratory wheezes. Her air entry was not good. There was prolongation of the expiratory phase of respiration. There were no inspiratory rales or rhonchi. Her chest was hyperresonant.

Abdomen: No abdominal masses, no tenderness.

Musculoskeletal system and C.N.S.: Grossly normal.

Rectal and pelvic exams: Not done.

IMPRESSION:
Chronic obstructive lung disease with asthmatic component. There is a mild bronchitis at the present time which does not seem to be bacterial. It may be as much due to irritation of a post-nasal drip as actual infections.

B.M. Good, M.D.

/lbp
copies: Dr. J.E. Plunkett
           Dr. E.J. Pelham

D:
T:

**Illustration 11.26   History and Physical Report — Modified Block Style**

| | |
|---|---|
| **NAME:** Green, Elizabeth | **DOB:** _____  **SEX:** F |
| **ADDRESS:** _____ | **HOSPITAL NO.** 202030 |
| **ADMISSION DATE:** _____ | **DOCTOR:** J.B. Lazary |

PHYSICAL EXAMINATION

Reveals a pale looking _____-year-old lady who on occasion demonstrates a flapping of her arms with excitement. She holds her eyes tightly closed, but responds to questions and to commands.

HEAD AND NECK: Reveals ear, nose, and throat to be normal. Her pupils are equal and react to light and accommodation. External ocular muscle movements are normal. Her fundi were difficult to assess.

CHEST: Clear. Heart sounds are normal. Blood pressure 150/80.

ABDOMEN: Unremarkable.

NEUROLOGICAL: Reveals her deep tendon reflexes to be 2-3+ and symmetrical. Plantars were upgoing with fanning of toes. She demonstrated marked neck stiffness, although she was able to, on the second occasion, bend her chin and touch her chest. Straight leg raising, however, is normal. She is able to move all her limbs voluntarily. Sensation is grossly normal.

ADMISSION
DIAGNOSIS: Possible C.V.A.
Possible subarachnoid hemorrhage.
Possible migraine headache with hysterical reaction.

She will be seen by Dr. Moore and assessed.

J.B. Lazary, M.D.

/cfb

copies to: Dr. R.M. Moore
　　　　　Dr. J.E. Plunkett
　　　　　Dr. E.J. Pelham

D:
T:

**Illustration 11.27   History and Physical Report — Indented Style**

---

NAME: ___Thompson, Mel_____   DOB: _____ SEX: _M_____

ADDRESS: _____   HOSPITAL NO. _346790_____

ADMISSION DATE: _____   DOCTOR: _T. Kerr_____

---

### HISTORY

CHIEF COMPLAINT:   This elderly gentleman has noticed increasing shortness of breath for the past 48 hours. This has not been associated with any chest pain. He has also been quite upset and nervous during this period as his wife has been ill and was admitted to hospital apparently yesterday.

PAST HISTORY:   Is well outlined in his previous admissions, as is his family history.

CARDIOVASCULAR SYSTEM:   He has had no chest pain. He has had no peripheral or sacral edema.

G.I.:   He has had no nausea or vomiting. He had a bout of diarrhea 48 hours ago, but this has subsequently subsided and was not associated with any bleeding or abdominal pain.

### PHYSICAL

A small, pale somewhat hard of hearing 74-year-old gentleman.

H.E.E.N.T.:   Pupils were equal and reactive to light. He has bilateral arcus senilis. No abnormalities were noted in the ears, nose, or throat.

NECK:   Trachea was midline. He has a scar from a possible previous tracheostomy, although the patient could not give a history to this.

CHEST:   Respiratory rate of 24. Chest showed good air entry in upper lobes, but rale in both bases, and dullness to percussion on the right.

CARDIOVASCULAR SYSTEM:   Blood pressure 100/70. Pulse 78. He had no jugular venous distention at 40°. Heart sounds were normal. No murmurs could be heard, but the heart sounds were somewhat diminished.

ABDOMEN:   He has scars from his previous surgery.

RECTAL:   Not done.

CLINICAL IMPRESSION:   An elderly gentleman with previous history of left ventricular failure who has been off medication and has probably again slipped into left ventricular failure. He will be digitalized and diuressed.

_____
T.A.W. Kerr, M.D.

/lbp

D:                     T:

**Illustration 11.28  History and Physical Report — Word Processing Style**

---

**NAME:**  Peters, Tim

**ADDRESS:**

**HOSPITAL NO:**

**DATE OF ADMISSION:**

**DOB:**                                    **SEX:**  M

**DOCTOR:**  S. Lawren

---

HISTORY

CHIEF COMPLAINT:   Acute onset, severe chest pain, and indigestion.

PRESENT ILLNESS:   This gentleman has had several bouts of prolonged heaviness and pressure across his chest which were eventually relieved by nitroglycerin. He has also complained of increasing shortness of breath and sputum production with no fevers, chills, or pleuritic chest pain. He is also complaining of decreased urine output and bilateral low back diffuse pain. His energy seems to be stable. He has had no syncopal episodes, nausea, or vomiting. He has had no burning, frequency, or urgency. His bowels seem to be working all right.

PAST HISTORY:   He has had osteomyelitis of the right leg. Appendectomy. He had a lymph node removed from his right groin in his early 30s which was possibly thought to be Hodgkin's and he received radiotherapy for this.

PHYSICAL

GENERAL:   The patient is an alert, cooperative male, clutching at the chest at times during the interview. He says that this is still uncomfortable. Pulse: 93 and irregular. Temperature 98.6.

HEENT:   React to L & A, no AV nicking. Ears are normal. Pharynx is normal. No thyroid enlargement or bruit noted.

CHEST:   Barrel shaped with a decreased air entry but no crackles or wheezes appreciated. Normal S1 S2 with faint heart sounds.

ABDOMEN:   Soft with no hepatosplenomegaly or tenderness.

RECTAL:   Deferred.

ANALYSIS AND PLAN:   It would appear that this man is having bouts of prolonged angina. He may have an acute exacerbating of his C.O.L.D. and he may have anuria secondary to his renal failure. He will be admitted to hospital, some basic tests will be done, and he will be observed over the next two to three days. If all is well, he will be sent back home to his apartment.

S. Lawren, M.D., C.C.F.P.

/lbp
copies to: R.W. Parker
          E.J. Pelham

D:
T:

**Assignment 11.2**

Produce a copy of each of the four illustrated History and Physical Report styles. Using the current date for admission, and matching birthdates with patients already on record, complete the personal information.

For Assignments 11.2 through 11.9 you may use the blank forms found in the Working Papers (pp. 78–95), or you may wish to produce word processing macros to complete the assignments.

**Assignment 11.3**

Complete the following History and Physical Report using style 2 (modified block). Send appropriate copies.

Patient: Peter J. Scott — Admit today. The dictating physician is Paul T. Scole, M.D. The family doctor is Dr. Plunkett. The tape was dictated two days ago. Hospital no. 357914. His chief complaint is diarrhea and vomiting over the past 24 hours. Present Illness: This __-year-old was perfectly well yesterday but awoke during the night with diarrhea and vomiting. There is severe cramping in the lower abdomen. Patient's last normal bowel movement was yesterday morning. His mother reports that he was at the movies yesterday and ate a large box of popcorn. Past History: Patient was born at Ottawa General Hospital — delivery uncomplicated. All childhood immunizations have been administered. He had a tonsillectomy at age 4 years and broke his right middle finger at age 7. Family History: Mother is 37 years old and is presently undergoing treatment for breast cancer. She reports that she had surgery and is on chemotherapy at the present time. Father is age 42 and well. They both had appendectomies, one of which ruptured. A maternal great niece, uncle, and grandmother have had diabetes. No diabetes in the immediate family and no other history of familial disorders. Personal History: Allergic to morphine, is not on any medication at the present, is attending school, an excellent student. His hobbies include stamp collecting, hockey, water skiing, and cross-country skiing. Systemic Review: HEENT: There has been a muscle in one eye that has been off for years; his vision is good, hearing normal; CR: No known murmurs. No chronic cough, no recent cough, no dyspnea. N.P.: No history of head injury, no history of polio, paralysis, meningitis. Analysis and Plan: The patient will be admitted to hospital and examined further for possible appendicitis.

**Discharge Summary/ Final Note**

A Discharge Summary/Final Note is prepared when a patient is discharged from the hospital. It is a summary of the treatment and medicine regimen during the patient's hospital stay and generally includes a final diagnosis of the illness. It is generally produced in block style, single-spaced, with double spacing between paragraphs. The title is centred and set in all capitals. Headings, such as Summary and Final Diagnosis, are typed in capital letters and underlined. The Final Diagnosis appears after the Summary.

A sample Discharge Summary/Final Note appears in Illustration 11.29.

**Illustration 11.29   Discharge Summary/Final Note**

---

**FINAL NOTE**

**Patient Number:**   987654-32                                   **DOB:** _____

**Patient Name:**   Shultz, Erik                                  **Admitted:** _____

**Address:** _____                       **Discharged:** _____

---

This _____-year-old man was admitted to hospital on the eighth day of August, 1982 with chest pain. The patient has a past history of possible pulmonary embolus and had surgery for carcinoma of the right ilium in 1979.

He was admitted to hospital with pain in the chest, and in the right foot. He had E.C.G. done which showed no abnormality.

SUMMARY

Serum enzymes were done and there was some elevation of the SGOT, but the CPK was normal.

BUN was normal. Alkaline phosphates was elevated to 204. Lung scan was done which showed a low to moderate possibility of embolism. Chest X-ray showed no significant abnormality.

The patient has now been up and around and has no further pain. He developed a bout of gout while in hospital, which was treated with indocid. He is to be allowed home and his condition followed with office visits.

A liver scan has been ordered but is not yet reported.

FINAL DIAGNOSIS

Acute gout, and chest pain with elevated liver enzymes, possible metastatic disease following carcinoma of the right ilium.

_____
R.M. Mann, M.D.

lbp
copies to: Dr. C.H. Hamblin
          Dr. R.M. McLeod

---

Produce a copy of the Discharge Summary appearing in Illustration 11.29.      **Assignment 11.4**

## Consultation/ Admission Note

A Consultation/Admission Note is generally completed when a second opinion is sought, or when a doctor other than the family physician admits a patient to the hospital. This report can follow any of the styles illustrated in the History and Physical section if a complete examination is undertaken. The Consultation Note, however, usually takes the form of a general report. Headings, if used, are at left margin, and the body is single-spaced with double spacing between paragraphs. The consulting doctor signs the note. A Consultation Note appears in Illustration 11.30.

## Assignment 11.5

Produce a copy of the Consultation/Admission Note in Illustration 11.30.

**Illustration 11.30    Consultation Note**

CONSULTATION NOTE

PATIENT'S NAME: _Bell, Thomas_ _____

ADDRESS: _____

DOCTOR: _____

DATE: _____

MEDICAL RECORD NO: _356428_

ROOM OR WARD: _316-A_

DOB: _____

This _____-year-old man was previously seen by myself, back in 1972. At that time he had lower abdominal suprapubic aching discomfort and low back pain. Also at that time, associated with the discomfort, he had some degree of daytime and nighttime frequency. His I.V.P. was normal. It was felt then, that he was suffering from prostatitis and was placed on some nitrofurantoin and butazolidin for a period of two weeks. His symptoms completely subsided.

He remained well as far as the urinary tract is concerned, up until about two weeks ago, when he developed a similar discomfort felt in the suprapubic area, but not, on this occasion, radiating down into the testicles or into the lower back. In addition, on this occasion he has had no frequency of urination. He claims to still void with a good urinary stream, but no gross haematuria, and no dysuria.

Arrangements had been made for me to see him in my office this afternoon, but last night he was admitted to hospital under Dr. Sprong following a seizure. He has a previous history of glioma from about eight years ago. He is currently under investigation for this problem.

While in hospital, we will carry out some further investigation, including an I.V.P., if this can be arranged, and urine cultures. We will treat him as if he has prostatitis, as long as this does not interfere with his other problems.

R.A. Beams, M.D., F.R.C.S.

/lbp

copies to: Dr. R.J. Sprong
Dr. E.J. Pelham

An Operative Record form is preprinted with headings as follows:       **Operative Record**

1. Preoperative Diagnosis
2. Postoperative Diagnosis
3. Operation
4. Procedure, or Findings and Procedure

   Some variations of style follow:

1. Double-space after each heading, and align left margin with heading.
2. Begin keying on the same line as the heading, leaving two spaces after the colon. The second and succeeding lines are aligned under the heading.
3. Follow the same procedure as (2), except second and succeeding lines are indented five spaces under each heading.

   A sample of an Operative Record is shown in Illustration 11.31.

Produce a copy of the Operative Record shown in Illustration 11.31.       **Assignment 11.6**

A Delivery Report is produced with dates and times in chronological order       **Delivery Report**
each time the patient is examined. Each date and time appears as a heading at
the left margin. Examine the Delivery Report shown in Illustration 11.32.

Produce a copy of the Delivery Report shown in Illustration 11.32.       **Assignment 11.7**

In a hospital environment, all investigations must be documented. These documentations are made in report form and vary according to specific requirements. Some reports are issued on carbon-pack preprinted forms with the regular patient, hospital, and physician information at the beginning of the report. The carbon packs are multicoloured with a specific colour representing a particular area; for example, a Form 3 Coroner's Investigation Statement has white, yellow, blue, and pink copies. The original white copy is sent to the chief coroner's office; the yellow copy is forwarded to the crown attorney's office; the blue copy is kept for the investigating coroner's files, and the pink copy, also kept by the investigating coroner, is to be made available to the deceased's immediate family, if requested.

**Illustration 11.31    Operative Record**

---

**OPERATIVE RECORD**

Patient:    Smith, Heather

Date:
Room:    Ward 457C
DOB:

PREOPERATIVE DIAGNOSIS:

Surgeon:        Dr. W.B. Bell

Epigastric pain with
regurgitation and heartburn

Assistant:      Dr. J.E. Plunkett

POSTOPERATIVE DIAGNOSIS:

Anaesthetist:   Dr. E.J. Pelham

Oesophagitis, 1 to 2+, patulous
oesophagogastric junction

Date:           08 12 __

OPERATION:

Oesophagogastroduodenoscopy

PROCEDURE:

The patient was sedated before coming to the operating room and this was further supplemented with demerol 80 mg and valium 10 mg I.V. The throat was sprayed with Xylocaine. Satisfactory sedation was obtained. An 18 levin tube was inserted into the stomach and 10 cc of mucus with brownish curds was aspirated. The scope was introduced without difficulty down to the lower end of the oesophagus. At the oesophagogastric junction there was some superficial erosion. Some reddening came up into the oesophagus, particularly in the lower half. No fissures or superficial ulceration above the oesophagogastric junction. The antrum and body of the stomach appeared normal. I was able to get into the duodenum with ease and into the second part of the duodenum; it was difficult to get good visualization. There was a rather sharp turn between the first and second parts of the duodenum. I did not see any abnormality and in the duodenal cap it looked quite normal. The scope was withdrawn and a U-turn was done in the body of the stomach. The fundus, oesophagogastric area, and lesser curvature were quite normal. The scope was withdrawn and the patient was taken to the recovery room in good condition.

On talking to the patient, I understand she has been on tagamet for about three years. She is having rather persistent difficulty. I'll have to find out when she had her last cholecystogram or ultrasound of the gallbladder. If the symptoms continue, I think the patient would be benefitted by an antireflux procedure.

_____

W.B. Bell, M.D.

/lbp
cc: J.E. Plunkett, M.D.
    E.J. Pelham, M.D.

D: 10 12 __
T: 11 12 __

**Illustration 11.32   Delivery Report**

---

**DELIVERY REPORT**

| | |
|---|---|
| **Name:** Davis, Hazel | **No.:** 8765233 |
| **Address:** | **Date:** |
| | **Doctor:** R. Smock, M.D. |
| **Date of Birth:** | **Ward No:** 557 |

---

1500:   Patient admitted to labour ward section with severe contractions q.10 minutes and slight red bloody show. Patient is a gravida 2, eight days past term. Head not engaged on admission.

1550:   Seconal 100 mg.

1800:   Continuous epidural established by doctor. Cervix 8 cm but presenting part still spines minus 2.

2035:   Membranes ruptured spontaneously. Some meconium staining but fetal monitor good. Head still above ischial spines.

2335:   Fully dilated.

0120:   Difficult mid forceps rotation from R.O.P. to L.O.A., L.M.L. episiotomy with left vaginal vault tear. A female child approximate weight 7 pounds, Apgar 8/9. Stiff traction for delivery.

0124:   Placenta removed manually. Cervix inspected and intact. Left sulcus tear repaired with continuous interlocking oo plain catgut and routine episiotomy repair.

Estimated blood loss 200 cc.

R. Smock, M.D.

/lbp
cc: J.E. Plunkett

---

Some forms are preprinted with headings for specific information, and may be computer generated, while others simply have preprinted areas for patient and hospital information, and a blank space for the report documentation.

If specific headings are not preprinted on the form, the following general rules can be used for keying the body of the report:

1. Single-space for the body of the paragraph; double-space after headings and between paragraphs.
2. Triple-space before headings.

3. Side margins approximately 4 cm (1½ inches), line length 15 cm (6 inches), and bottom margin 2.5 to 3 cm (1 to 1¼ inches).

4. Specific headings should be placed at the left margin, all capital letters, and underlined.

5. Number the second and consecutive pages on Line 7 at the right margin, or centred 2.5 cm (1 inch) from the bottom of the page, depending on the type of report.

6. Leave sufficient space at the bottom of the report for the name and title of the reporting physician; key a line of underscores from the centre to the right margin, leave one line of space, and key the physician's name and title. The reporting physician signs on the line of underscores.

The above rules should be considered as general guidelines. Format rules will vary according to the reporting physician's requirements.

Illustration 11.33 is an example of a Pathologist's Report. Note the preprinted areas for information required by the hospital, such as Laboratory no. and Admission no., the area for names of the physician(s) performing the autopsy, and the patient information.

## Assignment 11.8

Produce the following reports on the appropriate forms provided.

1. A Coroner's Investigative Statement — Dr. R.J. Browning, Area No. 12, has investigated the death of __-year-old Mr. Thomas Bell. The death occurred on October 14, 19__, and was reported to the coroner on that day. The patient was dead on arrival (DOA) at Ottawa General Hospital. The patient died from a possible ruptured aortic aneurysm, by natural means. A post-mortem was not performed.

The investigation revealed:

The death of this __-year-old man was reported to me by Dr. Plunkett when the patient arrived, dead on arrival, at Ottawa General Hospital at approximately 0900 hours. His pupils were fixed and dilated. Dr. Plunkett had seen this patient only one time, and that was the night before, at which time he made a house call to the son's home, where the patient was visiting. At that time he had experienced abdominal pain for 24 hours, and after careful examination and finding the patient in no great distress, Dr. Plunkett gave him some mild sedation. He was to be seen the following day. When the family went in the next morning to find him, he was obviously dead and they rushed him to Ottawa General Hospital where he was pronounced dead by Dr. Plunkett.

After discussion with the family, and because there was no evidence of any foul play, it was felt that an autopsy was not entirely necessary, and

**Illustration 11.33   Pathologist's Report**

---

**PATHOLOGIST'S REPORT**

**Department of Pathology**                                          **Ottawa General Hospital**

**Laboratory No:** 6578-DP 56789              **Date:**                       **Adm. No:** 3546

**Name:** Steed, Robert                                 **Age:** 75      **Sex:** Male

**Surgeon:** Dr. Roger Jamieson                                      **Room No:** 304B

**Material:** Needle biopsy prostate. Prostatic tissue              **Date Rec'd:** 04/10/84

---

GROSS:

The specimen is received in formalin in two containers. The first is labelled needle biopsy of prostate. The specimen consists of six needle cores of white to tan prostatic tissue. A total length is approximately 7 cm. The biopsies are quite slim and are submitted in block A.

The second is labelled prostatic tissue. The specimen consists of 12 g of prostatic curettings with a somewhat nodular outline. The tissue is pink to tan in colour, a small amount of clot is received with the curettings. The tissue is submitted in toto in blocks B, C, and D.

MQ/hmb

MICROSCOPIC:

Multiple step sections of needle biopsy of prostate demonstrate in two fragments an adenocarcinoma of moderately well differentiated type associated with a marked chronic inflammatory cell infiltrate, lymphocytes being so numerous as to almost completely obliterate in some areas the markedly atypical glands. The remaining tissue shows predominantly fibromuscular bands in which large nerve fibres are identified.

Blocks B, C, and D. Multiple sections of curettage biopsy and prostate demonstrate a nodular outline in which hyperplastic gland elements are noted. A prominent feature is a marked granulomatous inflammation with central caseation. GMS, PAS, and ZN stains have been done but all are negative for identification of pathogenic organisms. It is, therefore, likely that these are the result of rupture of large ducts. In the fibromuscular stroma and areas away from the caseation there is moderate chronic inflammation. A single area in block D shows gland crowding. However, the glands are lined by a double layer of glandular epithelium and are AB PAS negative.

DIAGNOSIS:

1.   Adenocarcinoma in needle biopsy of prostate.
2.   Granulomatous inflammation in prostatic curettings.

Martin Quigg, M.D.

---

accordingly, following their wishes, we did not proceed with an autopsy. This man also had had chronic obstructive pulmonary disease for many years and known arteriosclerotic heart disease. It was felt death may have been due to something such as a rupture of an abdominal aortic aneurysm, and in view of the lack of any suggestion of foul play, the body was released for burial without autopsy or inquest being needed.

2.   Tissue Pathology Report from Ottawa General Laboratory No. S78-885, patient Timothy Peters, Admission No. 25403, Room 5G, Age __. Surgery

performed by Drs. D. Myles and R. Parrott on October 12, 19__, material was received on October 12, 19__, consisting of sigmoid polyp, appendix, and sigmoid. No preop, postop, and frozen section diagnoses are reported.

Gross — The first specimen is labelled sigmoid polyp and this polyp which is lobulated reddish, glistening firm, and finely granular with an ovoid outline is 1 × 1 × 0.6 cm with a stalk covered by purplish-grey finely granular glistening mucosa with a length of 1.3 cm, and its base measures 1 × 0.3 cm. The tissue is bisected in the long axis and both halves embedded. The stroma of the stalk is congested.

The second specimen is labelled appendix. The appendix is received with slightly congested fatty mesoappendix up to a depth of 2.3 cm attached. The appendix itself, which is curved in the long axis with a slightly congested pink glistening surface, is 5.5 cm long with a width varying between 0.7 and 1 cm and is firmly fluctuant and slightly expanded at the tip where grey creamy puslike material is presented within the distended lumen. More watery pink-tinged mucoid or purulent material is present within the proximal lumen and the mucosa appears somewhat flattened throughout the length. Representative transversely cut blocks are embedded.

The third specimen is labelled sigmoid and consists of a segment of colon 18 cm long, and at the one end the circumference is 3.5 cm and at the opposite end, which appears to be upper rectum, the circumference is 8 cm. At a distance 6 cm from the broader end there is an area of hemorrhage and granularity on the antemesenteric surface of the colon, and the tissue here feels palpably firmer. On opening the specimen it completely encircles the tumour with an ulcerated inner surface present. It occupies the length of the bowel for 5.5 cm and has characteristic overhanging margins. The inner surface of the remainder of the segment of bowel is unremarkable. Transverse cutting through the centre of the area of ulceration reveals a greyish-tan granular infiltration apparently the full thickness of the wall, which at this point measures up to 1 cm in thickness. Representative blocks from the tumour are embedded as C. Blocks from the lower line of resection are embedded as D. Serial cutting of the external congested fatty tissue reveals firm to hard slightly to moderately enlarged pinkish-grey lymph nodes which are embedded as E. The largest node found measures approximately 1.5 × 1 cm on its cut surface, and lymph node tissue taken from the mesentery tissue of the sigmoid colon are embedded as F. These are smaller and softer up to about 0.3 cm diameter. A fragment of apparently fatty tissue which feels somewhat indurated is also embedded as F. Final inspection of the colonic mucosa reveals two diverticulae 4 cm from the proximal line of resection and a final block taken through these embedded also as F.

Microscopic — Sections of the polypoid lesion reveal an active chronic inflammation and foci of in-situ carcinoma where there is stratification of the epithelium and a back-to-back arrangement of variable sized glands and variable sized nuclei, many of which have prominent nucleoli. The congested stalk stroma is edematous and free of infiltrating tumour and the marginal epithelium is normal.

Sections of the appendix reveal some inflammatory exudate present in the lumen and hyperplasia of lymphoid tissue present in the mucosa and a congested serosa in which scatterings of chronic inflammatory cells are present. In places, some of these are neutrophil polymorphs. Within the submucosa there is some fatty change and some increase of fibrous tissue with partial replacement of the somewhat thinned inner muscle coat where the lumen is distended.

Sections of the tumour confirm it as a moderately well differentiated infiltrating adenocarcinoma with transmural infiltration and a quite marked desmoplastic reaction with active chronic inflammation present in the pericolonic fibrofatty tissue and ulceration of the inner aspect.

Sections embedded as D from the line of resection show it to be free of tumour but the lymphoid component is hyperplastic in the mucosa.

Sections of lymph nodes reveal hyperplasia and edema but no tumour infiltration.

Diagnosis 1. Sigmoid polyp. Adenocarcinoma. In-situ.
2. Appendix. Active chronic periappendicitis.
3. Sigmoid colon. Ulcerated infiltrating stenosing adenocarcinoma. Lymph nodes negative for tumour.

Dr. H.A. Montmorency was the reporting pathologist.

3.  Tissue Pathology Reports for the following patients (Dr. Cranston is pathologist, Dr. Ling and Dr. McKenzie are the surgeons.)

a.  Elizabeth Green at O.G.H. Lab No. S78885, Adm. No. 76279, Room No. 361, operation on October 14, 19__, material received on that day consisting of uterus with resected right and left ovaries and oviducts.

Gross — The specimen consists of a uterus with cervix and resected right and left ovaries and oviducts. The uterus is anteroverted, somewhat nodular and it measures 5 × 5 × 3.5 cm. In the right cornu there is a subserosal nodule 3.5 cm in diameter. The serosa is otherwise pinkish and smooth. The cervix measures 4 cm in length × 3 cm in diameter. The portio-vaginalis is pinkish smooth and shiny up to 2.6 cm in width. The external os is a short transverse slit 0.7 cm in width. The endocervical canal measures 4 cm in length, is pinkish, smooth, and moderately trabeculated. The endometrial cavity measures 4.5 × 1.5 cm. The endometrium is thin, pinkish, and soft. The myometrium measures 1.4 cm, and it is pinkish and fibrous throughout. The nodule described on the external description is made of intertwined fibrous tissue and it reveals multiple hemorrhagic dots. On further sectioning of the myometrium, a small intramural fibroid, 0.5 cm in diameter, is noted on the anterior wall of the uterus. Two sections of cervix are embedded in A, two of endometrium in B, and three of the nodule are embedded in block C.

Separately submitted is the right oviduct. The right ovary is not received. The oviduct measures 7 cm in length. The two proximal thirds have an external diameter of 0.5 cm and the distal third is dilated to 1 cm. The serosal is pinkish and smooth, and the fimbriated end is patent. There is moderate amount of fibrous tissue attached to the oviduct but no ovarian tissue is recognized on gross examination. Multiple representative sections are embedded in block D.

Separately submitted is the left ovary with attached oviduct. The ovary is ovoid and measures 4 × 3 × 2 cm. The albuginea is in part tan pink and gyriform and in part covered with a yellowish fibrous tissue. On serial sectioning of the ovary there is a cyst 1 cm in diameter with a pinkish smooth internal lining and filled with clear fluid. Also noted under the area covered with fibrous tissue is a focal blackish blue stony nodular lesion a few millimetres in diameter. The oviduct is distorted and adherent to the ovary, and it measures 0.5 up to 0.8 cm. The fimbriated end is patent.

Microscopic — There is basal cell hyperplasia of the lower endocervical canal with infiltration of the stroma by moderate numbers of chronic inflammatory cells. The portio-vaginalis shows increased parakeratosis. The endometrium is moderately thin and made up of round glands lined with mitosing regular columnar epithelium. In focal areas the glands are moderately hyperplastic and somewhat crowded. The appearance is that of a proliferative endometrium. The nodule described in the right cornu is made up of intertwined myometrium in which islands of endometrial glands supported by endometrial stroma are present.

Sections of the right oviduct reveal attached fibrous and muscular tissue in which islands of endometriosis are present. Ovarian tissue is not identified in these sections.

Sections of the fibrous and fatty tissue attached to the left ovary reveal again islands of endometriosis. The right ovary contains several corpora atetrica and a cystically dilated follicle with a fibrous wall. Other sections of the ovary reveal old hemorrhage and areas of calcification and ossification.

Diagnosis 1. Total hysterectomy with right salpingectomy and left salpingo-oophorectomy.

2. Chronic cervicitis.

3. Proliferative endometrium.

4. Adenomyosis.

5. Small intramural leiomyomas.

6. Endometriosis of right oviduct and left ovary and oviduct.

b. Amelia Jackson at Ottawa Civic, Lab. No. T33992, Adm. No. 13776, Room No. 293. Operation on October 18, 19__, material received October 18 consisting of a left breast measuring 17 × 10 × 4 cm.

Gross — The specimen consists of a left breast removed at subcutaneous mastectomy. It measures 17 × 10 × 4 cm. On serial sectioning it is pinkish and fibrous throughout with moderate amount of yellow fatty tissue. In the area marked with a clamp there is an ovoid cyst measuring 3 cm in diameter with a pinkish thin smooth and moderately trabeculated lining and filled with thin brownish fluid. Representative sections are embedded in blocks A, B, and C.

Microscopic — Sections reveal breast tissue with scattered mammary lobules exhibiting a variable degree of epithelial hyperplasia and ductal dilatation. An occasional lobule is lined with tall vacuolated cytoplasm while others reveal apocrine type of epithelium. A hint of intraduct papillomatosis is noted and there is minimal microscopic calcification of some of the ducts. In other areas the intralobular stroma is abundant and somewhat obliterates the lobule, and over extensive areas there is marked hyalinization of the stroma. The cyst described in the gross has a thick fibrous wall lined in part by a low regular cuboidal epithelium.

Diagnosis 1. Subcutaneous mastectomy.

2. Fibrocystic disease of the left breast.

On the X-ray forms provided, produce the following X-ray reports. (Dr. H. Lam is the radiologist.)

4. a. Mary Jane Brown — X-ray No. 3533-44, contract No. 88-99, X-ray of uterine cavity, outpatient.

Hysterosalpingogram — Two films were taken during the hysterosalpingogram. There is apparent spillage of dye into the vagina. The uterine cavity is not very well demonstrated.

There is a pocket of dye measuring approximately 2½ inches in length slightly to the right of the midline, which probably represents the uterine cavity, but it would indicate either anteversion or retroversion of the uterus and tilting of the uterus to the side.

There was spillage of dye into the peritoneal cavity indicating at least one patent fallopian tube. However, detail is not sufficient to identify both tubes well.

Impression — Since the uterine cavity is not very well outlined, it is difficult to say whether it is entirely normal. There is patency of at least one fallopian tube. There is probable retroversion or anteversion of the uterus.

b. Tim Peters has had a venogram of his right leg performed on November 13, 19__. He is an outpatient; X-ray No. 3567-92, contract No. 66-78.

Right Venogram — The tourniquet was applied above the right ankle. A needle was inserted into the dorsal veins of the right foot and 15 ml of Conray-60 were injected through the venous system of the right leg. This examination was then compared with the venogram of the same extremity dated May 7, 19__.

On the present examination, there is excellent filling of both superficial and deep veins of the right leg and no abnormalities are demonstrated. Specifically, I see no evidence of thrombophlebitis.

On reviewing the last examination, I think the nonfilled deep veins of the calf may have been related to compression of these veins during the examination, because on the present study, the patient's leg was both internally and externally rotated.

Impression — Normal right leg venogram.

c. William Harris has been a patient at O.G.H. Ward No. 346 for several days. An assessment of his left ear was made by the X-ray technician on X-ray No. 5542-57 and contract No. 69-08.

Mastoids and tomograms of left temporal bone — The mastoid air cells are symmetrically and normally developed bilaterally with delicate normal appearing bony septi between the air cells. No evidence of bone destruction is seen. The ossicles and attic spur on the left are intact with no evidence of erosion. The middle and inner ear structures are unremarkable. The atticus at antrum and the mastoid antrum on the left are well aerated. Opinion — No demonstrable abnormality of mastoids or left upper bone structures.

## Assignment 11.9

An Autopsy Report will be given to you by your instructor as a production assignment. You will be informed of the time allowed to produce the report. The patient's name is Mrs. Janet Bell. The student is responsible for making all necessary corrections in order to produce an acceptable document.

## Out-Patient Forms and Requisitions

In the medical office, the physician may request laboratory tests or X-rays. The medical administrative assistant is responsible for arranging appropriate times for these tests and completing the necessary requisition forms. In some instances, the patient may be required to fast, take laxatives, or supply a urine sample prior to a laboratory test or radiology examination. Most health care facilities have preprinted forms with specific instructions to the patient. The form is given to the patient sometime before the examination or test, with confirmation of the instructions given by the medical administrative assistant. The preprinted form may resemble Illustration 11.34, with the administrative assistant's check mark opposite the appropriate information.

Once again, accuracy in the completion of these forms is essential. If you are in doubt about specific orders, ask the physician to clarify the instructions. Many problems can be avoided by asking a simple question. Ensure that all orders for tests and X-rays are recorded in the patient's file, specifying the dates when the requisition was ordered and sent. The medical administrative assistant must always remember to record every procedure for future reference and also to avoid misunderstandings. Verbal orders do not have any follow-up. *Written records are the only answer.*

A physician may request home care, Victorian Order of Nurses care, private nursing care, or admission to a nursing home for a patient. In order to accomplish the request, completion of requisition forms or composition of letters may be necessary. The medical administrative assistant may act as liaison between the ordering physician's office and the institution or health care service. Accuracy of data is most important.

When tests are completed, the results are returned to the ordering physician's office. The medical administrative assistant receives the reports and therefore has access to the information. Sometimes, outsiders such as insurance companies and family members are interested in the test results. It is imperative that you never divulge medical information without specific instructions from the physician. It is good practice to refrain from giving information over the telephone. Someone could call and give false identification. If you are requested to give information over the telephone, inform the party that you will have to consult with the doctor and call back. By following this procedure, you will be sure that the correct party receives the information.

Malpractice suits are becoming more prevalent each year in Canada. The medical administrative assistant cannot be too careful when releasing information. The simplest request, even the results of a blood test, should not be divulged without the physician's approval and a signed consent from the patient.

Confidentiality must be stressed again and again to everyone involved in the medical profession.

# Completion of Requisition Forms in the Physician's Office

**Illustration 11.34    Patient Instructions**

## Mammography

☐ Do not use deodorant, talcum powder or any other ointment or cream on your breasts or underarms before your exam. Dress comfortably, preferably in a two piece outfit since you will be asked to undress above the waist for the procedure.

## Radiography

☐ **Upper GI Series:**  Do not eat or drink anything (including oral medications) after 10pm on the night before your appointment. Take any bedtime oral medications before 10 pm. Bring your morning oral medications to the hospital and take them after your test. Do not smoke or chew gum on the day of the examination.

☐ **Small Bowel Follow-Through:**  Do not eat or drink anything† after 10pm the night before your appointment. Expect to be in the department at least 2-3 hours.

☐ **Barium Enema:**

*Day 1:* Drink clear fluids only.‡ Take your oral medications with the fluids. Do not eat solid food.

*Day 2:* Drink clear fluids only.‡ Take your oral medications with the fluids. Do not eat solid food.

  Take one package of ROYVAC, following the manufacturer's enclosed instructions.

*Day 3:* Drink clear fluids only.† Report for your test.

☐ **Enteroclysis (small bowel intubation):**

*Day 1:* Drink clear fluids only.‡ Take two (2) ounces of castor oil at 2 pm. After 10 pm, do not eat or drink anything.

*Day 2:* Do not eat or drink anything.† Report for your test.

☐ **IVP:**

*Day 1:* At 2 pm, take 2 ounces of castor oil or 1 full container of X-PREP. After 2 pm, drink only clear fluids‡; do not take any solid food. You should take your normal oral medications with the clear fluids.

*Day 2:* Drink clear fluids only. You may drink as much of these as you like.‡ Report for your test.

## Ultrasound

☐ **Abdominal Ultrasound:**

*morning appointment:*  Do not eat or drink anything† after 10 pm on the evening before your test. Do not chew gum the day of the test.

*afternoon appointment:*  Do not eat or drink anything† after 8 am on the day of your test. Do not chew gum the day of the test.

☐ **Pelvic Ultrasound:**  Drink five (5) glasses of water (8 ounces each) before your test. You should be finished drinking this by one hour before your appointment time. Do not void after drinking this water as your bladder must be full for a successful test. In certain special circumstances, an ultrasound probe may be inserted internally.

☐ **Obstetrical Ultrasound:**

*before 20 weeks (4 1/2 months):*  Follow the instructions listed for pelvic ultrasound above.

*after 20 weeks (4 1/2 months):*  No preparation is required.

☐ **Other ultrasound tests:**  No preparation is required.

## Nuclear Medicine

**Nuclear medicine examinations require three possible stages:**

*First visit:*    You will be given a small injection after arriving for your test (see table).

*Delay:*    This is the waiting period between the 1st and 2nd visits. The length of time is different for each test (see table).

*Second visit:*    At this time, the pictures of your test are made (see table).

| Test | First Visit | Delay | Second Visit |
|---|---|---|---|
| ☐ Brain Scan & Flow Study | 20 minutes | 40 minutes | 20 minutes |
| ☐ Gallium Scan | 10 minutes | 1-3 days | 30 minutes |
| ☐ Liver/Spleen Scan & Flow Study | 45 minutes | none | none |
| ☐ Lung Scan (perfusion & ventilation) | 45 minutes | none | none |
| ☐ Renal Scan & Flow Study/GFR | 90 minutes | none | none |
| ☐ RBC Scan & Flow Study | 1 hour | 1-24 hours | 30 minutes |
| ☐ Testicular Scan & Flow Study | 60 minutes | none | none |
| ☐ Thyroid Scan | 1 hour | none | none |
| ☐ WBC Scan | 1 hour | 4, 18 & 24 hours | 1 hour |
| ☐ Whole Body or Regional Bone Scan | 20 minutes | 2-3 hours | 30 minutes |

†If you require heart medications, you should take these as per your normal routine, using very small sips of water.

‡Clear fluids include apple juice, clear jellies, consommé, water, and tea. They do not include milk, coffee, or orange juice.

If you require insulin injections, you should discuss this with your doctor prior to coming for your test. Please inform the technologist.

## In-Patient Forms and Requisitions

If hospital admission has been prearranged (elective), forms are sent or given to the patient, or the admitting department personnel will phone the patient to obtain the essential personal information. If hospital admission is not pre-arranged (emergency), the forms are completed on admission.

If surgery is to be performed, the patient must complete and sign a patient consent form.

Most provincial health care plans cover standard ward accommodation only. Hospitals generally have patients complete a request for accommodation form on admission which explains their responsibility for payment of the extra daily charges incurred for semi-private and private ward accommodation.

A Preadmission Form is shown in Illustration 11.35, a Consent Form in Illustration 11.11 (see page 164), and an Admission Insurance Form in Illustration 11.36. Examine each of these forms, taking note of the information required to complete each form.

---

**Assignment 11.10**

Assume that you are to be admitted to the hospital in one week's time to have your tonsils removed. Dr. Plunkett has explained the procedure to you and Dr. Pelham will be performing the surgery. Your hospital admission number is 998864. Complete the consent, preadmission, and admission insurance forms (Working Papers, pp. 96–101). Sign the documents; ask a classmate to witness your signature.

**Assignment 11.11**

This is a production assignment. Your instructor will provide you with the assignment material. Marks will be assessed for appearance, style, patient information, and ability to complete work in the allotted time. Patient's personal information can be obtained from the patient information forms in Chapter 3. Reports must be correlated with the patient list. Complete a preadmission form and a consent form for Jean Belliveau, inserting only information that you have available, and items 1 and 2 on day 1; items 3, 4, and 5 on day 2; items 6, 7, and 8 on day 3; items 9, 10, and 11 on day 4; and items 12, 13, 14, and 15 on day 5. Insert the completed assignment in your portfolio.

As the admitting doctor, Dr. Plunkett will do the History and Physical Reports; Discharge Summaries/Final Notes are signed by M. Brown, M.D., F.R.C.P.; Dr. Pelham completes Operative Records; Dr. W. Jarozenich completes Consultation Notes; and Dr. Emily Baret dictates the Delivery Report. All documents must be completed with all required information included.

**Illustration 11.35    Preadmission Form**

**REGISTRATION SHEET** — PLEASE COMPLETE & RETURN TO THE ADMITTING DEPT. OF THE APPROPRIATE HOSPITAL IMMEDIATELY.

DEAR PATIENT: YOU HAVE BEEN BOOKED FOR A PROCEDURE AT:

☐ ST. JOSEPH'S HOSPITAL & HEALTH CENTRE
384 ROGERS ST.
PETERBOROUGH, ONT. K9H 7B6
ADMITTING: TEL. (705) 740-8000 FAX (705) 740-8001

☐ PETERBOROUGH CIVIC HOSPITAL
ONE HOSPITAL DRIVE
PETERBOROUGH, ONT. K9J 7C6
ADMITTING: TEL. (705) 876-5068 FAX (705) 876-5107

☐ A.M. ADMIT
☐ IN–PATIENT
☐ SURGICAL OUT–PATIENT
☐ MEDICAL OUT–PATIENT

PATIENT'S NAME: _____ AGE _____

DATE OF ADMISSION: _____
Month    Day    Year

DATE OF PROCEDURE: _____
Month    Day    Year

ATTENDING DOCTOR: _____ ( )
INITIAL

FAMILY DOCTOR: _____ ( )
INITIAL

PROCEDURE: _____

| 1. LAST NAME | ALL GIVEN NAMES (No Initials) (Underline Name Used) | ANY PREVIOUS LAST NAME |
|---|---|---|
| | | |

| 2. HOME ADDRESS (STREET, R.R., BOX, APT.) | CITY/TOWN | POSTAL CODE | TOWNSHIP |
|---|---|---|---|
| | | | |

3. IF YOU ARE FROM: HOME FOR THE AGED_____NURSING HOME_____RESIDENTIAL FACILITY_____

NAME THE FACILITY _____

4. HOME TELEPHONE:

AREA CODE_____ - _____

DATE OF BIRTH:     MONTH   DAY   YEAR     AGE     SEX     MARITAL STATUS (Please Circle)

_____/_____/_____     __ M __ F     S    M    D    W    SEP    CL

5. RELIGION & _____

NAME OF CHURCH _____

IF YOUR "CLERGY PERSON" OR THE PASTORAL CARE DEPT. WERE TO INQUIRE, WOULD YOU LIKE THEM TO BE MADE AWARE OF YOUR HOSPITAL ADMISSION?

YES ☐     NO ☐

TO ENSURE THAT YOUR "CLERGY PERSON" IS AWARE OF YOUR ADMISSION, PLEASE CONTACT HIM/HER YOURSELF BEFORE COMING TO THE HOSPITAL.

6. NAME OF NEXT OF KIN OR FRIEND:

SPOUSE _____ TELEPHONE _____ ADDRESS _____

PARENT _____ TELEPHONE _____ ADDRESS _____

OTHER & _____ TELEPHONE _____ ADDRESS _____

RELATIONSHIP _____

7. IF WORKERS' COMPENSATION:     MON.    DAY    YR.

YES _____ NO _____     SIN # _____ _____ _____     DATE OF ACCIDENT _____/_____/_____     CLAIM # _____

NAME OF EMPLOYER _____ ADDRESS OF EMPLOYER _____

8. IS THIS HOSPITAL VISIT DUE TO COSMETIC SURGERY?   YES _____ NO _____     COVERED BY ONT. HEALTH INS.? _____

| 9. HEALTH CARE # : | VERSION CODE: | PLEASE BRING YOUR HEALTH CARD WITH YOU |
|---|---|---|
| \|_\|_\|_\|_\|_\|_\|_\|_\|_\| | \|_\|_\| 1 OR 2 LETTERS BOTTOM RIGHT OF CARD. | _____ |

10. PATIENT'S EMPLOYER: _____ ADDRESS: _____

(Please Circle)

11. IF YOU ARE ADMITTED DO YOU WISH A         STANDARD WARD         SEMI-PRIVATE         PRIVATE ROOM?
(YOU WILL BE RESPONSIBLE FOR SEMI OR PRIVATE ROOM CHARGES IF YOUR INSURANCE DOES NOT COVER THIS ACCOMMODATION REQUEST.)

12. ADDITIONAL INSURANCE FOR SEMI–PRIVATE:

NAME OF INSURANCE _____ NAME OF EMPLOYER _____
(IF A GROUP PLAN)

IDENTIFICATION / POLICY # _____ GROUP # _____

INSURANCE HOLDER'S NAME _____ INSURANCE HOLDER'S SIN # _____ _____ _____

13. ADDITIONAL INSURANCE FOR PRIVATE:

NAME OF INSURANCE _____ NAME OF EMPLOYER _____
(IF A GROUP PLAN)

IDENTIFICATION / POLICY # _____ GROUP # _____

INSURANCE HOLDER'S NAME _____ INSURANCE HOLDER'S SIN # _____ _____ _____

14. WHAT CONTACT HAVE YOU HAD WITH THE HOSPITALS?

PETERBOROUGH CIVIC     YEAR _____     PREVIOUS SURNAME _____

ST. JOSEPH'S     YEAR _____     PREVIOUS SURNAME _____

15. ALLERGIES:  FOOD _____    DRUG _____    NONE _____    UNKNOWN _____

FORM # 0505021 JF    (PAGE 2 OF 5)

**Illustration 11.36 Admission Insurance Form**

# ADMISSION INSURANCE FORM

St. Joseph's Hospital & Health Centre

Peterborough Civic Hospital

| WARD ☐ | SEMI-PRIVATE ☐ | PRIVATE ☐ |
|---|---|---|
| (3-4 patients per room) | (2 patients per room) | (1 patient per room) |
| | | (Room may not have private bathroom) |

Cost per day     Cost per day     Cost per day

☐ Covered by Health Card

☐ Non-Ohip   $_____    $_____     $_____

☐ Out of Province   $_____    ☐ Covered by insurance    ☐ Covered by Insurance

Health Card #_____    ☐ Self-Pay      ☐ Self-Pay

☐ Out of Country   $_____

Insurance Company Name: _____

Policy #: _____ Division #: _____ Certificate #: _____

Employer: _____

Employee/Certificate Holder: _____

For Work Related Injury? ☐ Yes ☐ No    W.C.B. Claim #: _____

S.I.N. #: _____    Date of Accident: _____

Employer: _____    Employer's Address: _____

The Hospital does not assume any responsibility for patient valuables. The Hospital does not assume any responsibility for the knowledge of your Insurance Coverage.

I acknowledge that if, for any reason, my Insurance agency (if applicable) does not honour my claim, I agree to make full and immediate payment for these charges.

Signature: _____

Date: _____

Witness: _____

White Copy: Business Office   Yellow Copy: Chart   Pink Copy: Patient

Form # 0072 (Oct. 94)

# Appendix A:  Common Abbreviations Used in the Health Care Field

A list of common abbreviations used in the medical profession appears below for your reference:

| | | | |
|---|---|---|---|
| ad | to; up to | EEG | electroencephalogram |
| abs. feb. | without fever | EKG | electrocardiogram |
| a.c. | before eating | EMG | electromyogram |
| adhib | to be administered | e.m.p. | as directed |
| ad lib. | as desired | ESR | erythrocyte sedimentation rate |
| agit | shake, stir | | |
| alt. dieb. | every other day | GI | gastrointestinal |
| alt. hor. | every other hour | gm | gram |
| alt. noc. | every other night | gr. | grain |
| aq. | water | grad. | by degrees |
| b.i.d. | twice daily | Gtt., gtt. | drops |
| b.i.n. | twice a night | h | hour |
| bis in 7d. | twice a week | HEENT | head, eyes, ears, nose, throat |
| BP | blood pressure | | |
| BUN | blood urea nitrogen | hgb | hemoglobin |
| c or c̄ | with | h.n. | tonight |
| C | Celsius | h.s. | at bedtime |
| ca. | about | hx | history |
| Ca | cancer | I.M. | intramuscular |
| cap. | capsule | IU | international unit |
| CBC | complete blood count | I.V. | intravenously |
| cc. | cubic centimetre | kg | kilogram |
| c.m. | tomorrow morning | L | litre |
| c.m.s. | to be taken tomorrow morning | liq. | liquid, fluid |
| | | mEq. | milliequivalent |
| c.n. | tomorrow night | mitt. | send |
| CNS | central nervous system | os. | mouth |
| comp. | compound | P | pulse |
| contra | against | PBI | protein-bound iodine |
| CV | cardiovascular | p.c. | after meals |
| d | day | p.o. | by mouth |
| /d | daily | ppm | parts per million |
| D | dose | p.r. | through the rectum |
| D&C | dilation and curettage | p.r.n. | as needed |
| dr. | dram | q.h | every hour |
| dx | diagnosis | q. 2h | every two hours |
| ECG | electrocardiogram | q. 3h | every three hours |
| ECT | electroconvulsive therapy | q.i.d. | four times a day |

| | | | |
|---|---|---|---|
| q.l. | as much as wanted | T | temperature |
| q.s. | as much as needed | tab. | tablet |
| R | respiration | t.i.d. | three times daily |
| RBC | red blood count | t.i.n. | three times a night |
| Rx | prescription | tinct. | tincture |
| s or s̄ | without | TKVO | to keep vein open |
| s.cut. | subcutaneously | ung. | ointment |
| SGOT | serum glutamic oxalacetic transaminase | ur | urine |
| | | top. | topically |
| SGPT | serum glutamic pyruvic transaminase | UV | ultraviolet |
| | | WBC | white blood count |
| stat. | immediately | Wt. | weight |
| suppos. | suppository | w/v. | weight by volume |
| syr. | syrup | | |

# Appendix B: Laboratory Medicine

## Biochemistry

**Biochemistry** — Analysis of routine, drug, and special testing on blood, urine, CSF (cerebrospinal fluid), and other fluids.

Following is a list of some laboratory tests and turnaround times for your reference.

| Test | Routine | Urgent | Emergent |
|------|---------|--------|----------|
| Acetaminophen | 24 hr | 3 hr | 90 min |
| Alkaline phosphate | 8 hr | na | na |
| Amylase | 8 hr | 2 hr | na |
| Barbiturates | 8 hr | 3 hr | 90 min |
| Bilirubin total | 8 hr | na | na |
| Calcium | 8 hr | 2 hr | 60 min |
| Chloride | 24 hr | na | na |
| CK (total) | 8 hr | 2 hr | na |
| CK-2 (MB) | 24 hr | na | na |
| Creatinine | 8 hr | 90 min | na |
| CSF — protein | na | 3 hr | 60 min |
| CSF — glucose | 3 hr | 90 min | na |
| Digoxin | 24 hr | na | na |
| Dilantin | 24 hr | na | na |
| Drug screen | 10 | na | na |
| Electrophoresis | 72 hr | na | na |
| Glucose | 8 hr | 2 hr | 60 min |
| HDL — C | 5 | na | na |
| Iron | 4 | na | na |
| Lithium | 2 | na | na |
| Magnesium | 8 hr | na | na |
| Occult blood | 24 hr | na | na |
| Osmolality | 8 hr | na | na |
| PH | 1 hr | 1 hr | 20 min |
| Phosphates | 8 hr | na | na |
| Potassium | 8 hr | 90 min | 60 min |
| Pregnancy test | 8 hr | 2 hr | 1 hr |
| Protein — CSF | na | 3 hr | 60 min |
| Protein — total | 8 hr | na | na |
| SGOT (AST) | 8 hr | na | na |
| Sodium | 8 hr | 2 hr | 60 min |
| Triglycerides | 8 hr | na | na |
| Urea (BUN) | 8 hr | 2 hr | na |
| Urate | 8 hr | na | na |
| Urinalysis | 8 hr | 60 min | na |

**Note:** Electrolytes = Sodium, Potassium, Chloride
Enzymes = SGOT, LDH, CK
BUN = Urea

The following information must be included when completing a biochemistry requisition.

Patient's name
Patient's birthdate
Patient's medical record number (if an in-patient)

**Illustration AB.1 Biochemistry I Requisition**

| RESULT | CHECK TEST | ✓ | REFERENCE RANGE |
|---|---|---|---|
| | UREA mmol/L | | 3.0 - 8.0 |
| | SODIUM (Na) mmol/L | | 135 - 146 |
| | POTASSIUM (K) mmol/L | | 3.5 - 5.0 |
| | CHLORIDE (CL) mmol/L | | 96 - 106 |
| | GLUCOSE mmol/L | | 4.0 - 6.0 |
| | | | |
| | CREATININE μmol/L | | M 60 - 120 F 50 - 100 |
| | BILIRUBIN μmol/L | | 3 - 20 |
| | DIRECT BILIRUBIN μmol/L | | < 6 |
| | MICROBILIRUBIN μmol/L | | < 240 |
| | CALCIUM mmol/L | | 2.20 - 2.60 |
| | PHOSPHATE mmol/L | | A 0.80 - 1.60 C 1.10 - 2.20 |
| | OSMOLALITY mmol/Kg | | 280 - 300 |
| | MAGNESIUM mmol/L | | 0.70 - 1.05 |
| | URATE μmol/L | | M < 450 F < 400 |
| | TOTAL PROTEIN g/L | | 60 - 80 |
| | ALBUMIN g/L | | 35 - 50 |
| | PROT. ELECT. | | |
| | | | |
| | | | |
| | | | |
| | AST (SGOT) U/L | | < 40 |
| | L.D.H. U/L | | 110 - 250 |
| | C K U/L | | M 25 - 210 F 25 - 175 |
| | CK-2 (MB) ng/mL | | |
| | RATIO CK-2(MB)÷TOTAL CK | | ≤ 0.05 |
| | ALK. PHOS. U/L | | A 35 - 120 C 100 - 360 |
| | GGTP U/L | | < 45 |
| | ACID PHOSPHATASE (TOTAL) U/L | | < 0.80 |
| | AMYLASE U/L | | < 130 |
| | | | |
| | ACETAMINOPHEN μmol/L | | 60 - 130 |
| | BARBITURATE SCREEN | | NEG. |
| | SALICYLATE mmol/L | | < 2.20 |
| | ETHANOL mmol/L | | < 1 |
| | DIGOXIN nmol/L | | 0.6 - 2.6 |
| | PHENYTOIN μmol/L | | 40 - 80 |
| | PHENOBARB μmol/L | | 65 - 172 |
| | CARBAMAZEPINE μmol/L | | 17 - 42 |
| | THEOPHYLLINE μmol/L | | 55 - 110 |
| | GENTAMICIN mg/L | | PRE < 2.0 POST 5.0 - 10.0 |
| | LITHIUM mmol/L | | 0.50 - 1.2 |

HOSP. NO.

PATIENT'S SURNAME

ADDRESS

DATE OF BIRTH — MO · DAY · YR.

SEX — ORIGINATING HOSPITAL

FAMILY/REFERRING PHYSICIAN(S)

MUNICIPALITY

GIVEN NAME/INITIALS

WARD ROOM

DATE — MO · DAY · YR

**BLOOD COLLECTION REQUEST:**

PLEASE CHECK

☐ SJH     ☐ COBOURG DISTRICT
☐ CMH     ☐ PORT HOPE & DISTRICT
☐ RMH

DATE:_____

☐ ROUTINE

☐ FASTING

☐ AT A SPECIFIC TIME

☐ AS SOON AS POSSIBLE/URGENT

☐ MEDICAL EMERGENCY

**ONLY THOSE TEST(S) HIGHLIGHTED BY RED BACKGROUND MAY BE ORDERED AS EMERGENCY/ASAP.**

LIST TEST(S) REQUIRED EMERGENCY/ASAP

CURRENT DIAGNOSIS:

ORDERING PHYSICIAN:

DATE & TIME OF LAST DOSE OF DRUG BEING REQUESTED:

| RESULT | TEST | REFERENCE RANGE |
|---|---|---|
| | | |
| | | |
| | | |
| | | |
| | | |

SPECIMEN COLLECTED

BY:                    TIME:

| DATE | TECH. |
|---|---|

PHONED TO:

BY:                    TIME:

DATE AND TIME RECEIVED IN LABORATORY

DATE AND TIME REPORT RELEASED

**BIOCHEMISTRY I     PETERBOROUGH CIVIC HOSPITAL**

**0505060**

**Illustration AB.2   Biochemistry II Requisition**

| RESULT | CHECK TEST | ✓ | REFERENCE RANGE |
|--------|-----------|---|-----------------|
| | h T.S.H. m U/L | | 0.45 - 5.0 |
| | THYROXINE(T₄) nmol/L | | 58 - 154 |
| | T-Uptake Units | | 0.72 - 1.24 |
| | FTI | | 64 - 154 |
| | T₃ (TOTAL) nmol/L | | 1.2 - 3.0 |
| | VIT. B₁₂ pmol/L | | 171 - 840 |
| | FOLATE (ser.) nmol/L | | 4.5 - 39 |
| | FOLATE (RBC) nmol/L | | 383 - 1600 |
| | CORTISOL A.M. nmol/L | | |
| | CORTISOL P.M. nmol/L | | |
| | | | |
| | | | |
| | IRON µmol/L | | 7 - 29 |
| | T I B C µmol/L | | M 47 - 72 F 47 - 80 |
| | IRON SATURATION | | 0.10 - 0.45 |
| | FERRITIN µg/L | | M 27 - 300 F 20 - 130 |
| | CHOLESTEROL mmol/L | | < 6.2 |
| | TRIGLYCERIDE mmol/L | | < 1.80 |
| | HDL - C mmol/L | | M 0.90 - 1.8 F 0.90 - 2.4 |
| | calculated LDL - C mmol/L | | < 4.1 |

GLUCOSE TOLERANCE   ☐ 75g   ☐ 50g screen   ☐ 100g

| | | |
|---|---|---|
| FASTING | | |
| ½ HOUR | | |
| 1 HOUR | | |
| 1½ HOURS | | |
| 2 HOURS | | |
| 3 HOURS | | |
| 4 HOURS | | |
| 5 HOURS | | |

FIO₂ _____   ☐ arterial   Pt. Temp
☐ capillary   ☐ venous   °C

| | | |
|---|---|---|
| pH | | a:7.35-7.45 v:7.32-7.42 |
| pCO₂ | | a:35-45 v:41-51 mmHg |
| pO₂ | | a:80-100 mmHg |
| ACTUAL HCO₃ | | 21 - 28 mmol/L |
| BASE | | ± 3.0 mmol/L |
| | | |

DATE _____   TECH. _____

PHONED TO: _____
BY: _____   TIME: _____

DATE AND TIME RECEIVED IN LABORATORY

DATE AND TIME REPORT RELEASED

HOSP. NO.

PATIENT'S SURNAME

ADDRESS

DATE OF BIRTH   MO   DAY   YR

SEX   ORIGINATING HOSPITAL

FAMILY/REFERRING PHYSICIAN(S)

MUNICIPALITY

WARD ROOM

GIVEN NAME/INITIALS

DATE   MO   DAY   YR

**BLOOD COLLECTION REQUEST:**

PLEASE CHECK
☐ SJH        ☐ COBOURG DISTRICT
☐ CMH        ☐ PORT HOPE & DISTRICT
☐ RMH

DATE: _____

☐ ROUTINE

☐ FASTING

☐ AT A SPECIFIC TIME _____ hr.

CURRENT DIAGNOSIS:

ORDERING PHYSICIAN:

| RESULT | TEST | REFERENCE RANGE |
|--------|------|-----------------|
| | | |
| | | |
| | | |
| | | |
| | | |
| | | |
| | | |
| | | |
| | | |
| | | |

SPECIMEN COLLECTED

BY: _____   TIME: _____

**BIOCHEMISTRY II      PETERBOROUGH CIVIC HOSPITAL**

**0505063**

**Illustration AB.3    Biochemistry III Requisition**

HOSP NO.

PATIENT'S SURNAME

ADDRESS

FAMILY/REFERRING PHYSICIAN(S)

DATE OF BIRTH

NO.  DAY  YR

SEX

ORIGINATING HOSPITAL

WARD ROOM

DATE

MO  DAY  YR

GIVEN NAME/INITIALS

MUNICIPALITY

**BLOOD COLLECTION REQUEST:**

PLEASE CHECK

☐ SJH        ☐ COBOURG DISTRICT
☐ CMH        ☐ PORT HOPE & DISTRICT
☐ RMH

DATE: _____

☐ ROUTINE

☐ FASTING

☐ AT A SPECIFIC TIME ____ hr.

SPECIMEN TYPE (IF NOT BLOOD):

DATE        TECH.

PHONED TO:

BY:        TIME:

DATE AND TIME RECEIVED IN LABORATORY

DATE AND TIME REPORT RELEASED

SPECIMEN COLLECTED

BY:        TIME:

**MISCELLANEOUS    PETERBOROUGH CIVIC HOSPITAL**

**BIOCHEMISTRY III        0505066**

Attending physician
Ordering physician
Tests required
Date and time of collection
Diagnosis or relevant clinical information

## Cytology

**Cytology** — Testing of gynecological cervical-vaginal specimens as well as a complete range of nongynecological specimens.

Following is a list of laboratory tests and turnaround times (if applicable) for your reference.

| Test | Routine | Urgent | Emergent |
|------|---------|--------|----------|
| Bronchial washing | | | |
| Broncho-alveolar lavage | | | |
| CMV — screen | | | |
| CSF (for malignant cells) | | | |
| Fine needle aspirates | | | |
| Gynecological smears | 5 | na | na |
| Pericardial fluid (for malignant cells) | | | |
| Peritoneal fluid (for malignant cells) | | | |
| Pleural fluid (for malignant cells) | | | |
| Sputum (for malignant cells) | | | |
| Urine (for malignant cells) | | | |

The following information must be included when completing a cytology requisition:

a.  Gynecological Requisition

Patient's name
Patient's birthdate
Ordering physician
Type of specimen
Date smear taken
Date of last menstrual period (LMP)
Relevant clinical information

b.  Nongynecological Requisition

Patient's name
Patient's birthdate
Ordering physician
Type of specimen
Date and time specimen taken
Relevant clinical information

**Illustration AB.4 Nongynecological Cytology Requisition**

USE BALL POINT PEN - YOU ARE MAKING MULTIPLE COPIES

☐ 175209

cash-drummond - HEALTH CARE DIVISION

**PLEASE PRESS FIRMLY ON A HARD SURFACE**

0505050

**PETERBOROUGH AND DISTRICT LABORATORY MEDICINE SERVICES**

**NON-GYNECOLOGICAL CYTOLOGY**

TEL. (705) 743-2121   EXT. 3073

☐ IN-PATIENT
☐ OUT-PATIENT
☐ REFERRED IN
☐ EMERG.

| LAB. NO. | NAME OF HOSPITAL |
|---|---|

PREVIOUS CYTOLOGY:   NO ☐   YES ☐

DATE/LAB. NO./DIAGNOSIS

HOSPITAL NO.                    WARD ROOM

PATIENT'S FULL NAME

ADDRESS                 CITY         POSTAL CODE

PREVIOUS PATHOLOGY:   NO ☐   YES ☐

OHIP NO.                    SEX | MARITAL STATUS | RELIGION

SUBSCRIBER'S NAME          OHIP INITIALS | RELATION PAT./ SUBSC.

SUBSCRIBER'S ADDRESS              POSTAL CODE

PREVIOUS SURGERY (SPECIFY)
NO ☐   YES ☐

IRRADIATION B
NO ☐   YES ☐

CHEMOTHERAPY:  NO ☐   YES ☐

DATE OF BIRTH   DAY | MO. | YR.   DOCTOR

DATE     DATE     AGENT

SPECIMEN TAKEN   DATE   TIME

SPECIMEN RECEIVED   DATE   TIME

**CLINICAL REMARKS & DIAGNOSIS**

| TYPE OF SPECIMEN | | SEROUS FL. | TRACHEO / BRONCHIAL (SPECIFY SITE; ONE COMPLETED REQUISITION PER EACH SPECIMEN) | FINE NEEDLE ASPIRATION (SPECIFY SITE; ONE COMPLETED REQUISITION PER EACH SPECIMEN) |
|---|---|---|---|---|
| SPUTUM | GENITO - URINARY | PLEURAL ☐ RT. ☐ LT. | | |
| FRESH | BLADDER < VOIDED ☐ CATHETERIZED ☐ | WASH ☐ | | |
| FIXED | WASH SPECIMEN ☐ | PERITONEAL ☐ | | |
| | URETERAL  RT. ☐  LT. ☐ | PERICARDIAL ☐ | OTHER | |

L E A V E   B L A N K

SPECIMEN DESCRIPTION

FOAMY ☐   CLEAR ☐   MUCOID ☐   CLOUDY ☐   BLOODY ☐   CLOTTED ☐   TISSUE FRAGMENTS ☐

MICROSCOPIC:   RBC   POLYS.   EOS.   LYMPHS.   PLASMAS   HISTIOS.   DUST CELLS

SUPERFICIAL SQUAMES < NUCLEATE / ANUCLEATE      IMMATURE SQUAMES < PARABASAL / METAPLASTIC

COLUMNAR CELLS      CILIATED CELLS      TRANSITIONAL EPITH.      MESOTHELIAL CELLS

BACTERIA      YEAST      PROTOZOA      PIGMENT      FOREIGN MATERIAL

**DIAGNOSIS & REMARKS**

NEGATIVE ☐   MILD ATYPIA ☐   INCONCLUSIVE ☐ (suggestive of malignancy; see below)   MALIGNANT CELLS ☐

**Illustration AB.5   Gynecological Cytology Requisition**

## USE BALL POINT PEN - YOU ARE MAKING MULTIPLE COPIES

R.L. CRAIN INC - HEALTH CARE DIVISION

### PLEASE PRESS FIRMLY ON A HARD SURFACE

0505049

PETERBOROUGH CIVIC HOSPITAL
DEPARTMENT OF LABORATORY MEDICINE
WELLER ST., PETERBOROUGH, ONT.  K9J 7C6
(705) 743-2121

☐ IN-PATIENT
☐ OUT-PATIENT
☐ REFERRED IN
☐ EMERG.

## GYNECOLOGICAL CYTOLOGY

**1** CYTOLOGY CONSULTATION
(PAP SMEAR)

LAB NO.

| A | DOCTOR | B | DATE SMEAR TAKEN | DAY | MO. | YR. |
|---|---|---|---|---|---|---|

PLEASE
PRINT
OR
TYPE

MISS. MRS. MS.    PATIENT'S LAST NAME (PRINT)                FIRST NAME

ADDRESS

PLEASE
COMPLETE
ITEMS
A - D

| C | PATIENT'S BIRTH DATE | D | PREVIOUS BIOPSY | | |
|---|---|---|---|---|---|
| | DAY   MO.   YR. | | DATE | LAB NO. | |

REPEAT EXAMINATION
WAS REQUESTED ☐

**2** CLINICAL REMARKS:

PREVIOUS CYTOLOGY DATE / NO.

CLINICAL DIAGNOSIS:

| **3** | AGE | PARA. | GRAV. | L.M.P. (FIRST DAY) | LAST PREGNANCY |
|---|---|---|---|---|---|
| | MENARCHE | CYCLE | DURATION | AMENORRHEA ☐   MENORRHAGIA ☐   DISCHARGE (TYPE) ☐ | |

**4** HORMONAL ℞
(SPECIFY TYPE, DOSAGE, DURATION)

**5** SPECIMEN TYPE:    VAGINAL ☐    CERVICAL ☐    COMBINED ☐    ENDOCERVICAL ☐
OTHER (SPECIFY) _____

MICROSCOPIC: ENDOCERVICAL CELLS        ENDOMETRIAL CELLS        POLYMORPHS
HISTIOCYTES        METAPLASTIC CELLS        R.B.C.        TRICHOMONAS        BACTERIA        YEAST

MATURATION INDEX:  PARABASAL        INTERMEDIATE        SUPERFICIAL

CYTO-HORMONAL
PATTERN
< CONSISTENT WITH DATA ☐
NOT CONSISTENT WITH DATA ☐

INTERP.
NOT
FEASIBLE ←
INSUFF. DATA ☐
ALTERED ☐
CERVICAL SMEAR ONLY ☐

☐ NO ABNORMAL CELLS        ☐ MILD DYSP.        ☐ MOD. DYSP.        ☐ SEVERE DYSP.        ☐ MALIGNANT CELLS (SEE BELOW)

☐ UNSATISFACTORY        ☐ MILD ATYPIA        ☐ INCONCLUSIVE (suggestive of malignancy; see below)

DIAGNOSIS & REMARKS

_____ CYTOTECHNOLOGIST                _____ CYTOPATHOLOGIST

C.H.P. < CONS. ☐
NOT CONS. ☐

_____ SCREENED BY

C.H.P.
INTERP
NOT
FEASIBLE
< INSUF. DATA ☐
ALTERED ☐
CX ONLY ☐

Haematology — Study of blood cells, bone marrow, and coagulation.

Following is a list of some of the laboratory tests and turnaround times for your reference.

a.   Haematology

| Test | Routine | Urgent | Emergent |
|------|---------|--------|----------|
| Leukocytes | 4 hr | 90 min | 10 min |
| Haemoglobin | 4 hr | 90 min | 10 min |
| Haematocrit | 4 hr | 90 min | 10 min |
| M.C.V. | 4 hr | 90 min | 10 min |
| Platelets | 4 hr | 90 min | 10 min |
| E.S.R. | 6 hr | na | na |
| Reticulocytes | 6 hr | na | na |
| Mono screen | 4 hr | 90 min | na |
| CSF count | 2 hr | 90 min | 60 min |
| CSF diff. | 3 hr | 2 hr | 90 min |
| Malarial parasites | 3 hr | 90 min | 60 min |
| Sickle screen | 3 hr | 90 min | 60 min |
| Kleihauer stain | 4 hr | na | na |
| Semen — fertility | 36 hr | na | na |
| Semen — post vasectomy | 6 hr | na | na |
| Bone marrow prep. | 24 hr | 2 hr | na |

b.   Haematology — Coagulation

| Test | Routine | Urgent | Emergent |
|------|---------|--------|----------|
| Prothrombin time | 4 hr | 90 min | 30 min |
| Pro-time — anticoagulant | 4 hr | 90 min | na |
| ACT P.T.T. — heparin | 4 hr | 90 min | 60 min |
| Bleeding time | 4 hr | na | na |
| Thrombin time | 4 hr | 2 hr | 60 min |
| Antithrombin III | 3 | na | na |
| Lupus anticoagulant | 4 hr | na | na |
| Protein C | 10 | na | na |
| Protein S | 10 | na | na |
| Platelet antibodies | 10 | na | na |
| Platelet count | 4 hr | 90 min | 10 min |

**Note:** CBC = Haemogram

The following information must be included when completing a haematology requisition:

Patient's name
Patient's birthdate
Ordering physician
Tests required
Date specimen to be taken
Relevant clinical information

**Illustration AB.6    Haematology Requisition**

# HAEMATOLOGY
### CODE DEFINITIONS FOR RESULTS

+ + + + + = Results over printable range
– – – – – = Results voted out
. . . . . = Incomplete computation occurred
R = Review results
\* = Abnormal condition caused other parameters to flag

L = Result is lower than lab action limit
H = Result is higher than lab action limit
+ = Result exceeds linearity
X = Abnormal condition
S = Suspect

184969

```
AFFIX
BAR CODE LABEL
HERE
```

| CASS. NO. | | | CHECK TEST REQUIRED | |
|---|---|---|---|---|
| TIME | | INITIALS | HEMOGRAM | ☐ |
| I.D. | | | (INCLUDES Lkcs, (WBC), Ercs (RBC) Hgb, Hct, MCV, MCH, MCHC, RDW, MPV Platelets) | |

| SA | OP. CODES | NORMAL VALUES | | |
|---|---|---|---|---|
| | | | DIFFERENTIAL | ☐ |
| | | Lkcs M 4.0-11.0 x 10⁹/L F 4.8-11.0 x 10⁹/L | CELL MORPHOLOGY | ☐ |
| • | | | E. S. R. | ☐ |
| • | | Ercs M 4.5-6.0 x 10¹²/L F 4.0-5.5 x 10¹²/L | RETICULOCYTES | ☐ |
| • | | Hb M 130-175 g/L F 120-155 g/L | MORPH. REPORT | |
| • | | Hct M 0.40-0.54 F 0.37-0.47 | | |
| • | | MCV M 80-100 fL F 80-100 fL | | |
| • | | MCH M 27.0-32.0 pg F 27.0-32.0 pg | | |
| | | MCHC M 320-360 g/L F 320-360 g/L | | |
| • | | RDW M 11.5-14.5 % F 11.5-14.5 % | | |
| • | | Plts M 150-450 x 10⁹/L F 150-450 x 10⁹/L | | |
| | | ESR M 0-10 mm/h F 0-20 mm/h | | |
| | | RETICS M 20-100 x 10⁹/L F 20-100 x 10⁹/L | | |

| | NORMAL VALUES | W | | | | |
|---|---|---|---|---|---|---|
| • | MPV M 8.9 ± 1.5 F 8.9 ± 1.5 | | LYMPHO-PENIA | | LYMPHO-CYTOSIS | |
| • | LYMPHS M 0.20-0.45 F 0.20-0.45 | W | NEUTRO-PENIA | | NEUTRO-PHILIA | |
| • | MONO M 0.02-0.10 F 0.02-0.10 | B | ATYP LYMPHS | | MONO-CYTOSIS | |
| • | NEUT M 0.40-0.75 F 0.40-0.75 | C | BLASTS | | EOSINO-PHILIA | |
| • | EOS M 0.01-0.06 F 0.01-0.06 | | IMMGRAN BANDS | | BASO-PHILIA | |
| • | BASOS M <0.02 F <0.02 | | NRBC | | ANISO | |
| • | LYMPH # M 1.5-3.5 x 10⁹/L F 1.5-3.5 x 10⁹/L | R B C | POIK | | MICRO | |
| • | MONO # M 0.2-0.8 x 10⁹/L F 0.2-0.8 x 10⁹/L | | RBC FRAG | | MACRO | |
| • | NEUT # M 2.0-7.5 x 10⁹/L F 2.0-7.5 x 10⁹/L | | RBC AGG | | HYPO | |
| • | EOS # M 0.04-0.4 x 10⁹/L F 0.04-0.4 x 10⁹/L | P L T | PLT CLUMPS | | LARGE PLTS | |
| • | BASOS # M <0.1 x 10⁹/L F <0.1 x 10⁹/L | | GIANT PLTS | | SMALL PLTS | |

| DATE/TIME REPORTED | TIME SPECIMEN RECEIVED |
|---|---|

| O.R. | DATE | TIME |
|---|---|---|

RESULTS PHONED

BY:                    TIME:

TO:

SPECIMEN TO BE TAKEN
M   D   YR.   TIME   INITIALS
ROUTINE
MEDICAL EMERGENCY
SPECIMEN COLLECTED
TIME:
BY:

CLINICAL INFORMATION

PATIENT'S LAST NAME (PRINT)

PATIENT'S FIRST NAME

ADDRESS

DOCTOR

## PETERBOROUGH HOSPITALS
0505056 JF REV. 3/95          PCH ☐     SJH&HC ☐

**Illustration AB.7    Haematology 2 Requisition**

REORDER FROM *cain-drummond* HEALTH CARE SYSTEMS

# HAEMATOLOGY 2

| CHECK TEST REQUIRED | RESULT | REFERENCE VALUES |
|---|---|---|
| ☐ PROTHROMBIN TIME | TIME<br>I.N.R. | 11.5 – 13.5 secs. |
| ☐ A.P.T.T. | | 25 – 40 secs. |
| ☐ THROMBIN TIME | | 11 – 15 secs. |
| ☐ BLEEDING TIME | | < 9 MINS. |
| ☐ D-DIMER(FDP$_3$) | | < 0.25 mg/L |
| ☐ OTHER COAGULATION | | |
| ☐ MONO SCREEN | | NEGATIVE |
| ☐ SICKLE SCREEN | | NEGATIVE |
| ☐ GLYCOSYLATED HAEMOGLOBIN (HB AIC) | | NON DIABETIC 3.5 - 6.1 %<br>CONTROLLED DIABETIC 6.2 – 9.0 %<br>UNCONTROLLED DIABETIC > 9.0 % |
| ☐ OTHER (Specify) | | |

LABORATORY COMMENTS

DATE/TIME REPORTED

TIME SPECIMEN RECEIVED

O.R.    DATE    TIME

RESULTS PHONED

BY:    TIME:

TO:

SPECIMEN TO BE TAKEN

M    D    YR.    TIME

INITIALS

ROUTINE

MEDICAL EMERGENCY

SPECIMEN COLLECTED

TIME:

BY:

PATIENT'S LAST NAME (PRINT)

PATIENT'S FIRST NAME

ADDRESS

DOCTOR

CLINICAL INFORMATION

**PETERBOROUGH HOSPITALS**
0505057

PCH ☐    SJH&HC ☐

# Histology

**Histology** — Routine surgical pathology reporting.

Following is a list of some specimens that are analyzed in the histological division of a laboratory and laboratory turnaround times for your reference.

| Test | Turnaround Time |
| --- | --- |
| Intra-operative consultations<br>Prebooked elective<br>Nonprebooked (elective or otherwise) | 15–20 min variable |
| Surgical pathology (without special stains, consultations, etc.) | 24–36 hr |
| Fresh tissue for possible malignant lymphoma | 24 hr<br>48 hr (depending on time received by lab) |
| Estrogen receptors | 2 wk |
| Renal biopsies | May be sent to another facility |
| Muscle biopsies | May be sent to another facility |
| Unstained slides | 1–3 wk |
| Mammographically directed biopsies | 24–48 hr<br>48–72 hr (depending on time received by lab) |

The following information must be included when completing a histology requisition:

Patient's full name
Patient's birthdate
Sex
Type of specimen
Anatomic location
Pertinent history, including where and when previous diagnosis
was made.
Date of surgery
Preoperative diagnosis
Postoperative diagnosis
Submitting physician or surgeon

**Illustration AB.8**    Surgical Pathology Requisition

## PLEASE PRESS FIRMLY
### ↓ DO NOT LABEL REQUISITION ABOVE THIS PERFORATION ↓

| PETERBOROUGH CIVIC HOSPITAL ☐ | ST. JOSEPH'S GENERAL HOSPITAL, PETERBOROUGH ☐ | DISTRICT HOSPITALS ☐ |
|---|---|---|

**SURGICAL PATHOLOGY REQUISITION**    EMERGENCY DEPT. ☐    SURGICAL OUTPATIENT ☐    OTHER OUTPATIENT ☐    LAB. NO.

HOSP. NO.     WARD ROOM     DATE OF OPERATION

**SPECIMENS** (SPECIFY ANATOMIC SITE OF ORIGIN FOR EACH)

PATIENT'S SURNAME     GIVEN NAME/INITIALS

1. _____

ADDRESS     MUNICIPALITY

2. _____

3. _____

DATE OF BIRTH    SEX    ORIGINATING HOSPITAL

4. _____

DAY   MO.   YR.

| PREVIOUS PATHOLOGY | PATH./CYT. NO. | LMP (first day) |
|---|---|---|
| YES ☐   NO ☐ | | |
| PREVIOUS CYTOLOGY | | |

SURGEON     DATE/TIME SPECIMEN REC'D.

FAMILY/REFERRING PHYSICIAN(S)

| | RADIATION | CHEMOTHERAPY | HORMONAL |
|---|---|---|---|
| ℞ | YES ☐   NO ☐ | YES ☐   NO ☐ | YES ☐   NO ☐ |

PRE-OP DIAGNOSIS

POST-OP/QUICK SECTION DIAGNOSIS

CLINICAL HISTORY

GROSS DESCRIPTION (LAB USE ONLY)

0505018 8/87

# Microbiology

**Microbiology** — Testing and identification of bacteria, fungi, parasites, and viruses in patients' specimens.

Following is a list of some of the laboratory tests and turnaround times for your reference.

a.   Microbiology (Routine)

| Test | Turnaround Time |
| --- | --- |
| Abscess for C&S (culture & sensitivity) | 48 hr |
| Acid fast bacilli | 24 hr |
| Auger suction — C&S | 48 hr |
| Bile — C&S | 48 hr |
| Blood culture — C&S | 72 hr |
| Blood culture — mycobacteria | 8 hr |
| Bronchial washing — C&S | 48 hr |
| Bronchial washing — fungus | 4 wk |
| Bronchial washing — T.B. | 8 wk |
| Catheter tip — C&S | 48 hr |
| Chlamydia | 3–6 d |
| Corneal scrapings | 48 hr |
| CSF — C&S | 72 hr |
| CSF — routine gram stain | 24 hr |
| Fluid (body) — C&S | 48 hr |
| Genital swab — C&S | 48 hr |
| Genital swab — GC culture | 72 hr |
| Genital swab — gonorrhea | 72 hr |
| Gram stain — routine | 24 hr |
| Lung washing — G&S | 48 hr |
| Lung washing — fungus | 4 wk |
| Lung washing — T.B. | 8 wk |
| Mouth & gums | 48 hr |
| Mycology (skin scraping/hair) | 4 wk |
| Mycoplasma | 10–14 d |
| Nails — fungus culture | 4 wk |
| Nose — C&S | 48 hr |
| Parasitology | 7 d |
| Pinworm | 1 d |
| Rectal culture | 72 hr |
| Rectal culture — gonorrhea | 72 hr |
| Skin — C&S | 48 hr |
| Skin scrapings (fungus culture) | 4 wk |
| Stool — C&S | 72 hr |
| Stool — O&P | 7 d |
| Stool — RSV | 24 hr |
| Stool — Clostridium difficile | 48 hr |
| Throat | 48 hr |
| Throat washing — (virus) | 7–10 d |
| Tissue | 72 hr |
| Tuberculosis — respiratory | 8 wk |
| Tuberculosis — urine | 8 wk |
| Urine — culture & colony count | 48 hr |

b.   Microbiology (Medical Emergency Requests)

| Test | Turnaround Time |
| --- | --- |
| Blood gram stain | < 30 min |
| C.S.F. and body fluid — gram stain | < 30 min |
| Lower respiratory gram stain | < 30 min |
| Wound gram stain | < 30 min |

The following information must be included when completing a micro-biology requisition:

Patient's name
Patient's birthdate
Patient's medical record number (if an in-patient)
Attending physician
Ordering physician
Tests required
Date and time of collection
Diagnosis or relevant clinical information
Antibiotics currently being given or preferred by physician

**Illustration AB.9    Microbiology Requisition**

LAB. NO.

PETERBOROUGH HOSPITALS:

PETERBOROUGH CIVIC

ST. JOSEPH'S HOSPITAL & HEALTH CENTRE

DISTRICT HOSPITALS (specify) _____

HOSP. NO.

ROOM

[ ] IN-PATIENT          [ ] OUT-PATIENT          [ ] REFERRED-IN

PATIENT'S SURNAME          GIVEN NAME/INITIALS

NURSE:          DATE/TIME COLLECTED:

SPECIMENS (Specify Anatomic Site)

DATE OF BIRTH (M D Y)

RELEVANT CLINICAL INFORMATION:          ANTIBIOTIC GIVEN/PREFERRED

FAMILY/REFERRING PHYSICIAN(S)

**TEST REQUESTED:** [ ] CULTURE     [ ] G.C. CULTURE     [ ] TB

[ ] FUNGUS          [ ] PARASITES          [ ] OTHER (Specify)

## FOR LABORATORY USE ONLY

SPECIMEN REC'D.: (Date, Time, Initials)

SPECIMEN DESCRIPTION

[ ] NON SATISFACTORY     [ ] INADEQUATELY LABELLED     [ ] SALIVA ONLY

CULTURED.: (Date, Tech, Initials)

[ ] SPECIMEN LEAKING     [ ] REPEAT SPECIMEN REQUESTED     [ ] UNPRESERVED

RESULTS RELEASED (DATE & TIME)

[ ] SPECIMEN / ORGANISM REFERRED OUT

URINE COLONY COUNT     [ ] < 10 X $10^6$/L     [ ] 10 – 100 X $10^6$/L     [ ] > 100 X $10^6$/L

### ORGANISM(S) / SENSITIVITY *

1.

2.

3.                    3.  2.  1.

PENICILLIN

AMPICILLIN

OXACILLIN / METHICILLIN

ERYTHROMYCIN

CEFAZOLIN / CEPHALEXIN

TETRACYCLINE

BACTRIM / SEPTRA

GENTAMICIN / TOBRAMYCIN

AMIKACIN

CARBENICILLIN / PIPERACILLIN

NORFLOXACIN / CIPROFLOXACIN

NITROFURANTOIN

BETA-LACTAMASE

### MICROSCOPIC EXAMINATION          [ ] UNCENTRIFUGED SAMPLE

[ ] NO CELLS SEEN                    AFB - ABSENT/PRESENT

_____ PUS CELLS          _____ EPITHELIAL CELLS          _____ RBC

KOH PREP-MYCELIAL FILAMENTS - ABSENT PRESENT

_____ GRAM POSITIVE COCCI

_____ GRAM NEGATIVE DIPLOCOCCI   INTRA / EXTRACELLULAR

_____ GRAM NEGATIVE BACILLI          TRICHOMONAS - ABSENT PRESENT     CLUE CELLS - ABSENT PRESENT

_____ GRAM POSITIVE BACILLI

_____ NO BACTERIA SEEN          _____ YEAST          [ ] NO PARASITES SEEN

### CULTURE REPORT          [ ] REQUEST REPEAT SPECIMEN

[ ] NO GROWTH IN 24/48/72 HR.     [ ] NORMAL FLORA     [ ] NON-SIGNIFICANT GROWTH

[ ] MIXED FLORA     [ ] SKIN FLORA ISOLATED     [ ] FECAL FLORA ISOLATED

[ ] NO GROWTH OF N. gonorrhoeae          [ ] NO GROWTH AFTER _____ DAYS

### STOOL CULTURE

[ ] NO SALMONELLA, SHIGELLA, YERSINIA, E. COLI 0157 : H7 or CAMPYLOBACTER ISOLATED

REPORT PHONED BY:          DATE          TIME          REPORT RECEIVED BY:

LABORATORY COMMENTS:

DATE          TECHNOLOGIST

| * GROWTH | SENSITIVITY | MICROSCOPIC CELLS / HPF |
|---|---|---|
| 3 + Heavy | S = Sensitive | FEW < 1 / HPF |
| 2 + Moderate | I = Intermediate | 1 + 1-5 / HPF |
| 1 + Light | R = Resistant | 2 + 6-10 / HPF |
| | | 3 + > 10 / HPF |

[ ] PRELIMINARY REPORT          [ ] FINAL REPORT

FORM # 0505 036 J F

**MICROBIOLOGY REQUISITION**

**Blood Bank** — Performs pretransfusion compatibility testing before blood is issued. Serological testing is also performed to predict obstetrical sensitization and to aid in the diagnosis of certain immune disorders.

Following is a list of some laboratory tests and turnaround times for your reference.

| Test | Routine | Urgent | Emergent |
|---|---|---|---|
| Blood Grouping — ABO | 24 hr | 10 min | 10 min |
| — Rh | 24 hr | 10 min | 10 min |
| — other phenotypes | 24 hr | 30 min | 30 min |
| Antibody investigation — screen | 24 hr | 60 min | 60 min |
| — identification | 24 hr | 60 min | 60 min |
| Complex antibody identification | 4 d | na | na |
| Blood group & antibody screen | | | |
| T&S (type & screen) (Pre-op, prenatal, & poss. transfusion) | 24 hr | 60 min | 60 min |
| Investigation of autoimmune haemolytic anaemia | 24 hr | 2 hr | 20 min |
| Direct antiglobulin test | 24 hr | 2 hr | 20 min |
| Neonatal testing (D.A.T., ABO, & Rh) | 24 hr | 2 hr | 60 min |
| Compatability testing (ind. T&S) | 24 hr | 90 min | 60 min |
| Investigation of transfusion reaction (nonhaemolytic) | 24 hr | na | na |
| Immediate spin crossmatch after type & screen | na | 10 min | 5 min |
| Issue uncrossmatched group O blood (trauma) | na | na | 5 min |
| Group patient and issue uncrossmatched group compatible blood | na | na | 10 min |
| Investigation of suspected haemolytic transfusion reaction | na | 2 hr | 20 min |

The following information must be included when completing a blood bank requisition:

Patient's surname and given name (no abbreviation)

Medical record number for in-patients and birthdate for out-patients

Location

Sex

Ordering physician

Priority of red cell transfusion

Clinical information or surgical procedure "type and screen" — check this area except when there is an order to transfuse the products, when the MSBOS (maximum surgical blood order schedule) calls for a crossmatch, or when it is an emergency situation.

**Illustration AB.10    Blood Bank Test/Product Request**

## PETERBOROUGH HOSPITALS

**BLOOD BANK** TEST / PRODUCT REQUEST

☐ CIVIC    ☐ SJH & HC    ☐ MINDEN    ☐ HALIBURTON

| ORDERED BY DR. _ _ _ _ _ _ _ _ _ _ _ _ _ _ _ _ _ | | | | | ☐ ROUTINE |
| TIME | MONTH | DAY | YEAR | INITIAL | ☐ PRE-OP |
| | | | | | ☐ ✱ URGENT |

☐ TYPE AND SCREEN (RESERVE SERUM)

     OR

☐ CROSSMATCH _ _ _ _ _ _ _ _ UNITS PACKED CELLS

☐ SUPPLY OTHER PRODUCTS

☐ _ _ _ _ _ FFP        ☐ _ _ _ _ PLATELET/CONC.

☐ OTHER ✱
  (specify) _ _ _ _ _ _ _ _ _ _ _ _ _ _ _ _ _ _ _ _ _ _

✱ CHECK LAB/NURSING MANUAL FOR AVAILABILITY

ARM BAND CHECKED, BLOOD COLLECTED AND TUBES LABELLED BY

|  | TIME | DATE (M, D, YR.) |
| WHEN REQUIRED | | |

CLINICAL INFORMATION / OR OPERATION PLANNED

**N.B.**

| | | YES | DATE | NO | UNKNOWN |
| PREVIOUS < | TRANSFUSIONS | ☐ | | ☐ | ☐ |
| | PREGNANCIES | ☐ | | ☐ | ☐ |

TIME

| MO. | DAY | YR |
DATE STAMP

## ✱IN URGENT / EMERGENT SITUATIONS CALL BLOOD BANK STATING DEGREE OF URGENCY.

RECEIVED IN LABORATORY

**BLOOD BANK USE ONLY**

PREVIOUS GROUP _ _ _ _ _ _ _ _ _ _ SCREEN _ _ _ _ _ _ _ _ _ _

COMMENTS / INSTRUCTIONS
(over if necessary)

CURRENT GROUP _ _ _ _ _ _ _ _ _ SCREEN _ _ _ _ _ _ _ _ _

COMMENTS / INSTRUCTIONS
(over if necessary)

TESTED BY:        CHK. BY:

JF 0505037 (4/94)        TEST SITE ☐ CIVIC    ☐ SJH & HC

### OTHER IMMUNOHAEMATOLOGY TESTS

☐ DIRECT ANTIGLOBULIN TEST (DAT) ADULT

☐ COLD AGGLUTININS (KEEP SPEC. AT 37°C)

☐ CORD BLOOD GROUP AND COOMBS (DAT)

☐ CHECK FOR Rh IMMUNE GLOBULIN (Rh Neg. OR UNKNOWN)

☐ OTHER
  (specify)

**TOP COPY (IN PATIENTS) LEFT AT NURSING STATION AFTER SIGNED/DATED BY PHLEBOTOMIST**

**NOTE:**    *EXCEPT IN EMERGENCY, REQUISITIONS SHOULD BE OUT NOT LATER THAN THE 1330 COLLECTION ON THE DAY BEFORE BLOOD IS REQUIRED.*

## Computerized Reports

Many laboratory facilities now process their reports by computer. The three pages in Appendix E at the end of the book illustrate computerized forms for hematology, chemistry, and serology reports. You will notice the barcodes on the reports. These are used to identify the type of test requested. The patient's name, date of birth, and ordering physician must appear in the top left corner of each report. The information would be handwritten or stamped with the addressograph card referred to in Chapter 11.

# Appendix C: Pharmacology

Following is a list of the most commonly prescribed drugs by their generic names and brand names (where available) for your reference.

**Antibacterials** — Agents that have properties to destroy or suppress growth or reproduction of bacteria.

| Generic Name | Trade Name |
|---|---|
| Amoxicillin/potassium clavulanate | Clavulin |
| Azithromycin | Zithromax |
| Bacampicillin hydrochloride | Penglobe |
| Cefaclor | Ceclor |
| Cefixime | Suprax |
| Cefuroxime axetil | Ceftin |
| Cephalexin monohydrate | Keflex |
| Ciprofloxacin hydrochloride | Cipro |
| Clarithromycin | Biaxin |
| Doxycycline | Vibramycin |
| Erythromycin | Eryc, E-Mycin |
| Erythromycin estolate | Ilosone |
| Erythromycin ethylsuccinate | EES |
| Erythromycin ethylsuccinate | Pediazole |
| Metronidazole | Flagyl |
| Norfloxacin | Noroxin |
| Pivampicillin | Pondocillin |
| Phenoxymethyl penicillin | PenVee |
| Trimethoprim-sulfamethoxazole | Septra, Bactrim |

**Anticoagulants** — Agents that act to prevent clotting of blood.

| Generic Name | Trade Name |
|---|---|
| Warfarin sodium | Coumadin |
| A.S.A. | — |

**Antihypertensives** — Agents that control blood pressure.

| Generic Name | Trade Name |
|---|---|
| Acebutolol hydrochloride | Sectral, Monitan |
| Amiloride hydrochloride | Midamor |
| Amlodipine besylate | Norvasc |
| Atenolol | Tenormin |
| Captopril | Capoten |
| Diltiazem hydrochloride | Cardizem |
| Enalapril maleate | Vasotec |
| Fosinopril sodium | Monopril |
| Furosemide | Lasix |
| Metoprolol tartrate | Lopressor, Betaloc |
| Nifedipine | Adalat |
| Sotalol hydrochloride | Sotacor |
| Spironolactone | Aldactone |
| Triamterene | Dyrenium |
| Verapamil hydrochloride | Isoptin |

## Cardiac Therapy

| Generic Name | Trade Name |
| --- | --- |
| Digoxin | Lanoxin |
| Disopyramide | Rythmodan |
| Hydrochlorothiazide | Hydrodiuril |
| Isosorbide dinitrate | Isordil |

## Lipid Lowering Agents

(Lipid: heterogenous group of fats and fatlike substances)

| Generic Name | Trade Name |
| --- | --- |
| Cholestyramine resin | Questran |
| Lovastatin | Mevacor |

## Peripheral Vascular Disease Therapy

| Generic Name | Trade Name |
| --- | --- |
| Pentoxifylline | Trental |

## Analgesics — Agents that relieve pain.

| Generic Name | Trade Name |
| --- | --- |
| Diclofenac sodium | Voltaren |
| Flunarizine hydrochloride | Sibelium |
| Hydrocodone bitartrate | Hycodan |
| Hydromorphone hydrochloride | Dilaudid |
| Ibuprofen | Motrin |
| Ketorolac tromethamine | Toradol |
| Ketoprofen | Orudis |
| Morphine | Doloral Morphitec |
| Naproxen | Naprosyn |
| Naproxen sodium | Anaprox |
| Oxycodone | Percodan/Percocet |
| Sumatriptan succinate | Imitrex |

## Anticonvulsants — Agents that control seizures.

| Generic Name | Trade Name |
| --- | --- |
| Carbamazepine | Tegretol |
| Clobazam | Frisium |
| Clonazepam | Rivotril |
| Divalproex sodium | Epival |
| Gabapentin | Neurotin |
| Lorazepam | Ativan |
| Nitrazepam | Mogadon |
| Phenytoin | Dilantin |
| Valproic acid | Depakene |
| Vigabatrim | Sabril |

**Antidepressants** — Agents that prevent or relieve depression.

| Generic Name | Trade Name |
| --- | --- |
| Amoxapine | Ascendin |
| Fluvoxamine maleate | Luvox |
| Fluoxetine hydrochloride | Prozac |
| Doxepin hydrochloride | Sinequan |
| Moclobemide | Manerix |
| Paroxetine hydrochloride | Paxil |
| Sertraline | Zoloft |
| Trazodone | Desyrel |
| Trimipramine | Surmontil |

## Antiparkinsonian Agents

| Generic Name | Trade Name |
| --- | --- |
| Beniztropine hydrochloride | Cogentin |

**Antipsychotics** — Agents effective in the management of mood control.

| Generic Name | Trade Name |
| --- | --- |
| Chlorpromazine | Largactil |
| Haloperidol | Haldol |
| Perphenazine | Trilaton |
| Prochlorperazine | Stemetil |
| Risperidone | Risperdal |

**Anxiolytics** — Agents that relieve feelings of apprehension, uncertainty, and fear appearing without apparent stimulus.

| Generic Name | Trade Name |
| --- | --- |
| Alprazolam | Xanax |
| Chlordiazepoxide hydrochloride | Librium |
| Diazepam | Valium |
| Lorazepam | Ativan |
| Oxazepam | Serax |

## Hypnotics and Sedatives

| Generic Name | Trade Name |
| --- | --- |
| Chloral hydrate | Novo-chlorhydrate |
| Nitrazepam | Mogadon |
| Temazepam | Restoril |
| Triazolam | Halcion |

**Mania Therapy** — Agents that control mood swings.

| Generic Name | Trade Name |
| --- | --- |
| Lithium carbonate | Carbolith, Duralith |

## Asthma Therapy

| Generic Name | Trade Name |
| --- | --- |
| Beclomethasone dipropionate | Beclovent, Becloforte |
| Budesonide | Pulmicort |
| Hydrocortisone sodium succinate | SoluCortef |
| Ipratropium bromide | Atrovent |
| Ketotifen fumarate | Zaditen |
| Methylprednisolone sodium succinate | Solu-Medrol |
| Oxtriphylline | Choledyl |
| Prednisone | Deltasone |
| Salbutamol sulfate | Ventolin |
| Terbutaline sulfate | Bricanyl |
| Theophylline | TheoDur |

## Cough and Cold Preparations

| Generic Name | Trade Name |
| --- | --- |
| Dextromethorphan hydrobromide | DM |
| Guaifenesin | Robitussin |
| Naphazoline hydrochloride | Vasacon-A |
| Pseudoephedrine hydrochloride | Sudafed |
| Xylometazoline hydrochloride | Otrivin |

# Appendix D: Reference Sources

As a medical administrative assistant, you will need to be familiar with a wide range of reference material. You have already used some medical reference materials such as medical dictionaries, *The Medical Word Book*, and the *Compendium of Pharmaceuticals and Specialties* (CPS). There are, however, literally hundreds more books of various types that you may use from time to time.

**Dictionaries**

You are, of course, now familiar with the standard medical dictionary. There are many such dictionaries available, from small pocket-size to large multivolume editions. There are also many dictionaries available by specialty area. Some other types you should be familiar with are inverted dictionaries (where the definition is given in alphabetical order, followed by the appropriate medical term) and dictionaries of abbreviations and acronyms, syndromes, diseases, hospital terminology, and so on.

**Directories**

A directory is basically a list, and there are many lists available. The *Canadian Medical Directory*, published annually, lists most doctors practising in Canada. There are also international, national, and local directories of health organizations and institutions, hospitals, social agencies, and health care professionals. A directory can be anything from a large bound publication on a worldwide scale to a small pamphlet put out by your local association of pharmacists.

**Drug Publications**

There are several varieties of publications dealing with drugs, but the one most widely used in Canada is the *Compendium of Pharmaceuticals and Specialties* (CPS). This book lists drugs by generic name (penicillin), trade name or monograph (Valium), manufacturer, type (antihistamines, oral), and so on. You will find a CPS in every practising physician's office. The CPS is updated and published annually.

The CPS is divided into sections of different-colour pages as follows:

| | |
|---|---|
| Pink | Classification System Index |
| Green | Drug Listing of Brand and Nonproprietary Names |
| Glossy White | A picture guide to assist in the identification of products |
| Yellow | Manufacturers' Index |
| Mauve | Clinical information including: |
| |     Poison Control Centres |
| |     Selected Resource Agencies and Literature |
| |     Nonmedicinal Ingredients |
| |     Clinical Monitoring |
| Blue | Patient Information |

White    An alphabetical list of each drug by name, including the chemical make-up of the drug, its use, indications, and contraindications, any precautions necessary when administering the drug, adverse effects, overdose symptoms and treatment, and appropriate dosages.

## MOH Fee Schedules/ Diagnostic Codes

Published by the Ontario Ministry of Health, the Fee Schedules and Diagnostic Code Listings booklet can be obtained at the Ontario Government Book Store.

## Handbooks for the Administrative Assistant

Every medical administrative assistant should have at least one handbook close by for quick reference. There are several available in your school library, and you should take time to browse through them to familiarize yourself with the type of information that is at your disposal. If your office does not have at least one medical handbook available for your use, you should get one and use it frequently.

Whether you work in a one-doctor office or in a large hospital or clinic, you will be required from time to time to research certain information for your employer. The more familiar you are with the types of reference sources available to you, the more efficiently you will be able to find the information you need. Your school library has a large selection of medical reference material, and your reference librarian will be pleased to show you where this material can be found.

## A List of Some Important Reference Sources

*Dorland's Medical Dictionary*
Publisher: W.B. Saunders Company
     55 Horner Ave.
     Toronto, Ontario
     M8Z 4X6

*Taber's Cyclopedic Medical Dictionary*
Publisher: McGraw-Hill Ryerson Limited
     300 Water St.
     Whitby, Ontario
     L1N 9B6

*Canadian Medical Directory*
Publisher: Southam Business Communications Limited
     1450 Don Mills Road
     Don Mills, Ontario
     M3B 2X7

*The Medical Word Book* by Sheila B. Sloane
Publisher: W.B. Saunders Company
     address as above

*The Surgical Word Book* by Claudia Tessier
Publisher: W.B. Saunders Company
      address as above

*Medical Record Management* by Edna K. Huffman
Publisher: Physician's Record Company
      Chicago, Illinois

*Medical Transcription Guide*
Publisher: W.B. Saunders Company
      address as above

*Dictionary of Medical Acronyms & Abbreviations*
Publisher: C.V. Mosby Co.
      5240 Finch Avenue East
      Unit #1
      Scarborough, Ontario
      M1S 4P2

*Physician and Hospital Index*
Publisher: Ministry of Health

*A Syllabus for a Surgeon's Secretary* by Jeannette A. Szulec
Publisher: Medical Arts Publishing Company
      P.O. Box 8627
      Kensington Station
      Detroit, Michigan
      48224

*Compendium of Pharmaceuticals and Specialties* (CPS)
Publisher: Canadian Pharmaceutical Association
      101 – 1815 Alta Vista Drive
      Ottawa, Ontario
      K1G 3Y6

*Structure and Function in Man*
Publisher: W.B. Saunders Company
      address as above

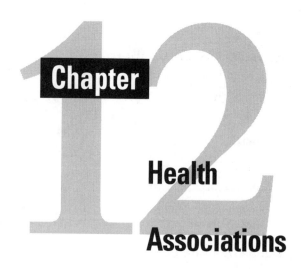

# Chapter 12

# Health

# Associations

**Chapter Outline**

- Associations of Importance to Medical Administrative Assistants

- Assignment 12.1
- Code of Ethics

**Learning Objectives**

To be aware of
- the existence of codes of ethics
- medical associations and organizations in Canada
- the College of Physicians and Surgeons
- the organizational structures of these associations

The range of health associations and organizations across Canada is extensive. There are associations relating to hospitals, physicians, medical secretaries, nurses, physiotherapists, nursing homes, health records administrators, diseases, and so on. It would be difficult to discuss in detail the purposes and bylaws of each association, so we will not do so. A few of the key associations will be dealt with later in the chapter.

## Codes of Ethics

Most health associations are guided by a code of ethics. An example is the Canadian Medical Association's Code of Ethics, which appears at the conclusion of this chapter.

## Organizational Structure

The organizational structures of health associations and organizations differ with the specific group. However, many associations have national, provincial, and regional branches. For example, many physicians in Canada are members of the Canadian Medical Association (CMA). The CMA is a national organization with twelve provincial medical association branches. But these

**Illustration 12.1    Provincial Health Associations in Canada**

CANADIAN MEDICAL ASSOCIATION
P.O. Box 8650
Ottawa, Ontario
K1G 0G8
(613) 731-9331

ALBERTA MEDICAL ASSOCIATION
9901-108 Street
Suite 300
Edmonton, Alberta
T5K 1G8
(403) 423-2295

BRITISH COLUMBIA MEDICAL ASSOCIATION
115-1665 West Broadway
Vancouver, British Columbia
V6J 1X1
(604) 736-5551

MANITOBA MEDICAL ASSOCIATION
125 Sherbrooke Street
Winnipeg, Manitoba
R3C 2B5
(204) 786-7565

NEW BRUNSWICK MEDICAL SOCIETY
176 York Street
Fredericton, New Brunswick
E3B 3N8
(506) 458-8860

NEWFOUNDLAND MEDICAL ASSOCIATION
164 MacDonald Drive
St. John's, Newfoundland
A1A 4B3
(709) 726-7424

NORTHWEST TERRITORIES MEDICAL ASSOCIATION
P.O. Box 1559
Yellowknife, Northwest Territories
X1A 2P2
(403) 473-5881

MEDICAL SOCIETY OF NOVA SCOTIA
6080 Young Street
Suite 305
Halifax, Nova Scotia
B3K 5L2
(902) 453-0205

ONTARIO MEDICAL ASSOCIATION
525 University Avenue
Suite 300
Toronto, Ontario
M5G 3K7
1-800-268-7215

PRINCE EDWARD ISLAND MEDICAL SOCIETY
279 Richmond Street
Charlottetown, Prince Edward Island
C1A 1S7
(902) 892-7527

QUEBEC MEDICAL ASSOCIATION
1010 Sherbrooke Street West
Suite 1010
Montreal, Quebec
H3A 2R7
(514) 282-1443

SASKATCHEWAN MEDICAL ASSOCIATION
211 Fourth Avenue South
Saskatoon, Saskatchewan
S7K 1N1
(306) 244-2196

YUKON MEDICAL ASSOCIATION
3089 Third Avenue
Whitehorse, Yukon
Y1A 5B3
(403) 668-4060

provincial branches also have municipal or regional medical association branches themselves (see Illustration 12.1).

## Associations of Importance to Medical Administrative Assistants

As a medical administrative assistant, you may be required at any time to write to or contact an organization or association relating to health care. At that time, you would use the information you have learned from this chapter as well as the reference sources available to you. There are, however, a few associations of direct significance to the medical administrative assistant.

### National, Provincial, and Local Medical Associations

**The Canadian Medical Association** — As the governing body of the provincial associations, the CMA deals with the federal government and acts as the national voice of medicine. A portion of the fees paid by provincial members goes to the CMA.

**Provincial Medical Associations** — The provincial medical associations are voluntary associations of provincial doctors. The bylaws of the associations differ among the provinces, but these differences are slight. For example, in one province membership is voluntary, but in another a fee is mandatory.

We will use the Ontario Medical Association (OMA) as an example to outline some of the points relevant to the provincial bodies. Membership in the OMA is open to all doctors in the province as well as medical graduates residing in Ontario and students enrolled in faculties of medicine at Ontario universities. Approximately 80 percent of practising physicians are members.

The objective of the OMA, broadly speaking, is to advance the practice and the science of medicine and the public health by working for the improvement of medical education, hospital and other health services, and medical legislation, through study, investigation, and research.

The OMA represents the medical profession to the Ontario government, offering recommendations about legislation and regulations affecting medical practice and the public health. The OMA produces a Schedule of Fees for medical services in Ontario and negotiates the Schedule of Benefits paid by the Ontario Ministry of Health. It publishes the *Ontario Medical Review*. The OMA also provides other services for its members, such as group insurance programs and support for continuing and postgraduate medical education.

**Municipal or Regional Associations** — The Ottawa Medical Association or the Edmonton Medical Association is simply a branch of the provincial association. Members generally meet on a regular basis to discuss issues relevant to their particular locality.

## The College of Physicians and Surgeons

Each province has its own College of Physicians and Surgeons. Established by provincial legislation, the College of Physicians and Surgeons is the official body that oversees the education, licensing, and discipline of doctors. In Ontario, as in other provinces, close liaison is maintained between the OMA and the College through a joint advisory committee of senior officers. These provincial colleges are completely separate and distinct from the provincial medical associations.

## Hospital Associations

Many provinces have established hospital associations. Today many of these provincial hospital associations have active memberships in other areas such as mental health centres, district health councils, institutional associate members, nursing homes, senior citizen homes, private hospitals, and some educational institutions that provide health care student programs. All members pay annual dues, and usually only active members have voting privileges and representations on boards of directors.

The fundamental objective of hospital associations is to stimulate, encourage, and assist in the provision of the highest possible standard of hospital and other health services to the people of the province.

## The Canadian Medical Protective Association

The Canadian Medical Protective Association is a mutual defence union of Canadian physicians. The association was founded in 1901 and had more than 47 000 members by January 1987. The purpose of the association is to provide its members with legal advice and counselling on any matters involving legal action. The association pays all legal costs incurred in the defence of such legal actions as well as any damages that the courts may award to the plaintiff. Members are also assisted with the defence of provincial governing body disciplinary actions, coroner inquests, and so on.

## Medical Secretaries' Associations

There are medical secretaries' associations located in some provinces in Canada. Local chapters of the provincial associations generally meet on a monthly basis. Their purpose is to improve the status and knowledge of all medical administrative assistants. Students who attend their local chapter meetings are provided with excellent exposure to the profession. Speakers' topics are varied and provide valuable information, the majority of which concerns health-related issues.

In 1990 the Ontario Medical Secretaries' Association Certification Program was affiliated with the Ontario Colleges of Applied Arts and Technology Office Administration — Medical Diploma Programs. Students who graduate with a 75 percent average mark from participating colleges can apply to the association for exemption from the certification examinations. For further information, contact the association's head office in Toronto.

**Assignment 12.1**

Investigate the local medical secretaries' association in your area. If there is no active chapter in your location, write to the Ontario Medical Secretaries' Association, 525 University Avenue, Suite 300, Toronto, Ontario M5G 3K7 to obtain information. This address is for use by students who do not live in a province where there is an active association. For those who live in a province where there is an active association, use an appropriate reference source to obtain the proper address for your association's provincial head office.

Write a report on the organization outlining the benefits to be derived from belonging to such a group. Prepare the report in proper form for submission.

This assignment should spark an interest in the association specifically related to your future profession. If there is no active chapter in your area, you may be interested in forming one after graduation. Ask your provincial head office for assistance. They will be only too happy to provide you with some guidance.

---

The Canadian Medical Association
Code of Ethics
April 1990

Principles of Ethical Behaviour
for all physicians, including those who may not
be engaged directly in clinical practice

I
Consider first the well-being of the patient.

II
Honour your profession and its traditions.

III
Recognize your limitations and the special skills of others
in the prevention and treatment of disease.

IV
Protect the patient's secrets.

V
Teach and be taught.

VI
Remember that integrity and professional ability should be
your best advertisement.

VII
Be responsible in setting a value on your services.

## Guide to the Ethical Behaviour of Physicians

A physician should be aware of the standards established by tradition and act within the general principles that have governed professional conduct.

The Oath of Hippocrates represented the desire of the members of that day to establish for themselves standards of conduct in living and in the practice of their art. Since then, the principles established have been retained as our basic guidelines for ethical living with the profession of medicine.

According to the Canadian Medical Protective Association, these principles are still followed by the majority of those in the profession.

The International Code of Ethics and the Declaration of Geneva (1948), developed and approved by the World Medical Association, have modernized the ancient codes. They have been endorsed by each member organization, including the Canadian Medical Association, as a general guide having world-wide application.

The Canadian Medical Association accepts the responsibility of delineating the standard of ethical behaviour expected of Canadian physicians.

An interpretation of these principles is developed in the following pages, as a guide for individual physicians and provincial authorities.

# Responsibilities to the Patient

An ethical physician

**Standard of care**

1. will practise the art and science of medicine to the best of his/her ability;
2. will continue self education to improve his/her standards of medical care;

**Respect for patient**

3. will practise in a fashion that is above reproach and will take neither physical, emotional, nor financial advantage of the patient;

**Patient's rights**

4. will recognize his/her professional limitations and, when indicated, recommend to the patient that additional opinions and services be obtained;
5. will recognize that a patient has the right to accept or reject any physician and any medical care recommended. The patient having chosen a physician has the right to request of that physician opinions from other physicians of the patient's choice;
6. will keep in confidence information derived from a patient or from a colleague regarding a patient, and divulge it only with the permission of the patient except when otherwise required by law;
7. when acting on behalf of a third party will ensure that the patient understands the physician's legal responsibility to the third party before proceeding with the examination;
8. will recommend only diagnostic procedures that are believed necessary to assist in the care of the patient, and therapy that is believed necessary for the well-being of the patient. The physician will recognize a responsibility in advising the patient of the findings and recommendations and will exchange such information with the patient as is necessary for the patient to reach a decision;
9. will, upon a patient's request, supply the information that is required to enable the patient to receive any benefits to which the patient may be entitled;
10. will be considerate of the anxiety of the patient's next-of-kin and co-operate with them in the patient's interest;

**Choice of patient**

11. will recognize the responsibility of a physician to render medical service to any person regardless of colour, religion, or political belief;

12. shall, except in an emergency, have the right to refuse to accept a patient;

13. will render all possible assistance to any patient, where an urgent need for medical care exists;

14. will, when the patient is unable to give consent and an agent of the patient is unavailable to give consent, render such therapy as the physician believes to be in the patient's interest;

**Continuity of care**

15. will, if absent, ensure the availability of medical care to his/her patients if possible; will, once having accepted professional responsibility for an acutely ill patient, continue to provide services until they are no longer required, or until arrangements have been made for the services of another suitable physician; may, in any other situation, withdraw from the responsibility for the care of any patient provided that the patient is given adequate notice of that intention;

**Personal morality**

16. will inform the patient when personal morality or religious conscience prevent the recommendation of some form of therapy;

**Clinical research**

17. will ensure that, before initiating clinical research involving humans, such research is appraised scientifically and ethically and approved by a responsible committee and is sufficiently planned and supervised that the individuals are unlikely to suffer any harm. The physician will ascertain that previous research and the purpose of the experiment justify this additional method of investigation. Before proceeding, the physician will obtain the consent of all involved persons or their agents, and will proceed only after explaining the purpose of the clinical investigation and any possible health hazard that can be reasonably foreseen;

**The dying patient**

18. will allow death to occur with dignity and comfort when death of the body appears to be inevitable;

19. may support the body when clinical death of the brain has occurred, but need not prolong life by unusual or heroic means;

**Transplantation**

20. may, when death of the brain has occurred, support cellular life in the body when some parts of the body might be used to prolong the life or improve the health of others;

21. will recognize a responsibility to a donor of organs to be transplanted and will give to the donor or the donor's relatives full disclosure of the intent and purpose of the procedure; in the case of a living donor, the physician will also explain the risks of the procedure;

22. will refrain from determining the time of death of the donor patient if there is a possibility of being involved as a participant in the transplant procedure, or when his/her association with the proposed recipient might improperly influence professional judgement;

23. may treat the transplant recipient subsequent to the transplant procedure in spite of having determined the time of death of the donor;

24. will consider, in determining professional fees, both the nature of the service provided and the ability of the patient to pay, and will be prepared to discuss the fee with the patient.

**Fees to patients**

## Responsibilities to the profession

An ethical physician

**Personal conduct**

25. will recognize that the profession demands integrity from each physician and dedication to its search for truth and to its service to mankind;

26. will recognize that self-discipline of the profession is a privilege and that each physician has a continuing responsibility to merit the retention of this privilege;

27. will behave in a way beyond reproach and will report to the appropriate professional body any conduct by a colleague that might be generally considered as being unbecoming to the profession;

28. will behave in such a manner as to merit the respect of the public for members of the medical profession;

29. will avoid impugning the reputation of any colleague;

**Contracts**

30. will, when aligned in practice with other physicians, insist that the standards enunciated in this Code of Ethics and the Guide to the Ethical Behaviour of Physicians be maintained;

31. will only enter into a contract regarding professional services that allows fees derived from physician's services to be controlled by the physician rendering the services;

32. will enter into a contract with an organization only if it will allow maintenance of professional integrity;

33. will only offer to a colleague a contract that has terms and conditions equitable to both parties;

**Reporting medical research**

34. will first communicate to colleagues, through recognized scientific channels, the results of any medical research, in order that those colleagues may establish an opinion of its merits before they are presented to the public;

**Addressing the public**

35. will recognize a responsibility to give the generally held opinions of the profession when interpreting scientific knowledge to the public; when presenting an opinion that is contrary to the generally held opinion of the profession, the physician will so indicate and will avoid any attempt to enhance his/her own personal professional reputation;

**Advertising**

36. will build a professional reputation based on ability and integrity, and will only advertise professional services or make professional announcements as regulated by legislation or as permitted by the provincial medical licensing authority;

37. will avoid advocacy of any product when identified as a member of the medical profession;

38. will avoid the use of secret remedies;

**Consultation**

39. will request the opinion of an appropriate colleague acceptable to the patient when diagnosis or treatment is difficult or obscure, or when the patient requests it. Having requested the opinion of a colleague, the physician will make available all relevant information and indicate clearly whether the consultant is to assume the continuing care of the patient during this illness;

40. will, when consulted by a colleague, report in detail all pertinent findings and recommendations to the attending physician and may outline an opinion to the patient. The consultant will continue with the care of the patient only at the specific request of the attending physician and with the consent of the patient;

**Patient care**

41. will co-operate with those individuals who, in the opinion of the physician, may assist in the care of the patient;

42. will make available to another physician, upon the request of the patient, a report of pertinent findings and treatment of the patient;

43. will provide medical services to a colleague and dependent family without fee, unless specifically requested to render an account;

44. will limit self-treatment or treatment of family members to minor or emergency services only; such treatments should be without fee;

**Financial arrangements**

45. will avoid any personal profit motive in ordering drugs, appliances, or diagnostic procedures from any facility in which the physician has a financial interest;

46. will refuse to accept any commission or payment, direct or indirect, for any service rendered to a patient by other persons excepting direct employees and professional colleagues with whom there is a formal partnership or similar agreement.

# Responsibilities to society

Physicians who act under the principles of this Guide to the Ethical Behaviour of Physicians will find that they have fulfilled many of their responsibilities to society.

An ethical physician

47. will strive to improve the standards of medical services in the community; will accept a share of the profession's responsibility to society in matters

relating to the health and safety of the public, health education, and legislation affecting the health or well-being of the community;

48. will recognize the responsibility as a witness to assist the court in arriving at a just decision;

49. will, in the interest of providing good and adequate medical care, support the opportunity of other physicians to obtain hospital privileges according to individual, personal, and professional qualifications.

*"The complete physician is not a man apart and cannot content himself with the practice of medicine alone, but should make his contribution, as does any other good citizen, towards the well-being and betterment of the community in which he lives."*

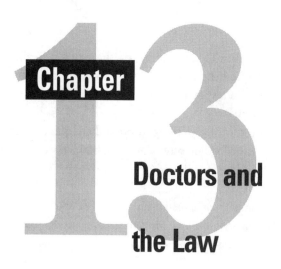

# Chapter

# 13

## Doctors and the Law

### Chapter Outline

- Responsibilities of the Doctor
- Responsibilities of the Medical Administrative Assistant
- Medico-Legal Problems
- Confidentiality

- Medical Records
- Medical Reports
- Miscellaneous
- Assignment 13.1

### Learning Objectives

To become familiar with
- the rules and regulations pertaining to the practice of medicine
- the proper names of various statutes that pertain to the medical environment
- reporting procedures
- various types of medico-legal problems
- the restrictions necessary to ensure patient confidentiality
- the minimum standards for medical records maintenance

Because a medical administrative assistant is acting on behalf of a doctor, the doctor may be held responsible for the consequences of the assistant's actions. Hence, an awareness of medico-legal problems is of great importance and is discussed in this chapter.

## Responsibilities of the Doctor

### Rules and Regulations

Just as all other disciplines and human endeavours are subject to rules and regulations, so is the practice of medicine. Doctors practise their profession under a well-defined and time-honoured ethical code. Even though doctors have the same general responsibilities as all citizens do, they have special additional responsibilities peculiar to their profession.

In order to practise medicine in Canada, a doctor must be licensed by the provincial College of Physicians and Surgeons or its equivalent, such as the Corporation Professionnelle des Médecins du Québec, the Provincial Medical Board of Nova Scotia, or the Newfoundland Medical Board. The profession and the college must operate under clearly defined rules as set out in the relevant provincial legislation and the regulations made under the medical acts. For example, the *Physicians' Administrative Manual* discusses statutes relevant to the practice of medicine in British Columbia. Every doctor and medical administrative assistant should obtain and read a copy of their legislation and regulations. Copies of regulations and pertinent provincial statutes can be obtained by contacting the Queen's Printer for the province, or the province's government book store.

Health care facilities have facility by-laws, medical staff by-laws, and medical staff rules. Any physician with privileges to practise within that facility must abide by these by-laws and rules.

## Other Statutes

Doctors should also be acquainted with other statutes that touch on or affect the practice of medicine in their province. Some of these statutes are the Child Welfare Act (now the Child and Family Services Act, 1984, in Ontario), the Coroners or Fatality Inquiries Act, the Health Services or Insurance Act, the Highway Traffic Act or Motor Vehicle Act, the Human Tissue Gift Act, the Mental Health Act, the Public Health Act (for example, the Ontario Health Protection and Promotion Act, 1983), the Vital Statistics Act, and so on.

Consideration should also be given to the fact that the practice of medicine may be controlled by certain federal statutes, most notably the Food and Drug Act, the Narcotic Control Act, and others.

## Reporting

Practising physicians should be particularly aware that several of the statutes mentioned above require mandatory reporting in certain circumstances. For example, reports may have to be submitted to the Children's Aid Society under provincial child welfare legislation, to the Registrar of Motor Vehicles under most Highway Traffic Acts or Motor Vehicle Acts, to the Workers' Compensation Board under the Workers' Compensation Acts and so on. If a doctor does not know how to go about reporting to these boards and agencies, a telephone call or letter to them will produce the desired procedures. A copy of the *Guide for Physicians in Determining Fitness to Drive a Motor Vehicle*, revised in 1981, can be obtained from the Canadian Medical Association, 1867 Alta Vista Drive, Ottawa, Ontario K1G 0G8. Information about reporting communicable diseases can be obtained by contacting the local, regional, or provincial health department.

**Responsibilities of the Medical Administrative Assistant**

Medical administrative assistants and other medical aides who are employees of doctors are usually considered to be doctors' agents. Doctors are likely to be held responsible for the acts of their agents. Therefore, when a medical administrative assistant or other assistant is acting on behalf of a doctor, the doctor may ultimately be responsible for the consequences of the actions. This puts a responsibility on the medical administrative assistant to be knowledgeable about the rules and regulations that govern the practice of medicine and the consequences that may occur if the rules are not followed. It should be noted that medical administrative assistants and other medical aides may also be held personally responsible for their own actions.

## Medico-Legal Problems

Doctors may be faced with a number of legal situations, such as partnership agreements, contracts with employees, estate planning, leases, and so on. And then there are the problems of a medico-legal nature. Rarely will a doctor face a criminal charge related to the practice of medicine. However, fraud, violations of the Narcotic Control Act, and allegations of sexual assault are examples of possible instances in which a doctor could be charged. A doctor is seldom charged with criminal negligence as a result of the professional care of a patient. (The term criminal negligence refers to reckless or wanton disregard for a patient's welfare.)

It is more common for physicians to face civil medico-legal problems. Medical malpractice actions can be brought against doctors in small claims or provincial courts or in courts of superior jurisdiction, such as the supreme courts or Court of Queen's Bench in each province. There may be one or several claims asserted for any one action.

A contract exists between a doctor and the patient. Although this does not take the form of a written document, a "contract" is implied when the patient requests from the doctor examination and treatment, and the doctor makes a commitment, probably unspoken, to treat the patient. Either party could breach the contract: a claim by the doctor against the patient is likely to be related to the financial aspect of the relationship; the patient may feel that the doctor has not met the patient's expectations and may be tempted to start a legal action. The patient may claim that the contract was breached because the result of treatment was not what the patient thought was promised by the doctor.

More often, however, a medico-legal action is commenced against a physician from allegations of negligence. What is negligence? Negligence is a term used to describe the alleged failure of a person to exercise a reasonable and acceptable standard of care, thereby causing harm or injury to another.

Malpractice actions alleging negligence generally fall into either of two categories. The first category includes those cases where a patient alleges that the treatment rendered by the doctor was negligent in a medical sense. For example, while undergoing surgery for removal of a gall bladder (cholecystectomy), the patient's bowel is punctured by the surgeon. The second category, increasing in frequency, includes claims by the patient that the physician was negligent by failing to disclose sufficiently the risks of the treatment beforehand. Claims of this nature come under the expression "lack of informed consent."

If patients feel that they have received treatment for which consent was not given, they may allege assault and battery. Recent case law has established that for there to be a claim for assault and battery, the treatment carried out must be wholly unrelated to or different from that treatment discussed earlier with the patient.

Other civil claims, in addition to medical negligence, lack of informed consent, or assault and battery, may be those that allege breach of medical confidentiality or defamation.

As well as, or perhaps instead of, suing a doctor, a patient may complain about the doctor's professional work. The complaint may be expressed directly to the doctor or to a member of the doctor's staff. It may be submitted to officials of the hospital, to the local academy of medicine or medical society, or to the College of Physicians and Surgeons or its equivalent.

Complaints or claims against doctors sometimes arise out of certain aspects of the practice of medicine with which medical administrative assistants have considerable involvement. The competent medical administrative assistant should pay heed to some of the following considerations.

## Confidentiality

Every patient has the right to expect that the information the doctor has obtained about him or her, on the basis of what the patient or others have told the doctor or what the doctor has discovered by examination and other means, will be kept confidential by the doctor. This duty applies also to the doctor's staff.

Information about a patient must never be revealed to anyone (except, of course, the patient) unless required by law or unless authorized by the patient or by the person legally responsible for the patient (in the case, for example, of a minor or developmentally handicapped patient). Unauthorized persons should not have access to appointment lists or other information and certainly not to patients' records or the information contained therein. Even the information that the patient was seen by the doctor should be considered as confidential.

A doctor or medical administrative assistant should not release medical information to a third party unless properly authorized in writing to do so. An authorization should state clearly what is intended, and it should be dated. (The date should be reasonably current.) The authorization should be kept in the doctor's possession in case it is later alleged that there was a breach of medical confidentiality.

If an inquirer, other than the patient, approaches a medical administrative assistant for information about a patient, it should be pointed out that the request for information should be put in writing and should be accompanied by an appropriate authorization, signed by the patient or the person responsible for the patient. Inquiries by the patient's lawyer, insurer, or employer should be in writing and should, like all other requests for medical information, be accompanied by the patient's signed authorization.

## Medical Records

Proper medical records are considered to be an essential component of the physician-patient relationship. The main reason for making and keeping records is to assist the doctor in the continuing care of the patient. The importance of complete and comprehensive records from a medico-legal point of view cannot be overemphasized.

In some provinces, the regulations or bylaws of the College of Physicians and Surgeons or its equivalent specify minimum standards for maintaining, organizing, and retaining medical records by physicians. For example, a section of the regulations under the Health Disciplines Act of Ontario requires that a member shall

"(a)  Keep a legible written or printed record in respect of each patient of the member setting out,
    (i)  the name and address of the patient,
    (ii)  each date that the member sees the patient,
    (iii)  a history of the patient,
    (iv)  particulars of each physical examination of the patient by the member,
    (v)  investigations ordered by the member and the results of the investigations,
    (vi)  each diagnosis made by the member respecting the patient, and
    (vii)  each treatment prescribed by the member for the patient;
(b)  keep a day book, daily diary, or appointment record setting out the name of each patient seen or treated or in respect of whom a professional service is rendered by the member."

Generally speaking, entries in a patient's record should be dated and clearly written or typed. All significant information should be put into the record, including personal and family data, the past and present history obtained by the doctor, the doctor's findings, advice and recommendations concerning investigation and treatment, discussion of risks of treatment, alternative forms of therapy, and any other pertinent information about the patient's medical management. Events that may or may not involve the doctor should also be noted in the record — for example, vital signs taken by the nurse, changed or cancelled appointments, the issuance of printed instructions or pamphlets to the patient, referral arrangements, and so on.

If a patient is thought to be allergic to certain medications, the office record should contain a clearly discernible warning to that effect, so that this important information is readily available whenever a prescription is given to the patient. Likewise, patient charts should be "flagged" when follow-up appointments, review examinations, and so forth are necessary.

Some doctors use "Problem Lists" in their records. These are a type of flow sheet on which diagnoses and other important clinical information are recorded. Such information is thereby readily available to the doctor for review at the time of each encounter with the patient.

Many doctors find it useful to keep in the patient's record a copy of each prescription given to the patient. A notation should be made in the record whenever a prescription is given or renewed by telephone.

## Retention of Records

The regulations under the Health Disciplines Act of Ontario require that a physician keep "each record for a period of six years after the date of the last entry in the record or until the physician ceases to be engaged in the practice of medicine, which ever comes first." Other provinces have similar requirements. Apart from these statutory requirements, it is wise for doctors to keep their medical records for as long as there is an appreciable risk that the records may be required for the purpose of defence against a complaint or claim. Clinical records are often the most important single factor in the defence of a lawsuit arising out of a doctor's work. They are also often necessary when dealing with a complaint to the provincial licensing authority. Because a doctor may be asked for information from the record years after the last contact with a patient, and because a patient may return to a doctor's practice after an absence of several years, records should be kept for a period longer than required by legislation. A doctor should maintain control over records as long as possible; they should never be destroyed before ten years have elapsed following the last entry date. Records relating to the treatment of minors should be retained until two years after the patients have reached the age of majority. There is always a slight possibility in some provinces that the doctor may be sued more than ten years after the last contact with the patient, even though the likelihood is remote.

When doctors leave practice because of retirement or for any other reason, or when they relocate their practices, they should ensure that their records are kept intact, that they have access to those records, and that the information contained in them is available to their patients' new doctors. When a doctor dies, the estate should make appropriate arrangements for the safekeeping of records until there is no likelihood that a claim will be made against the estate. It is prudent for physicians to include in estate planning provisions for the care of their medical records.

## Production of Records

It sometimes happens that patients or relatives of patients will ask for their records for one reason or another. It is generally considered that the record is the property of the doctor or clinic and not that of the patient. It is possible that future legislation might be enacted that could have a bearing on the rights of patients to obtain copies of their clinical records. Such legislation already exists in Quebec. The patient does have rights, however, to the information contained in the medical records. The regulations under the Health Disciplines Act of Ontario require that, on a patient's request, a doctor must provide a report of the relevant information in the record, but not necessarily the actual record or a photocopy of it.

Medical administrative assistants should not give the doctor's office record (or a photocopy of it), or the information contained in the record (including consultants' reports, laboratory and X-ray reports, and so on), to a patient or a relative to read. Such records and reports frequently require interpretation for the patient, and the doctor's administrative assistant should arrange for the patient to have time with the doctor to discuss the information in the record.

Of course, if the doctor is presented with a court order to produce a patient's record, the doctor must comply, but steps should be taken to ensure that a duplicate copy of the record is kept by the doctor. The doctor should also keep the court order.

A second exception to releasing patients' records might arise when the doctor is served with a subpoena or summons requiring submission of evidence in any legal action or other proceeding. The doctor may have to bring along a copy of the patient's office record. On occasion, a doctor may also be directed to forward to the College of Physicians and Surgeons or its equivalent a copy of a patient's record.

If a lawyer requests records, the physician can only send patient records that apply to the physician's direct patient care. Consultation notes, correspondence, and such from other physicians involved in the patient's care *must not* be released.

## Transfer of Records

If a patient is transferring to another doctor's practice, the patient may ask the first doctor to forward the record to the second doctor, or the new doctor may ask for the record. A doctor should comply with such a request by sending a summary of the record or, if the first doctor prefers, a photocopy of pertinent portions of it. The first doctor should keep possession or control of the actual record. (On occasion, a doctor may have custody of another provider's record. Before transmitting such records or photocopies, the doctor might like to obtain medico-legal advice.)

The doctor should obtain appropriate authorization from the patient (or the patient's legal guardian) even when transferring medical information or clinical record material to the patient's new doctor.

When a summary or photocopy of the record is sent to another doctor, a notation should be made in the record indicating when and to whom it was sent.

## Medical Reports

The Code of Ethics of the Canadian Medical Association adopted in most provinces states, "An ethical physician will, on the patient's request, assist him by supplying the information required to enable the patient to receive any benefits to which the patient may be entitled." This ethical duty is also effected in the province of Ontario by the regulations under the Health Disciplines Act, which require the doctor to provide within a reasonable time "any report or certificate requested by a patient or his authorized agent in respect of an examination or treatment performed by the member." There is, therefore, a clear obligation, imposed ethically and by law, for a doctor to provide the patient or the patient's authorized agent with a report when requested to do so.

Unless reporting is required by legislation, as mentioned earlier, a doctor should obtain a signed authorization from the patient before releasing medical information. In other words, if a doctor is going to provide information about a patient to a third party, appropriate authorization must be obtained before doing so. When the information contained in the report is of a particularly sensitive nature, the patient should be alerted to the contents of the report. Whenever a doctor prepares a report, issues a certificate, or completes a form, a copy should be filed in the patient's chart. In many situations the patient will not be entitled to receive a copy of the report from the physician and should be so advised.

A special kind of report is a medico-legal report, that is, one that is requested by a lawyer. The College of Physicians and Surgeons expects a doctor to provide a patient's lawyer with a report if requested to do so. It is preferable that the lawyer's request be written, outlining specifically what information is required. It is likely that the lawyer will provide the doctor with an appropriate authorization, signed by the patient or, if the patient is deceased, by the executor or administrator of the patient's estate. If a proper authorization (sometimes called a "direction" or "release") does not accompany the lawyer's request, the doctor should ask the lawyer for one before submitting a medical report. The doctor's report should be forwarded to the lawyer within a reasonable period of time. The doctor should keep a copy of the report.

If the doctor has reason to believe the patient consulted a lawyer because of dissatisfaction with the doctor's care, the doctor may wish to seek the advice of a medical defence organization before responding to the lawyer.

## Miscellaneous

Problems that may have legal implications may arise from the day-to-day events in doctors' offices and clinics.

Each medical administrative assistant should discuss with the doctor the type of advice he or she may give by telephone as well as the doctor's instructions about dealing with requests for appointments, referrals, reports, and so on.

Problems may be averted by an efficient system for handling incoming telephone calls and noting in patients' records the nature of the calls.

Medical administrative assistants who witness patients signing consent for treatment forms should assure themselves that the description of the proposed treatment on the form is correct. They should also satisfy themselves with the identity and competence of the patients who sign such forms. Should a patient have questions about the proposed procedure, the doctor should be specifically notified that the patient has unanswered questions and concerns.

Bookings for operative and investigative procedures should be exact and clear. Copies of booking slips should be retained. Notations should be made in patients' records about the arrangements that have been made.

Injuries sustained by a patient in a doctor's office can lead to a claim for damages. Those who work in medical offices should always be alert to situations that could put patients' safety in jeopardy.

Medical administrative assistants are important members of the health care team. A knowledgeable and caring medical administrative assistant can play a significant role in the interaction between patients and the providers of medical care.

Historically, the medical profession has been very aware of the confidentiality of patient information. The recent enactment of federal and provincial freedom of information legislation reinforces the importance of confidentiality. Before releasing any information concerning a patient, it is imperative that you secure in writing the permission of the patient. Illustration 13.1 is a sample of a release of information form.

## Assignment 13.1

The material for this test assignment will be provided by your instructor

**Illustration 13.1   Authorization for Release of Patient Information**

AUTHORIZATION FOR RELEASE OF PATIENT INFORMATION


I hereby authorize _____
                    name of facility releasing the information

to release the following information_____

_____
         description of information to be disclosed

to_____
         name and address of person / agency requesting the information

from the records of _____  _____
                        name of patient            date of birth


                    _____
                         address of patient

concerning treatment on _____
                            dates of contact / hospitalization

I understand that this information is to be used by the recipient for the purpose of:

_____

_____



_____        _____
   Witness                            Signature of patient or person having
                                      lawful custody of patient*

Expiry date of
authorization_____     _____
                                      * Relationship to patient

                                      _____
                                           Date

**Notes:**
1. This authorization must contain the original signature of:
   (i) the patient;
   (ii) where the record is of a former patient who is deceased, the personal
        representative of the patient;
   (iii) the parent or person who has lawful custody of an unmarried patient
        under **sixteen** years of age;
   (iv) where the patient is unable to consent in writing by reason of mental or
        physical disability, the person having lawful custody of the patient.

2. This authorization may be rescinded or amended in writing at any time prior to the
   expiration date, except where action has been taken in reliance on the authorization.

**Ref.** Reg. 518/88 made under the Public Hospitals Act, Sec. 21 (4) (c); Sec. 25(1) (c)


6519 JF
June 1989

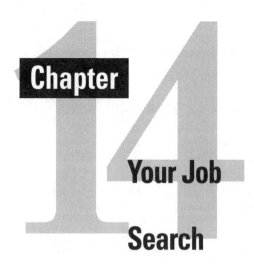

# Chapter

# Your Job

# Search

## Chapter Outline

- Assignment 14.1
- Assignment 14.2
- Assignment 14.3

## Learning Objectives

To
- identify entry-level positions
- identify considerations for job search
- learn the importance of the letter of application and résumé

Your medical administrative assistant program has taken you through all the basic requirements for a position in a medical office. The next step is to find the "right" job. In today's society, education and experience are generally listed as requirements of the position in job advertisements. You have the education, but how do you gain the experience?

## Entry-Level Positions

Most entry-level positions, such as file clerk and receptionist, do not require the same level of experience that would be required for, say, a medical office administrator position in a hospital emergency ward. It may be necessary for you to begin your career as a file clerk or a receptionist in order to gain the experience that will allow you to advance to a higher-level job.

Entry-level positions allow you to gain valuable knowledge and experience without having the responsibilities of a more senior job. You have the opportunity to observe and learn the activities in your environment. You will receive ideas and constructive criticisms from your administrators and peers that will help you to grow in the knowledge and requirements of your chosen career.

It is essential that you always practise the points covered in Chapter 1 concerning personal qualities and appearance, customer service, and skills.

## Where to Find Job Leads

Several months before graduation, you should begin thinking about sources of information for your job search.

Most colleges have a placement office that publishes notices on a bulletin board or advises program instructors of employment opportunities. Job opportunities are advertised in the classified section of the newspaper. Employment agencies servicing the medical profession will also be interested in your résumé.

Networking is often the best way to secure a job. Inform your doctor that you will soon be graduating. Attend the Medical Secretaries' Association meetings if there is a chapter in your city. The OMSA has a job bank that you can access if you are a student member. Write to the association for more information.

## What to Consider

When beginning your job search, it is important to consider your expectations, needs, and abilities. For example, if you had difficulty with medical machine transcription, it would be unwise to seek a job as a transcriptionist. If you have a very pleasing personality, a pleasant smile, and enjoy meeting people, a job in the admitting office in your local hospital might be of interest to you.

Another important point to consider is whether it may be necessary for you to relocate in order to get a job. Administrative skills are very portable. Can you think of any business that does not require some type of office skills? Providing there is no language barrier, your skills are required in all parts of the world. Of course, you may not have to move to the other side of the continent to get a job. However, if there is a shortage of jobs in your city, you may have to consider an alternative. And if you are adventurous, you may find yourself in another country.

Investigate the salary level, skill requirements, location, benefits, and working hours of the position you want. Are the services provided by the organization in your area of interest? Is there room for advancement in the organization? Will the salary level allow you to reach a goal you have set, such as to buy a car or move into your own apartment? All of these things must be considered, because if you accept a position and you are not happy, you will not work to your potential.

Because of today's job market, it may be necessary to accept a job that is not exactly what you want; however, work with the idea that you are gaining valuable experience that will provide you with the necessary qualifications when the right job comes along.

When you are invited for an interview, be prepared. You will be assessed on your ability to communicate (maintain eye contact, use appropriate grammar, do not continually answer questions with "yes" or "no"), on your appearance (dress in appropriate business attire), and on your attitude (be courteous and positive).

Ask a peer to give you a mock interview. The person may point out mannerisms or nervous habits that are distracting, for example, finger tapping, voice inflections, or constant throat clearing. Be ready to sell yourself. Tell the interviewer about your achievements. Following the interview, send a thank-you letter.

## Your Letter of Application and Résumé

Colleges often provide instruction in communication classes for writing letters of application and résumés.

When preparing your letter of application and résumé, talk to your peers and instructors and get their ideas. Research formats in textbooks. However, when you put all of the facts and ideas together, make certain that the finished product projects *you*. Do not copy from a textbook illustration. The person reading the application wants to know about you, not a textbook character.

For students who have not had formal instruction on the preparation of a letter of application and résumé, we have provided a job advertisement (Illustration 14.1), a letter of application responding to the advertisement (Illustration 14.2), and some examples of résumés (Illustrations 14.3, 14.4, and 14.5).

In developing your résumé, you should use a format that best reflects your skills and abilities and emphasizes the particular requirements of your job targets.

The following examples of résumés respond to the ad listed in Illustration 14.1. The "before" résumé in Illustration 14.3 does provide an account of the applicant's academic and work history. However, it doesn't effectively reveal to its fullest potential the applicant's skill level, strengths, and attributes.

The following examples have been created using two common formats: chronological and functional/combination.

In Illustration 14.4, the chronological résumé outlines the applicant's background in reverse order beginning with the most recent and working back to previous experiences. This format emphasizes career progression and/or job continuity in the same or related field. It is best used when the job target is directly in line with your work history.

**Illustration 14.1    Job Advertisement**

Medical Administrative Assistant required for busy family physician's office. Sound knowledge of terminology and anatomy, and office procedures (reception, appointment booking, billing, and records management) as applied to a medical office environment. Excellent communication, word processing, medical machine transcription, time management and problem-solving skills are essential. Apply to Dr. Jasbir Sandhu, 310 O'Connor Street, Ottawa, Ontario J5Z 2X8.

**Illustration 14.2    Letter of Application**

1356 Gloucester Drive
Ottawa, ON
Z8X 1X9

October 21, 1995

Dr. Jasbir Sandhu
310 O'Connor Street
Ottawa, Ontario
J5Z 2X8

Dear Dr. Sandhu:

Subject: Application for a Medical Assistant Position

You can meet your requirement for a Medical Administrative Assistant as listed in the (paper) on (date) by positively considering my application. The enclosed résumé outlines my skills and experience that are most relevant in securing a clerical position in the medical environment.

Excellent administrative skills, a sound knowledge of medical terminology and anatomy, and demonstrated computer abilities will allow me to effectively meet the challenges of a busy family physician's office. Demonstrated time management and problem-solving skills combined with my high energy level and positive, progressive attitude will provide you with a cooperative member of your health-care team.

My education, background, and keen desire to succeed have prepared me to approach future challenges with enthusiasm and determination. A progressive and efficient family practise such as yours will enable me to work at my best while achieving your organizational goals.

I would appreciate a personal interview to allow a detailed discussion of my future contribution to your organization. I can be reached at (613) 555-0000.

Sincerely,


Daphne Smith

Attachment: Résumé

**Illustration 14.3   Résumé (Before)**

DAPHNE R. SMITH
1356 Gloucester Drive
Ottawa, Ontario
Z8X 1X9
613-742-9856

SUMMARY OF JOB RELATED SKILLS

- High-level typing speed and accuracy
- Effective communication skills
- Ability to recognize problems and reach satisfactory solutions
- Effective time management
- Excellent people skills

EDUCATION

- Anytown Business College

    Graduate of the two-year Office Administration — Medical Programme in May, 19__
    Recipient of Medical Secretarial Association Outstanding Graduate Award

  Subjects studied include:

| | |
|---|---|
| Medical Typewriting (70 wpm) | Organizational Behaviour |
| Medical Machine Transcription | Communications |
| Paramedical Studies | Anatomy and Physiology |
| Medical Terminology | Medical Office Procedures |
| Computer Software Applications | Accounting |
| Introduction to Data Processing | Government of Canada |
| Word Processing (Wang and Word Perfect) | Shorthand (100 wpm) |

- Anytown Collegiate and Vocational School

    Honours Secondary School Graduation Certificate (First Class Honours), 19__
    Provincial Scholar
    Gold Letter Recipient
    Valedictorian

EXPERIENCE RELEVANT TO A MEDICAL POSITION

- Anytown Hospital

    Volunteer Candystriper
    Responsibilities:   transport newly admitted patients to rooms
    transport patients for tests
    provide errand service for nurses                                    19__ to 19__

- Anytown Medical Centre

    Part-Time Office Worker
    Responsibilities:   answer telephone
    prepare billing information for computer
    computer input
    assist nurses
    filing                                                                            19__ to 19__

- Doctor J.E. Plunkett's Office

    Two-Week Field Placement in conjunction with College Programme
    Responsibilities:   answer telephone
    book appointments
    computerized billing
    reception
    patient flow
    assist physician with some tests

**Illustration 14.3   Résumé (continued)**

EXTRACURRICULAR ACTIVITIES

- Medical Secretaries' Association
  Student member
  Assisted with organization of 19__ Clinic Day
- Anytown Curling Club
  President — Junior Section
  Certified Curl Canada Instructor
- Anytown Church
  Sunday School Instructor — Junior Department
  Choir member

RECREATIONAL ACTIVITIES

Squash, jogging, curling, skiing, singing, and crafts

REFERENCES

Mrs. Jean Bowen
Anytown Business College
135 Main Street
Anytown, Ontario Z5X 1X5

Doctor J.E. Plunkett
278 O'Connor Street
Ottawa, Ontario
J5Z 2X8

Rev. George Smith
Anytown Church
158 Main Street
Anytown, Ontario
Z5X 1X6

**Illustration 14.4    Résumé (Chronological)**

---

DAPHNE R. SMITH
1356 Gloucester Drive
Ottawa, Ontario
Z8X 1X9

SUMMARY OF JOB-RELATED SKILLS

- Work effectively in a busy medical office environment
- Knowledge of medical procedures, terminology and anatomy
- Familiar with computers and business machines
- Effective communication skills
- Ability to recognize and solve problems
- Effective time management

EDUCATION

Anytown Business College                                                                                    19__ to 19__
Office Administration — Medical Programme Diploma

- Recipient of Medical Secretarial Association Outstanding

Graduate Award for academic excellence

   *Acquired Skills:*

- Knowledge of medical terminology, anatomy and physiology, and paramedical studies
- Exceptional keyboarding skills, machine transcription, and office procedures
- Computer software applications, data processing and word processing (Wang and Word Perfect)
- Effective communications skills through report writing and class presentations

Anytown Collegiate and Vocation School                                                          19__
Honours Secondary School Graduation Certificate

- Gold Letter and First Class Honours Recipient
- Provincial Scholar and Class Valedictorian

RELEVANT EXPERIENCE

Dr. J. E. Plunkett Medical Office                                                                       19__
Office Assistant (Two-Week Field Placement)

- Performed reception duties and secretarial functions: medical machine transcription, filing medical documents, answering telephones, and scheduled appointment bookings
- Prepared computerized billing and transmitted electronically to Ministry of Health using "xxs" system
- Entered and retrieved data on IBM-PC; ran spreadsheet reports of daily bookings
- Prepared consultation notes and medical correspondence
- Effectively monitored patient flow and ensured records management
- Assisted physician with medical tests

Anytown Medical Centre                                                                                 19__ to 19__
Office Worker

- Handled high volume of bookings and all routine work for medical office including filing, reception, telephones
- Input patient records, prepared and handled billing documentation for computer input on IBM
- Completed hospital requisitions and reports
- Accurately transcribed medical dictation
- Organized and maintained a workable filing system of over 400 medical files respecting patient confidentiality
- Assisted nurses with routine medical procedures
- Handled high pressure situations and deadlines

Anytown Hospital                                                                                           19__ to 19__
Volunteer Candystriper (Volunteer)

- Assisted nurses with errand service
- Transported newly admitted patients to rooms and patients for tests

**Illustration 14.4   Résumé (Chronological) (continued)**

MEMBERSHIPS/CERTIFICATION

Medical Secretaries' Association
- As student member, assisted with organization of 199_ Clinic Day

Anytown Curling Club
- President — Junior Section
- Certified Curl Canada Instructor

RECREATIONAL ACTIVITIES

Squash, jogging, curling, skiing, singing, and crafts

REFERENCES

Available upon request

The functional/combination résumé in Illustration 14.5 highlights the applicant's skills, strengths, and accomplishments that target specific job and work objectives. Work experience and abilities are listed by key functional areas in the order that best meets the requirements of the job. Those wanting to draw attention to a strong skill set required by a specific job and away from limited work experience, career change/redirection, or re-entry into the job market will benefit from this format.

**Assignment 14.1**

If you have not been required to do so in another course, select an advertisement from the "Help Wanted" section of your local newspaper and prepare a letter of application and résumé.

Ask your instructor to assess the finished product and make suggestions for improvement, if necessary.

**Assignment 14.2**

Extract from your portfolio the rating sheet you completed in Assignment 1.3. Would your ratings in any of the categories change?

**Assignment 14.3**

Extract from your portfolio the skills and personal qualities inventory sheet completed in Assignment 1.4. Reassess your skill levels. Have you acquired any new skills? How would you rate those skills? Have any of your skills improved; how much?

Reassess your personal qualities. Would you rate any of your personal qualities stronger?

**Illustration 14.5   Résumé (Functional/Combination)**

DAPHNE R. SMITH
1356 Gloucester Drive
Ottawa, Ontario
Z8X 1X9

SUMMARY OF JOB-RELATED SKILLS

- Work effectively in a busy medical office environment
- Knowledge of medical procedures, terminology and anatomy
- Familiar with computers and business machines
- Effective communication skills
- Ability to recognize and solve problems
- Effective time management

SKILLS AND ABILITIES

Medical Administrative Support:

- Performed reception duties and secretarial functions: medical machine transcription and typing, filing medical documents, answering telephones, and scheduled appointment bookings
- Effectively monitored patient flow and ensured records management
- Knowledge of medical terminology, anatomy and physiology, and paramedical studies
- Exceptional keyboarding skills, machine transcription, and office procedures
- Accurately transcribed medical dictation
- Completed hospital requisitions and reports
- Organized and maintained a workable filing system of over 400 medical files respecting patient confidentiality
- Assisted physician with medical tests and nurses with routine medical procedures and errand service
- Transported newly admitted patients to rooms and patients for tests

Computer Knowledge:

- Computer software applications, data processing and word processing (Wang and Word Perfect)
- Prepared computerized billing and transmitted electronically to Ministry of Health using "xxs" system
- Entered all patient records on an IBM-PC, retrieved data from patient database, and ran spreadsheet reports of daily bookings
- Input patient records, prepared and handled billing documentation for computer input on IBM
- Composed correspondence, prepared reports, completed hospital requisitions, merged letters with labels for mailing of 500

Time Management/Problem Solving:

- As Receptionist, answered and redirected heavy load of incoming calls and relaying messages to staff
- Handled high volume of patients while meeting appointment booking schedule
- Effectively handled high pressure situations and office procedures; met all billing deadlines
- Greeted patients and suppliers in a friendly and courteous manner.

RELEVANT EXPERIENCE

| | |
|---|---|
| Dr. J.E. Plunkett Medical Office<br>Office Assistant (Two-Week Field Placement) | 19__ |
| Anytown Medical Centre<br>Office Worker (Part-Time) | 19__ to 19__ |
| Anytown Hospital<br>Volunteer Candystriper (Volunteer) | 19__ to 19__ |

EDUCATION

| | |
|---|---|
| Anytown Business College<br>Office Administration — Medical Programme Diploma | 19__ to 19__ |

- Recipient of Medical Secretarial Association Outstanding Graduate Award for academic excellence

| | |
|---|---|
| Anytown Collegiate and Vocation School<br>Honours Secondary School Graduation Certificate | 19__ |

- Gold Letter and First Class Honours Recipient
- Provincial Scholar and Class Valedictorian

**Illustration 14.5   Résumé (Functional/Combination) (continued)**

MEMBERSHIPS/CERTIFICATION

Medical Secretaries' Association
- As student member, assisted with organizing 19__ Clinic Day

Anytown Curling Club
- President — Junior Section
- Certified Curl Canada Instructor

RECREATIONAL ACTIVITIES

Squash, jogging, curling, skiing, singing, and crafts

REFERENCES

Available upon request

# Part 2

# Document Processing for the Canadian Medical Administrative Assistant

## A Reference for Formats of Business Memos, Letters, Envelopes, and Financial Reports

The purpose of this part of the book is to provide a reference and/or instructional guide for producing memos, letters, envelopes, and financial reports. It is assumed that students have had previous instruction on the appropriate formats for these documents. If you have not, however, we have provided practice exercise assignments. Some of these assignments contain deliberate errors, which the student is expected to correct.

Instructions on how to use a typewriter to centre and to complete forms with lines and boxed spaces are also included.

Most tasks that were once performed on a typewriter are now prepared using computer software, such as word processing programs and integrated packages that include spreadsheets, word processing, data base, medical billing, appointment booking, and others. In a medical environment, however, there are still some documents such as autopsy reports that are in carbon-pack form and must be completed on a typewriter. It is hoped that the guidance on typing on lines and in boxes and on correct centring methods will be helpful.

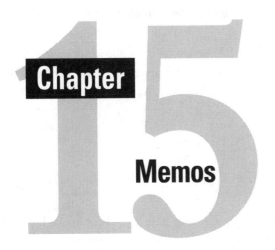

# Chapter 15

## Memos

### Chapter Outline

- Styles of Memos
- Assignment 15.1

### Learning Objectives

To review
- the purpose of a memo
- different styles of memo format

The most informal type of written communication is a memo. Three acceptable memo styles will be reviewed in this chapter. A memo can be a handwritten note scribbled on a piece of paper. Producing the note with the name of the sender and receiver formalizes the message.

Most business organizations send informal messages on a memo form, which could be a computer-generated macro or a preprinted carbon-pack. This allows the original to be sent to the recipient of the message and a copy kept by the sender for future reference and filing. Some preprinted forms contain two copies for the recipient of the message: the second copy is used to write a reply.

Although there are several acceptable styles for memo headings, most headings consist of "To" (the name of the recipient); "From" (the name of the sender); "Date" (the date the message is produced); and "Subject" (what the message is about).

The body of the memo is generally single-spaced, but can be double-spaced if the message is short. (If double-spaced, indent the beginning of each paragraph five spaces.) Initials of the person who produced the memo appear at the left margin, a double space below the last line of the message.

If four or five people are to receive the memo, key all names on the memo, and place a check mark or an arrow opposite the appropriate name when distributing or mailing the finished memo.

Headings and body styles of the following memo forms can be interchanged to produce a style that is appealing and acceptable to your employer/physician.

# Styles of Memo

## Style I

The headings are placed flush with the left margin with enough space allowed for the rest of the information (names, date, and subject) to be blocked as well. Double-space between heading lines and triple-space before the memo message. Single-space the body (double-space if the message is short) and double-space between paragraphs. Initials are typed at the left margin, a double space below the last line of the message.

Note that there is no formal signature line on a memo because the sender's name appears in the memo headings. A memo produced on 21.5-cm (8½-inch) paper usually has approximately 4-cm (1½-inch) margins.

Style I is shown in Illustration 15.1.

## Style II

Headings are placed as in Style I, except the longest line (subject) is keyed flush with the left margin and the last letters of the heading titles are aligned. The body is single-spaced with five-space paragraph indentation.

Style II is shown in Illustration 15.2.

## Style III

"To" and "Subject" are placed flush with the left margin; "From" and "Date" begin at the centre point. The headings can be rearranged, for example, "To" and "From" at the left margin and "Subject" and "Date" at the centre. Note that, depending on its length, a memo can be double-spaced. Paragraphs would then be indented five spaces at the beginning (see Illustration 15.3).

**Illustration 15.1    Memo Style I**

TO:        Dr. J.E. Plunkett

FROM:    Dr. M.C. Scott

DATE:      (current date)

SUBJECT: Mrs. Hazel Davis

Thank you for referring Mrs. Davis, who certainly appears to have an epidermoid cyst behind the right ear.

I will be making an arrangement for the removal of this, under general anaesthesia as an outpatient at the Ottawa General Hospital.

/ti

**Illustration 15.2    Memo Style II**

TO:     Dr. E.J. Pelham

FROM:     Dr. M.C. Scott

DATE:     (current date)

SUBJECT:     Mrs. Hazel Davis

Mrs. Davis is scheduled to have an epidermoid cyst removed from behind her right ear. Surgery is scheduled for September 30, 19___ at 9 a.m. in operating room 4 at Ottawa General Hospital.

I would appreciate it if you would administer the anaesthetic during surgery. Please advise if the date and time fit in with your schedule.

/ti

**Illustration 15.3    Memo Style III**

TO:     Dr. M.C. Scott        FROM:     Dr. E.J. Pelham

SUBJECT:     Mrs. Hazel Davis        DATE:     (current date)

I will be pleased to administer anaesthetic on Mrs. Hazel Davis during surgery and will be in

operating room 4 at O.G.H. on September 30, 19___ at 9 a.m.

/ti

---

**Assignment 15.1**

Produce the following memo using each of the three different styles. Check for correct spelling and paragraphing.

Dr. Plunkett has asked you to send a memo to the Ottawa Hospital Board of Directors informing them that the annual board dinner meeting will be on December 1, 19___, at the Holiday Inn in the Wilfrid Laurier Room. Dinner will be served at 6 P.M.; meeting at 8 P.M. Members are asked to be prepared to present their annual reports.

Compose the memo and present it in an appropriate style.

Submit the assignment for assessment.

**Assignment 15.2**    Produce the following memos using Style I for the first memo, Style II for the second, and Style III for the third.

Memo to JEP From Dr. W. Parks Subject: Bob Baxter.

Thank you for referring the above named patient who certainly appears to have an infected chilagion on the right upper eyelid. I have as of the present time treated him with antibiotics and will be reviewed in a week's time. He also has been booked for some cutaneous excisional surgery as an outpatient at O.G.H.

To. Dr ESP From Dr. T Hicks Sub. L. Elliott

Mrs. Elliott was reviewed in my off. today after being referred by Dr. ~~Elmer~~ Plunkett. At this time she has a large ulceration on the lateral aspect of her left leg, just above the lateral malleous. I will arrange to have her admitted for surgery next week. Will you be available to administer anaesthetic?

Write a memo to above stating I will be available any day next week except. Wed.

ESP.

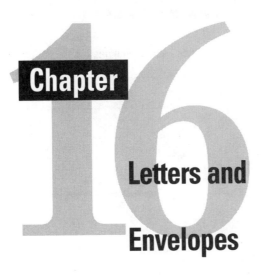

# Chapter 16

# Letters and Envelopes

## Chapter Outline

- Letters
- Parts of a Business Letter
- Assignment 16.1
- Envelopes
- Assignment 16.2
- Assignment 16.3

## Learning Objectives

To review
- letter styles: block, modified block, and modified block with paragraph indentation
- parts of a business letter
- punctuation styles: all-point (closed), two-point (mixed), and no-point (open)
- preparing envelopes

The purpose of this chapter is to review letters styles, punctuation styles, parts of a business letter, envelope addressing, and folding and inserting. The material used will allow the student to observe how medical correspondence is composed and how medical terminology is applied to communication documents.

## Letters

### Letter Styles

Several styles of letters have been used over the years. At one time, the very formal indented style was used extensively. Since the advent of the computer, letter styles have become more simplified and the indention of paragraphs is seldom used.

**Block Style** — This is the easiest style to remember. All lines begin at the left margin. Illustration 16.1 is an example of the block format.

**Illustration 16.1   Block Letter Style — Open Punctuation**

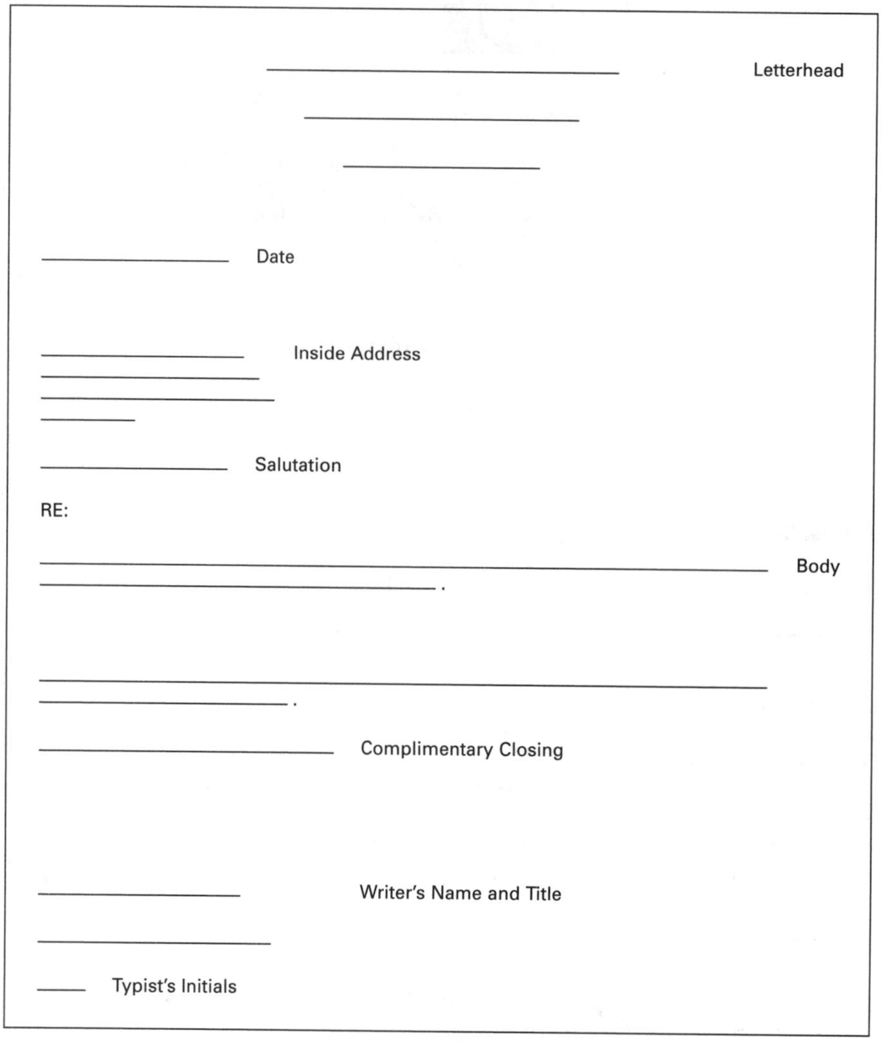

_____  Letterhead

_____  Date

_____  Inside Address

_____  Salutation

RE:

_____  Body

_____  Complimentary Closing

_____  Writer's Name and Title

_____  Typist's Initials

**Modified Block Style** — The body, inside address, and salutation of the letter are identical to the block style. But the date, complimentary closing, writer's name, and title all begin at the centre of the page (see Illustration 16.2).

The simplified letter is yet another style, but it is not used in a medical environment.

## Spacing

A letter properly arranged on the page should resemble a picture in a frame. This effect is achieved by using proper line lengths and by correctly spacing between parts of the letter.

The letterhead usually occupies the first ten to twelve lines of the paper. Depending on the length of the letter, you may prefer to begin the date on the fourteenth or fifteenth line and adjust your spacing between the date and the inside address, or you may adjust the position of your letter by always

**Illustration 16.2  Modified Block Style — Mixed Punctuation**

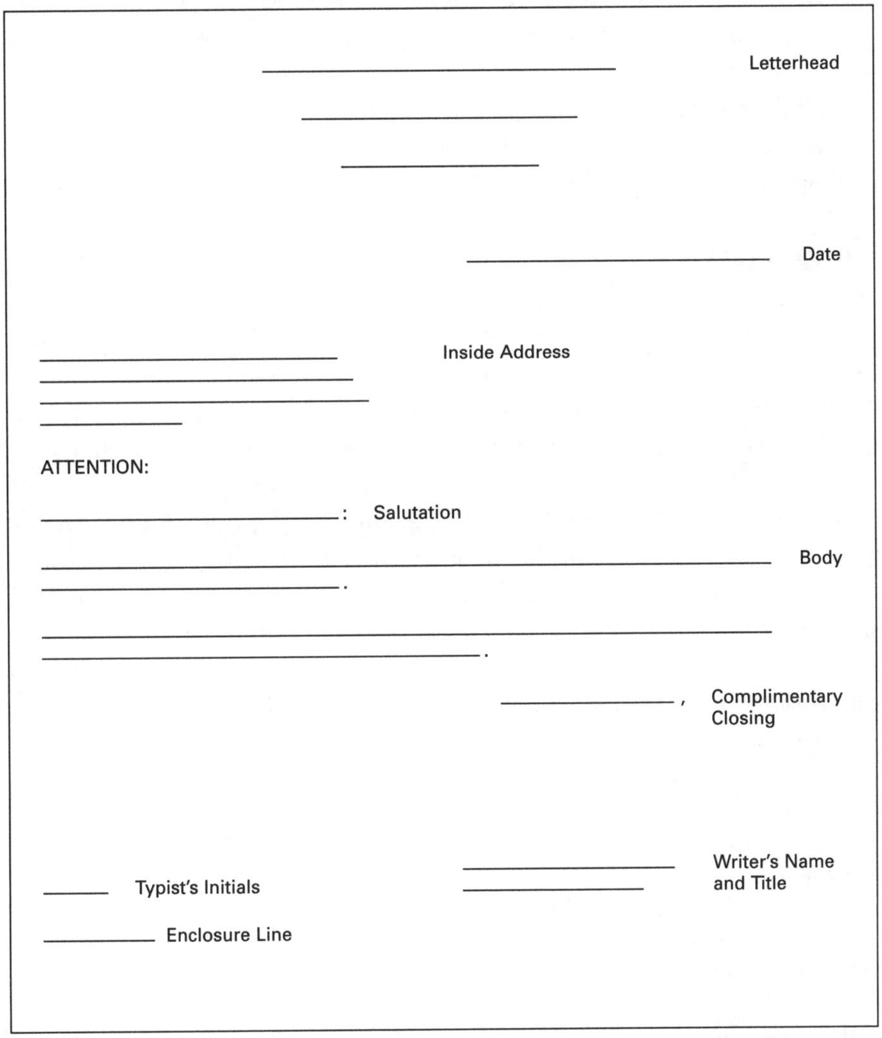

leaving five or six spaces between the date and inside address and placing the date according to the length of the letter.

*An efficient administrative assistant does not spend time calculating line lengths and spaces. You should assess the letter to be produced and position it according to your assessment.*

## Punctuation Styles

The two accepted styles of punctuation are open (no-point) and mixed (two-point). Punctuation styles do not pertain to the body of the letter. They deal only with the date, inside address, salutation, complimentary closing, and the writer's name and title lines (all short lines).

**Open Punctuation** — This is also referred to as no-point because there is no punctuation after any short line. This style is generally used with the block style shown in Illustration 16.1.

**Mixed Punctuation** — This style, or two-point punctuation, means there is punctuation at two points in the letter: a colon after the salutation and a comma after the complimentary closing. Mixed punctuation can be used with any style of letter (see Illustration 16.2).

While it is acceptable to use any style of punctuation with any style of letter, general practice is to use the simplest style (open) with block style letters and mixed with the block and modified styles.

## Two-Page Letters

When producing letters with more than one page, place the name of the recipient, the page number, and the date at the top of the second and succeeding pages. If referring to a patient, replace the recipient's name with "Re (patient's name)" or keep both names. If the second page is preprinted with the company name, begin keying three or four lines below the heading. If plain paper is used for the second page, begin keying on line 6 or 7. Triple-space before continuing with the body of the letter.

If the block or modified block style is used, place the name, page number, and date at the left margin, single-spaced, as shown in Illustration 16.3.

**Illustration 16.3   Second Page — Block or Modified Block Style**

```
Name
Page Number
Date
```

# Parts of a Business Letter

## Letterhead

The essential parts of the letterhead are the name and address of the firm and can also include the telephone number, telex number, executives, branches, products manufactured, and so on. Most businesses use good-quality bond paper on which the letterhead is preprinted. Many companies have preprinted second-page stationery as well. (The second page is usually preprinted with only the firm's name.)

## Date

The date is generally placed three or four lines below the letterhead and includes the month, day, and year.

## Inside Address

This is placed at least four and as many as ten or twelve lines below the date, depending on the length of the letter. The inside address consists of the recipient's name, title (if any), street address, city, province, and postal code.

## Attention Line

Some letters are addressed to a firm and sent to the attention of a specific person in the organization. The attention line is double-spaced below the last line of the inside address and placed at the left margin. The position of the attention line is shown in Illustration 16.2.

## Salutation

The salutation is double-spaced after the last line of the inside address or attention line, if used. When a letter is addressed to a company and/or contains an attention line, the salutation is usually Gentlemen, Ladies and Gentlemen, or Dear Sir or Madam. When the letter is addressed to an individual, the salutation is Dear Mr. Smith, Dear Ms. Jones, or Dear Jim.

## Subject or Reference Line

Some writers identify the letter's subject in a reference line, which appears a double space below the salutation. The reference line is placed at the left margin (see Illustration 16.1). In the medical environment, letters contain the patient's name and date of birth in the reference line. Any other pertinent identifying information, for example, a workers' compensation claim number, should follow the date of birth.

## Body

The body of the letter begins a double space below the reference line (or the salutation if there is no reference line). The body is generally single-spaced with a double space between paragraphs. The body of the letter should contain at least two paragraphs.

## Complimentary Closing

The closing is placed two spaces below the last line of the body of the letter. "Yours truly" and "Sincerely" are the most commonly used closings for business letters. Only the first word of the closing is capitalized.

## Signature Block

This contains the writer's name and title. A space (not less than three or more than five spaces) after the complimentary closing is left for the signature, and the writer's name is placed below this space. The title line(s) should be single-spaced after the writer's name. A doctor's name is usually followed by his or her degree but not preceded by "Dr."

## Reference Initials

There are several styles used when keying reference initials. At one time, the writer's initials followed by the typist's initials was the preferred style, as in

ABC/DEF or ABC:def. However, since the writer's name is already at the end of the letter, the initials of the person producing the letter are all that are required (/def, :def, or def.). Initials are placed at the left margin, usually two spaces below the signature block.

## Enclosures

If a document is enclosed with the letter, a reference to the enclosure is made either single- or double-spaced below the reference initials. If more than one document is enclosed, the number may appear after the word "enclosures." Some styles of enclosure lines follow:

Enclosure
Encl.
Enclosures (3)
Enclosures — Policy
               Cheque
               Questionnaire

## Copy Notations

If copies of a letter are being sent to people other than the addressee, a copy notation must be included. Copy notations are placed a double space below the last line of a letter, that is, the producer's initials or enclosure line. The copy notation comes before the postscript.

Occasionally the originator of a letter will send copies to associates and request that the copy notation not appear on the original letter. Such copies are referred to as blind or silent copies. After the original letter is completed, a blind copy notation is made on any additional copies of the letter. Illustration 16.4 shows an example of the method for making copy and blind copy notations.

## Postscript

The postscript can be used to express an important afterthought. The postscript appears at the very end of the letter, a double space below the last keyed line.

**Illustration 16.4    Carbon Copy and Blind Carbon Copy Notations**

```
lbp
Enclosure


c:    J.E. Smith — Accounting Dept.
      R.S. Green — Bell Clinic

bc:   Dr. M.R. Dantzer — Psychiatric Department
```

Produce the following letters on appropriate letterhead. For Letter 1 use block style, open punctuation; for Letter 2 use modified block style, mixed punctuation; and for Letter 3 use block style with open punctuation.

## Assignment 16.1

## Letter 1

From Doctor Pelham to Dr. H.A. Schmidt, 33 Block Avenue, Ottawa, Ontario, J5Z 3Y7. Reference Mrs. Lisa Basciano. Mrs. Basciano whom we thought had an acute carpal tunnel syndrome on the right wrist was reviewed in my office today. I presume you have the E.M.G. report with you and those indicate normal tracing with no evidence of any compression of the median nerve at the wrist. Also, clinically today, when I examined her, she seems to have normal sensation but with the occasional pain and tenderness whenever she lifts heavy objects. I think she should be left alone and periodically reviewed.

## Letter 2

From Doctor Plunkett to Dr. R.J. Mahon, Bell Clinic, 377 Unger Street, Ottawa, Ontario, J5Z 5X8. Subject Peter J. Scott. Thank you for referring me to see Peter John who certainly has a lesion on his upper lip, as well as a possible intradermal naevus on the temporal areas. I will be making an arrangement for the removal of this under local anaesthesia (L/A) as an out-patient at the O.G.H. I am enclosing a reference report on this patient.

## Letter 3

From Doctor Pelham to Heavenly Haven Home for the Aged, R.R. 3, Kars, Ontario A7W 5S3. Attention: Mr. R.J. Seymour, Administrator. Re: Mr. Mel Thompson. Mr. Thompson was reviewed in my office today, regarding his persistence of having an operative procedure of blepharoplasty done on his lower eyelids. I certainly appreciate the baginess of his bilateral lower eyelids, and he tells me they are impairing his vision because they are dragging his lower eyelids down. Dr. Blenkan, medical consultant for MOH, did phone me that it has been approved in May 19__ and I could carry out the procedure of bilateral lower blepharoplasty with this approval. I will be making an arrangement for him to be admitted to the Ottawa General Hospital and carry out the procedure of bilateral blepharoplasty and reconstruct the orbital septum.

Produce Letter 4 using modified block style and mixed punctuation, Letter 5 using block style and open punctuation, and Letter 6 using block style and mixed punctuation. Use proper sentence structure and paragraphing. Correct *all* spelling errors.

Keep Letters 1 to 6 for use in Assignment 16.2.

**Letter 4**

Dear Dr. Pelham / ▸Subject Latent Syphilis

It has been brought to my attention by the Ont. Min. of Health that many cases of latent syphilis are becoming evident in your ₙpeople. These are persons who have been treated for

Insert ▸ gonorrhaie but without having blood taken
* for possible syphilis being present concurrently. By doing syphilis serology (when positive) adequate dosages of antibiotics can be administered which will control together both gonorrhaea and syphilis. This will prevent the later fatal complications of syphilis, including neurosyphilis. It will also prevent the further spread of syphilis which is increasing each year.

Your cooperation will be of great assistance.

*Insert - treatment for gonorrhaea above is at a level which temporarily can mask syphilis but not control it

JN Brownd MDCN
DOH
Med. Off. of Health

**Letter 5**

From Med. Off. of Health as above to Dr. Plunkett.
Re. Birth Control Clinics. Recently it was
suggested to us by the Ont. Min. of Health
that we open a birth control clinic with
spec. emphasis on our teenage pop. The abortion
rate in Ontario arising at an alarming rate.
Since ab. as ~~togi~~ a failure of birth
control the best method of avoiding abortion
is to give instr. on b.c. At its last meeting
our Bd. of Health approved the opening of a b.c.
Since in our health unit. This clinic will
open in ~~Spt~~ Oct. We shall be asking our
physicians to man this clinic since it
will be on Wed. afternoon. There is
remuneration for each case attended. For
full details will you please call
Elizabeth Myles at 745-7677.

## Letter 6

**To**: Kenmar Ins.
Co. Ltd.

327 Crown Dr.
Ottawa

**Re**: Lois Elliott
Accident Feb. 9,
19___

(This letter was
actually mailed by a
medical secretary)

Thank you for your letter dated May 6, 19___ regarding _____ _____. I had seen her in the Emergency Department at the Ottawa General Hospital on February 9, 19___, at the request of Dr. _____. She was involved in a motor vehicle accident with crush avulsion injury involving the forehead along with multiple pieces of glass (foreing bodies) in the skin and subcutaneous tissues. She was taken to the operating room the same day and the procedure of debridement and plastic reconstruction along with removal of the foreing

She was kept in the hospital from February 9, 19___ to February 13, 19___. During this period, she did well, with good recovery, along with good wound healing. She was reviewed after being discharged from the hospital in my office for a follow-up. The sutures were removed, the wound was healing well and naturally the scars were visible. She had a palpable, tender, painful foreign body in the form of a glass piece in the forehead and she was taken to the O.R. on September 12, 19___ and this was removed under general anaesthesia (G/A) as an out-patient at the O.G.H. Since then, she has been followed up and her progress has be satisfactory.

She was reviewed in my office on May 28, 19___ for the purpose of this information to you. Mrs. _____ says that _____ complains of headaches, dizziness, occassionaly. To my knowledge, she did not have any head injury at the time of the accident. I attribute this headache and dizziness symptoms are probably due to the lacerations she had sustained to the forehead. However, if the symptoms persist and she continues to have problems and a neurological consultation is necessary. The scars are visible and she likes to have the forehead scars covered by a type of hairdo.

She feels the scars are rough and visible. On examination she has a visible scar which is irregular and almost resembles a hockey stick running from right side forehead hairline and obliquely towards nose and then turning horizontally above the nose in the center of the forehead then again up toward the scalp. The whole area approximately measures 7-8 cm in oblique pattern. There is still marked roughness and irregularity on her forehead. The area is hyperaemic and and certain parts break open due to the instability of the epithelium. This, I think, will gradually epithelialize in time. The irregularity of the area may be improved by the way of dermabrasion in about 6 months or 1 year's time. She does not appear to have numbness or a tingling sensation distal to the laceration indicating that the nerves on her forehead are intact and injuries were mostly superficial in the way of abrasion of skin and subcutaneous tissue only.

## Letter 6 (continued)

> The skull bones and facial bones are all intact and normal. The maxilla and mandibles are also intact and with good occlusion of the teeth.
>
> In summary, this young lady was involved in a motor vehicle accident and injuries were confined to her forehead. There were abrasions and lacerations which were treated and repaired. There were foreign bodies removed and repaired. She is still left with a visible, irregular, rough, scar on her forehead. I think in 6 months to a year's time, she needs to be re-assessed and if I thing she needs to have any dry skin surface abrasion surgery, I will be considering it. The disability at the resent time is a visible, irregular, roughened scar on the forehead. There will be some of this persistent for a long time.
>
> I hope this report will be of help to you and accompanied is the account in the amount of $_____.

# Envelopes

The two sizes of envelopes most commonly used are no. 8 and no. 10. A no. 8 envelope measures approximately 16.5 cm × 9 cm (6½ inches × 3⅝ inches) and a no. 10 envelope is approximately 24 cm × 10.5 cm (9½ inches × 4⅛ inches).

When keying the address on any envelope, the first line should begin approximately one line below and five spaces to the left of the centre point. On a no. 8 envelope, space down approximately twelve spaces, and for a no. 10 envelope, thirteen or fourteen spaces. The address on the envelope should duplicate the letter both in name and address and in punctuation style.

Most addresses are single-spaced. The address consists of the name of the recipient, the title (if any), street address or post office box number, city or town, and province. The postal code is keyed two spaces after the province on the same line. Regardless of the style of punctuation used, there is no punctuation after the postal code. Nothing should be placed opposite, or in the space below the postal code. Special mailing instructions, attention lines, and so on are usually placed two or three spaces below the return address. See Illustration 16.5.

When folding a letter for insertion into a no. 8 envelope, place the letter on the desk facing you and fold from bottom to top to within roughly 0.5 cm (¼ inch); fold from the right one-third to the left and fold from the left to within roughly 1 cm (½ inch) of the right edge. With the envelope opening facing you, insert left creased edge first with the open side facing toward you.

**Illustration 16.5    Envelope Set-Up**

| | |
|---|---|
| _____ | Return Address |
| _____ | |
| _____ | |
| | |
| Airmail, Special Delivery | |
| Attention Line, etc. | |

Stamp
Area

_____

_____        Mailing
Address

City,   Province   Postal Code

Nothing should be
keyed in this area

When folding a letter for insertion in a no. 10 envelope, you may do as follows: with the letter on the desk facing you, fold from bottom to top one-third of the way and from top to bottom to within roughly 1 cm ($\frac{1}{2}$ inch) of the first creased edge. Insert the last creased edge toward the bottom of the envelope. Or, with the letter on the desk facing you, fold from bottom to top one-third of the way, turn the letter over and fold the top edge down over the first crease approximately 1 cm ($\frac{1}{2}$ inch). Insert with the overlap to the top of the envelope.

The second method of folding eliminates the risk of the recipient cutting the letter in two with a letter opener.

Remember to insert any required enclosures before sealing the envelope.

## Assignment 16.2

Prepare envelopes for the letters you produced in Assignment 16.1 (use the envelopes in the Working Papers [pp. 118–23] or produce computer-generated envelopes). Produce two no. 8 envelopes and four no. 10 envelopes. Attach two blank folded sheets to your envelopes, one folded for a no. 8 envelope and one folded for a no. 10 envelope.

## Assignment 16.3

Dr. Plunkett has sent the following letter to Mr. Ronald Gilmour, 3279 Circle Square, Ottawa, J5X 7W4. Mr. Gilmour is about to be discharged from the hospital following a heart attack. Dr. Plunkett has asked you to send a copy of the letter to Dr. Pelham and to Dr. E.S. Langan at the heart clinic. He has also requested that a blind copy be sent to Mr. E.S. Hicks, Mr. Gilmour's boss. Produce the required copies.

Once you are discharged from the hospital, you should continue to add activities according to the schedule I have given you. It would be helpful to yourself if you established realistic weekly goals of activity or other alternatives of lifestyle which are important for your heart's health. For example, make a contract with a family member that you will lose one kilogram each week for a month, or you will walk a set distance every day, reduce cigarette consumption by one cigarette per day until you stop. You may help someone else besides yourself! Continue with your activity program even after complete recovery. Whatever form of activity you choose, remember, it must be performed a minimum of three times a week to be of any benefit. You are well on the way to recovery and if you follow the instructions I have given you, a full recovery and resumption of normal activities is expected.

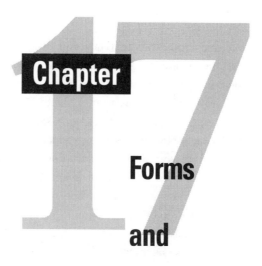

# Chapter 17

# Forms

# and

# Requisitions

## Chapter Outline

- Assignment 17.1
- Assignment 17.2
- Assignment 17.3

## Learning Objectives

To review
- the proper placement of typing on lines
- the proper placement of typing in boxed areas

Many medical offices will produce computer-generated macros for forms and requisitions. However, medical forms remain that must be produced on a typewriter, for example, autopsy reports. The main point of instruction here is to learn to type properly on lines and in spaces.

## Typing on Lines

The proper placement for typewritten information in relation to a line is as follows:

TOO HIGH
_____

TOO LOW
_____

CORRECT
_____

All typists should know their own typewriter and where a line of typing displays in relation to the alignment scale. On some typewriters, the characters sit on the alignment scale line; on others the characters may be slightly above or below (see Illustration 17.1). If you are familiar with your typewriter, you can very quickly adjust for proper placement on a line.

**Illustration 17.1 Typewriter Alignment Scale Line**

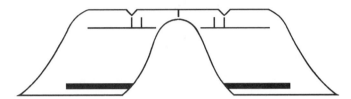

The variable line spacer is used to adjust the paper up or down until the exact position is reached (see Illustration 17.2).

**Illustration 17.2 Variable Line Spacer**

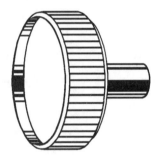

## Assignment 17.1

Complete the following questions by typing your answers correctly positioned on the lines. The blank forms can be found on pp. 102–103 of the Working Papers.

What is your name? _____

What is your address? _____

What school do you attend? _____

Do you have a part-time job? _____

If so, where? _____

Fill in the blanks in the following paragraph:

Today's date is _____ in the year _____. Christmas day is on _____ this year. The Prime Minister of Canada is _____. The President of the United States is _____. The date of my birthday is _____.

Were you able to place your typing characters correctly in relation to the line? If you are still having difficulty, ask your instructor for extra help.

You may also be required to type in a boxed or columned area. If you are typing in columns, try to centre your characters within the column lines. Examine Illustration 17.3.

**Illustration 17.3    Type in a Columned Area**

| Date | Reference | Charges | | Payments | | Balance | |
|---|---|---|---|---|---|---|---|
| | **THIS** | | | | | | |
| 10 01 96 | Balance Forward | | | | | 35 | 00 |
| 10 03 96 | Physical Examination | 26 | 80 | | | 61 | 80 |
| 10 05 96 | Received Payment | | | 35 | 00 | 26 | 80 |
| | **NOT THIS** | | | | | | |
| 10 01 96 | Balance Forward | | | | | 35 | 00 |
| 10 03 96 | Physical Examination | 26 | 80 | | | 61 | 80 |
| 10 05 96 | Received Payment | | | 35 | 00 | 26 | 80 |

The same principle applies when you are typing in boxed areas, such as those on a health claim card. Examine Illustration 17.4.

**Illustration 17.4    Type in a Boxed Area**

**THIS**

| P | L | U | N | K | E | T | T | | L | B |
|---|---|---|---|---|---|---|---|---|---|---|

**NOT THIS**

| P | | U | N | K | | T | | | | B |
|---|---|---|---|---|---|---|---|---|---|---|

**Assignment 17.2**

Jodi Campbell, R.R. 2, Anytown, Ontario, was given a Pap smear test on December 16, 19__. She is a health insurance plan subscriber under no. 3423352735. Her birthdate is May 18, 1960. Dr. Pelham performed the test. The lab number is 33657. Mrs. Campbell is experiencing abnormal bleeding. The test was a combined smear. The charge for the service was $17.50. Fill in the appropriate blanks on the gynecological form (Illustration 17.5) found on pp. 104–105 of the Working Papers.

**Illustration 17.5   Gynecological Form**

| PATIENT'S LAST NAME – PRINT: | | PATIENT'S FIRST NAME | YEAR OF BIRTH |
|---|---|---|---|
| ADDRESS | HEALTH NO. | | CHARGE   $ |

| DOCTOR | DATE | PCH LAB NO |
|---|---|---|

CLINICAL DIAGNOSIS

IF PREVIOUS ABNORMAL CYTOLOGY GIVE NAME OF
EXAMINING LABORATORY

☐ P C H

CLINICAL DATA

D L M P _____ MENOPAUSE ☐

PREGNANT ☐ _____ MONTHS

POST-PARTUM ☐ _____ WEEKS

HORMONE Rx ☐

SPECIFY

ABNORMAL BLEEDING ☐

| COMBINED SMEAR ☐ | CERVIX ONLY ☐ | VAGINA ONLY ☐ |
|---|---|---|
| ASPIRATION ☐ | CANAL ☐ | CAVITY ☐ |

LAB USE ONLY

CANCER DIAGNOSIS

NEGATIVE
☐

COMMENTS

TRICHOMONAS
PRESENT ☐

YEAST
PRESENT ☐

INFLAMMATORY
EFFECTS ☐

PATHOLOGIST

**Assignment 17.3**

On the memo form provided by your instructor, type a memo to Dr. Pelham from Dr. Plunkett informing her that he is performing a hysterectomy on Krista Peters (Tim Peters's wife) at Ottawa Civic Hospital on January 4, 19__. Dr. Plunkett would like Dr. Pelham to administer the anaesthetic and wonders if she will be available on that date. The time of surgery has been booked for 1000 in operating room no. 7.

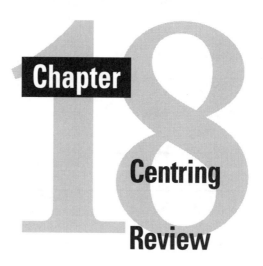

# Chapter 18

## Centring Review

**Chapter Outline**

- Assignment 18.1
- Assignment 18.2

- Assignment 18.3

**Learning Objectives**

To review
- vertical centring
- horizontal centring
- block centring

The advent of the computer has, in most cases, eliminated the necessity of understanding how to centre material on a page. There may be occasions, however, when the medical administrative assistant may be producing material on a typewriter that requires centring. We have included appropriate centring methods for your reference.

## Vertical Centring

On most typewriters, six single-line spaces can be typed in 1 vertical inch (2.3 single-line spaces in 1 vertical centimetre). On a standard 21.5 cm × 28 cm sheet, 64 single-line spaces (28 × 2.3) can be typed. Using the linear measure equivalent, 66 single-line spaces (11 × 6) can be typed on a standard 8½ inch × 11 inch sheet.

In order to centre an item vertically on a piece of paper, you would calculate the number of single-line spaces available (A); subtract the number of typing lines and spaces in the exercise (B); divide your answer by 2 and add 1. Your answer (C) would be the number of times you return you carriage (single-spacing) before beginning to type the article.

Centring Equation: $[(A - B)/2] + 1 = C$

Examine Illustration 18.1.

**Illustration 18.1   Vertical Centring**

| | | |
|---|---|---|
| 1 | | MEDICAL TERMINOLOGY |
| 2 | | |
| 3 | | (2 single-line spaces) |
| 4 | Word | Meaning |
| 5 | | (1 single-line space) |
| 6 | Gastric | Pertaining to the stomach |
| 7 | Mucosa | Mucous membrane |
| 8 | Virus | A minute infectious agent |
| 9 | Chronic | Persisting for a long time |
| 10 | Hiatus | Gap, cleft, opening |
| 11 | Dermatitis | Inflammation of the skin |
| 12 | Neuralgia | Pain in a nerve |
| 13 | Arthritis | Inflammation of a joint |
| 14 | Phlebitis | Inflammation of a vein |
| 15 | Ecchymosis | Escape of blood into tissue |
| 16 | Periorbital | Around the eye socket |
| 17 | Transverse | Extending from side to side |
| 18 | Epistaxis | Hemorrhage from the nose |
| 19 | Asymptomatic | Showing no symptoms |
| 20 | Palpate | To feel with fingers or hand |
| 21 | Jaundice | Yellowness of skin and eyes |
| 22 | Protrusion | Extension beyond the usual limit |
| 23 | Bowel | The intestine |
| 24 | Cephalic | Pertaining to the head |
| | | (Total of 24 line spaces) |

Using our mathematical equation, let us assume we are typing the illustrated material on a page 8½ inches × 11 inches.

## Horizontal Centring

Centring lines horizontally is a very simple task if you let your typewriter do the work. In order to centre a line horizontally on a page, you find the centre of the paper, place the paper in your typewriter with the centre aligned with the centre of the typewriter, and backspace once for every two letters and spaces; for example, in order to centre the words "medical administrative assistant," centre the paper in the typewriter and, using the backspace key, backspace as follows:

ME DI CA Lspace AD MI NI ST RA TI VE
bs  bs  bs   bs   bs  bs  bs  bs  bs  bs  bs

AS SI ST AN T
bs  bs  bs  bs

Note that the last three letters are incorporated into one backspace. If a single letter remains, the backspace key is not depressed for that letter.

There may be occasions when you wish to emphasize a specific line in a typewritten display. In order to accomplish this, you may use extended centring (one space between letters, three spaces between words). If you wish to spread-centre the words "medical administrative assistant," centre the paper in the typewriter and backspace once for each letter and space:

<u>M</u> <u>E</u> <u>D</u> <u>I</u> <u>C</u> <u>A</u> <u>L</u> space <u>A</u> <u>D</u> <u>M</u> <u>I</u> <u>N</u> <u>I</u> <u>S</u> <u>T</u> <u>R</u> <u>A</u> <u>T</u> <u>I</u> <u>V</u> <u>E</u>
bs bs bs bs bs bs bs   bs   bs bs bs bs bs bsbs bs bs bs bs bs bs

<u>A</u> <u>S</u> <u>S</u> <u>I</u> <u>S</u> <u>T</u> <u>A</u> <u>N</u> <u>T</u>
bs bs bs bsbs bs bs bs

Do not backspace for the *last* letter in the line.

As you type, press the space bar once after each letter and three times between words.

---

**Assignment 18.1**

Using the backspace method for horizontal centring, centre the following exercise vertically and horizontally on 21.5 cm × 14 cm (8$\frac{1}{2}$ inch × 5$\frac{1}{2}$ inch) paper. Display it attractively in invitation format.

The Medical Secretaries' Association invites you to attend WHAT'S NEW WITH YOU on Saturday, April 1, 199__, at 9 A.M. at Trent University Great Hall. Admission is $15.

---

## Block Centring

Another method of centring is called block centring: the longest line in the exercise is the only line exactly centred horizontally. After using the backspace method to centre the longest line, set the left margin at the stopping point of the carriage. All lines in the exercise are then typed at the left margin. Examine Illustration 18.2.

### Illustration 18.2    Block Centring

<u>Major Purchases</u>
1981-82

Two Ventilators
Operating Table
Two Anaesthetic Tables
Code IV Cart
Autoclave
Neo-Med Bovie Machine
Complete Laparoscopic Setup
Bronchoscope

"Complete Laparoscopic Setup" is the longest line in Illustration 18.2. Centre the paper in the typewriter and place the carriage at the centre point. Backspace once for every two letters and spaces in "Complete Laparoscopic Setup." When backspace centring is complete, set the left margin where the carriage is positioned. Return to the beginning of the list, "Two Ventilators," and type each line flush with the left margin.

On a full sheet of paper, double-spaced, type the following department list (use block centring); centre vertically and horizontally.

**Assignment 18.2**

Department ~~Index~~ List : Building Services;
Laboratory ; Nuclear Medicine; Pharmacy;
Radiology, Psychiatry; Pycology; Ambulance;
Diet Clinics; Financial Services; Food
Service, Housekeeping; Department of
Medicine ; Department of Anaesthesia;
Medical Records : Admitting; Purchasing;
Supply, Processing and Distribution;
Electroencephalography; Infection Control;
Respiratory Technology; Physiotherapy.

**Assignment 18.3**

Type the following notice, centred vertically and horizontally on a full sheet.

(Extended Centering) → Job Posting

Required immediately: SECRETARY – STENO III

Qualifications ← (block caps)

Must have good typing skills, a sound knowledge of medical terminology, and the ability to deal with co-workers and patients in an efficient and friendly manner  } block centre

Resumes should be sent to:

Robert Johnstone
Human Resources Dept.
Room 3400, Main Building  } block centre

Deadlines for application: November 1, 19—

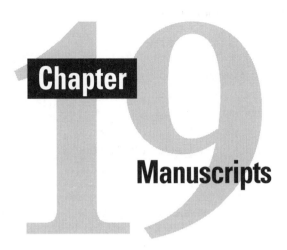

# Chapter 19

# Manuscripts

**Chapter Outline**

- Assignment 19.1
- Assignment 19.2
- Assignment 19.3

**Learning Objectives**

To review
- manuscript-formatting rules
- parts of a manuscript
- title pages
- use of notes
- bibliographies

From time to time, you may be required to produce a copy of a speech, an educational submission, or the text of a medical manual. The information for such documents is generally in rough-draft handwritten form, or on a tape. Your responsibility is to decipher the rough draft and produce a readable document.

If the information is easy to decipher, you can produce a finished copy from the original draft. Because of very poor handwriting, unfamiliar terminology, and so on, you may wish to type a draft and have the author proofread it before the final copy is produced. If you produce a draft, leave ample space (triple space) for the author to make corrections and additions. Check that spelling, grammar, punctuation, paragraphing, and form are correct, and ask the author for confirmation of any questionable areas. Make an effort to decipher as much of the original rough draft as possible so that the draft will require little revision. When producing the rough draft, you don't have to be specific about form.

## General Rules for Producing a Manuscript

1. The title should be placed at least ten and not more than thirteen lines from the top of the page, centred, and in block capitals.
2. Use only one side of the page.

3. Use standard 21.5-cm × 28-cm (8½-inch × 11-inch) paper.

4. Manuscripts are usually double-spaced, although one and one-half or single spacing may be requested by the author.

5. Indent the first line of each paragraph five spaces.

6. Top-bound and unbound manuscripts should have 3 cm (1¼ inches) left and right margins (i.e., a 15-cm or 6-inch line). If the manuscript is bound on the left, move the line spacing roughly 1 cm (½ inch) to the right. The line length is still 15 cm (6 inches); however, the left margin is 4.5 cm (1¾ inches) and the right margin is 2 cm (¾ inch) wide. The centre point of the page is also moved roughly 1 cm (½ inch) to the right.

7. Leave a 2.5- to 4-cm (1 to 1½ inches) margin at the bottom of each page; be consistent. Second and succeeding page numbers are usually placed on line 5 or 6, centred, or at the right margin for side-bound and unbound documents. If a manuscript is top-bound, the page number should be centred at the bottom of the page. Using the pagination function of your word processor will automatically number pages.

8. Triple-space after the title and each page number.

9. If the copy is a draft, the word "DRAFT" should appear across the top of every sheet. This will avoid confusion and the possibility of draft pages being mixed with finished copy.

## Parts of a Manuscript

In order to produce a readable, easily understood document, various headings are used. General rules are given as a guideline. You may wish to alter these somewhat; however, consistency is important. For example, if the first sub-heading is centred and underscored, *all* subheadings must be centred and underscored.

## General Rules for Producing Manuscript Headings

1. Title
   - centre
   - use block capitals
   - can be spread-centred
   - triple-space after

2. Subheading for principal subdivision
   - centre
   - use initial capitals and lower case
   - underscore
   - triple-space before
   - double-space after

3. Side heading
   - second most important subdivision
   - use block capitals or normal upper and lower case

- underscore
- triple-space before
- double-space after

Note: If only one type of heading is required, side headings are generally used.

4. Paragraph (or run-in) heading used to identify material in the paragraph
   - usually is a part of the first sentence in the paragraph
   - underscore the key words

Illustration 19.1 is an excerpt from a manuscript and shows the heading and subheading styles.

**Illustration 19.1   Heading and Subheading Styles in a Manuscript**

HEADACHES

Have you ever "seen the sun" inside the house minutes before the onset of a blinding headache; or felt like dying because your head hurt so much you couldn't stand it? These are symptoms of chronic, debilitating headaches.

Migraines

The first symptom is a migraine symptom. A migraine is a very severe headache caused by the swelling of blood vessels. The pain is usually experienced on one side and is sometimes preceded by warning symptoms, such as visual changes or numbness in the extremities.

Cluster Headaches

The second symptom is indicative of a cluster headache. The victim experiences severe stab-like pain around the eye area. The attacks occur daily and last for long periods and then disappear.

Tension Headaches

Tension headaches are not imagined by the sufferer. Emotional upsets can produce physiological and biochemical changes. The body's painkilling chemicals — endorphins — may be reduced, resulting in more severe pain.

Depression Headaches

Conflict and stress resulting in depression can create problems. Many people suffering from depression headaches treat the discomfort with over-the-counter drugs. This condition should be assessed by a physician and treated.

Diagnosing the Cause
Sometimes diagnostic procedures are fairly simple. Minor nervous upsets are often the cause; however, such problems as allergies, sinusitis, improper diet, poor posture, and low-grade fevers can be the culprit.
The medical field now recognizes that there are different forms of headaches and that they are caused by many variables. This, together with new drugs, relaxation and biofeedback techniques, and special diets, has resulted in much-needed relief for the headache sufferer.

## Title Page

Some reports and manuscripts require a title page. The title page includes such information as the title of the report, the author's name, the date of printing, and the city and province of the author. Some title pages may include the purpose of the document. All of this information should be vertically and horizontally centred on a full page to produce an attractive presentation.

Notice that the manuscript in Illustration 19.1 uses one and one-half rather than double spacing.

## Assignment 19.1

This is a production assignment, and your instructor will provide you with the required material. You will be given a specific amount of time to complete the document. Assume the article was written by Dr. Zarstell this year. Produce the manuscript and prepare a title page.

## Reference Notes

If a reference source is quoted in the body of a printed document, the author must acknowledge the reference. The general format of presentation is as follows:

1. The author's name is first, followed by the title. Articles or chapters are placed in quotations; books or magazines are underscored.
2. The name of the publishing house, its location, the date of publication, and the page number of the reference follow the title.

Styles of punctuation and order of presentation of item (2) may vary. Using commas to separate each section of the reference note is acceptable. Some manuals dictate a period after the book title, a colon after the location of the publishing house, and commas in all other areas. It doesn't matter which style you choose, but you must be consistent. Do not mix styles.

There are four ways to present notes in a text:

1. The most common method is to place a superscript (a number placed one-half line above the keyed line) immediately following the words cited; double-space after the last line on the page and place fifteen underscore characters; double-space, indent five spaces, place the identical superscript one-half line above and one space before the first character in the footnote; key the footnote. This method is convenient for the reader.
2. Place the note immediately following the reference. A solid line of underscores is placed between the right and left margins, the footnote is

keyed below the solid line, and another solid line of underscores is placed below the note. This method is convenient, but if several references appear on one page, the document may appear disjointed and confusing to read.

3. Notes may appear at the end of the document (sometimes referred to as *endnotes*).

4. Place the notes in parentheses, immediately following the last word in the reference. This method is becoming more popular because the reference source is immediately available to the reader. This method is called *journal footnoting* or *parenthetical notation*.

---

Go to the library and select a book or article that has illustrated notes. In order to complete the assignment you will have to make three exchanges with fellow classmates. You will be working with four books or articles in total, including your own selection.

**Assignment 19.2**

Note the variety of methods publishers use to illustrate notes.

From each of the four books or articles, select one paragraph with a superscript and produce the accompanying note using each of the four methods just described. Do the endnote method on a separate sheet of paper.

---

## Bibliographies

A bibliography is a list of books, magazines, and articles used for reference when writing a paper and should be included at the end of the document.

The following is a general outline for producing bibliographies:

1. The first line is flush with the left margin.
2. Second and succeeding lines are indented five spaces.
3. The last name of the author appears first, followed by a comma and the author's given name(s).
4. As in footnotes, titles of articles or chapters appear in quotation marks; book and magazine titles are underscored.
5. Publisher's name, location, and date of publication follow the title.
6. Punctuation styles and order of presentation after the title may vary. (The guidelines given for footnotes may be followed.)
7. Bibliographies are always produced with the author's last names listed in alphabetical order.

---

Produce a bibliography of *all* textbooks and *all* medical reference books used in your courses.

**Assignment 19.3**

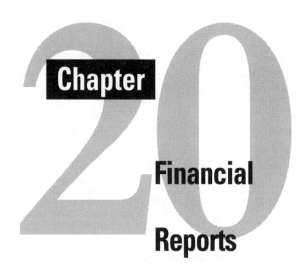

# Chapter 20

## Financial Reports

**Chapter Outline**

- Assignment 20.1

**Learning Objectives**

To review
- the proper format for financial reports
- the use of open and closed leaders

Although medical administrative assistants are usually not responsible for the production of financial statements, it is wise to have a general idea of their content and format. There are several methods used to produce financial statements so that they are clearly presented on the page. Illustrations 20.1 to 20.5 are examples of common financial statements.

Remember, when producing any financial statement, figures must be aligned at the decimal point.

Illustration 20.1 shows the owner's equity portion of a balance sheet. Produce a copy of the illustration.

**Illustration 20.1   Owner's Equity Portion of a Balance Sheet**

OWNER'S EQUITY

| | | |
|---|---|---|
| John Brown Capital, November 30, 19___ | | $10,550.00 |
|    Net Profit, December 31, 19___ | $4,625.00 | |
|     Less Drawings for December | 2,782.00 | 1,843.00 |
| Total Owner's Equity | | $12,393.00 |

There are several types of financial statements including balance sheets, income statements, trial balances, and bank reconciliation statements. Headings for most statements answer the questions "Who?" (name of company or individual), "What?" (type of statement), and "When?" (date of statement). These three identification headings should be centred and double-spaced with the "Who?" statement in block capitals. It is unnecessary to centre a financial statement vertically, although to do so is acceptable. If vertical centring is not used, begin on lines 8 to 10.

A trial balance (Illustration 20.2), balance sheet (Illustration 20.3), income statement (Illustration 20.4), and bank reconciliation statement (Illustration 20.5) are displayed for your perusal and study.

Note the following details:

1. The placement of main headings, side headings, and indentations.
2. A dollar sign is placed at the *beginning* of each money column, and repeated only after an addition or subtraction line, or to begin a new section of the statement.
3. Leaders may be used to help read the numbers. A leader is a line of periods, and is usually preceded by a space and followed by a space. Leaders may be open (a space between each period) or closed (no spaces). When using open leaders, note if the periods are placed on the odd or even spaces. Illustrations 20.2 and 20.3 are produced without leaders; Illustration 20.4 uses open leaders, and Illustration 20.5 uses closed leaders.
4. Thousand units may be separated by a comma or by leaving a space.
5. At the completion of the report, double underscores are placed immediately below the amount columns.

**Illustration 20.2   Trial Balance**

**ANYTOWN GENERAL HOSPITAL**
**Trial Balance**
**November 30, 19___**

| | | |
|---|---:|---:|
| Cash | $ 14,000.00 | |
| Accounts Receivable | 22,000.00 | |
| Land | 300,000.00 | |
| Buildings | 800,000.00 | |
| Furniture and Office Equipment | 170,000.00 | |
| Accounts Payable | | $ 60,000.00 |
| Mortgage Payable | | 100,000.00 |
| Retained Earnings | | 104,712.00 |
| Prescription Revenue | | 50,729.00 |
| Out-Patient Revenue | | 125,000.00 |
| Ward Revenue | | 572,399.00 |
| Private Ward Revenue | | 435,123.00 |
| Semiprivate Ward Revenue | | 768,421.00 |
| Salaries Expense | 750,000.00 | |
| Heat and Hydro | 25,928.00 | |
| Telephone Expense | 13,767.00 | |
| Office Supplies Expense | 35,297.00 | |
| Interest Expense | 10,000.00 | |
| Maintenance and Repair Expense | 75,392.00 | |
| | $ 2,216,384.00 | $ 2,216,384.00 |

**Note:** At the completion of the report, place double underscores immediately below the amount columns.

**Illustration 20.3   Summary Balance Sheet**

---

**EVERYTOWN GENERAL HOSPITAL**
**Summary Balance Sheet**
**As at November 30, 19___**
**(Expressed in 000s)**

### ASSETS

| | | |
|---|---:|---:|
| Current Assets | $ 2,350 | |
| Assets Held for Capital Purposes | 310 | |
| Property, Plant & Equipment | | |
|    at Cost Less Accumulated Depreciation | 8,411 | |
| Other Assets | 10 | |
|    TOTAL ASSETS | | $ 11,081 |

### LIABILITIES

| | | |
|---|---:|---:|
| Current Liabilities | $ 1,848 | |
| Capital Liabilities | | |
|    Short-term | 243 | |
|    Long-term | 1,072 | |
|    TOTAL LIABILITIES | | $   3,163 |

### SHAREHOLDERS' EQUITY

| | | |
|---|---:|---:|
| Total Shareholders' Equity | | 7,918 |
|    TOTAL LIABILITIES & SHAREHOLDERS' EQUITY | | $ 11,081 |

**Illustration 20.4   Income Statement**

**ALLTOWN GENERAL HOSPITAL**
**Income Statement**
**For the fiscal year ended June 30, 19___**
**(Expressed in 000s)**

REVENUE

| | |
|---|---|
| Short-term stay | $ 3 500 |
| Long-term stay | 2 800 |
| Out-patient | 1 728 |
| Pharmacy | 1 262 |
| TOTAL REVENUE | $ 9 290 |

EXPENSES

| | |
|---|---|
| Laundry | $   382 |
| Office Supplies | 17 |
| Salaries | 3 053 |
| Telephone | 63 |
| Heat | 1 239 |
| Taxes | 728 |
| Hydro | 62 |
| Depreciation | 11 |
| Maintenance and Repair | 302 |
| Drugs | 1 627 |
| Surgical Supplies | 1 329 |
| TOTAL EXPENSES | 8 813 |
| NET INCOME | $   477 |

**Illustration 20.5    Bank Reconciliation Statement**

### J.E. PLUNKETT, M.D.
### Bank Reconciliation Statement
### November 30, 19___

Balance as per bank statement, October 31, 19___ .........................$ 2,741.16

    Add bank deposit October 30, 19___ not recorded ......................     290.00

Adjusted bank balance .............................................................          $ 3,031.16

Deduct Outstanding Cheques:

    No. 35 ..........................................................................$     19.75

    No. 39 ..........................................................................      75.80

    No. 41 ..........................................................................      68.30

    No. 43 ..........................................................................     127.50

        TOTAL OUTSTANDING CHEQUES ......................................          291.35

        Bank Balance ................................................................          $ 2,739.81

Balance as per Cash Record October 31, 19___ ............................$ 2,808.56

    Add Bond Interest on Bonds .................................................      37.50

Adjusted Cash Record ..............................................................          $ 2,846.06

Deduct:

    Debit memo for safety deposit .................................................$      7.50

    N.S.F. Cheque patient #327 ....................................................      50.75

    Bank Interest ......................................................................      10.00

    Service charge for month ........................................................       2.00

    Error on cheque #42 ..............................................................      36.00

        TOTAL DEDUCTIONS ............................................................          106.25

        Cash Record Balance .......................................................          $ 2,739.81

## Assignment 20.1

Dr. Pelham has asked you to produce the following information into correct format for her balance sheet and income statement. Her year end is June 30, 19__.

Balance Sheet

Assets

Current Assets: cash $1 522.25; accouts receivable 10 268; deposits 99.50.

Fixed Assets: furniture $10 616.25; equipment 4 000.00; less accumulated depreciation 3 082.

Liabilities

Bank indebtedness $8 800; accounts payable and accrued liabilities 1 361; income taxes payable 375.

Owner's Equity: J.E. Pelham capital June 30, 19__, $5 000; net profit 23 511; drawings 15 623; capital June 30, 19__, 12 888.

Income Statement

Revenue: $119 833.

Expenses: accounting fees $3 600; automobile 806; bank charges and interest 1 840; business taxes 2 594; capital tax 1 050; drugs and medical supplies 6 167; fees, books, and conventions 2 348; general office 4 203; insurance 1 115; legal fees 1 100; postage and stationery 2 052; rent 16 000; salaries and benefits 37 293; telephone 2 571; depreciation 2 408; total expenses 85 147.

Income before taxes $34 686; income taxes 11 175.

# Part 3

# Timed Writings and Speed, Accuracy, and Terminology Development Exercises

Timed writings and speed, accuracy, and terminology development exercises form Part 3 of the book. These drills are excerpts from actual medical situations. The purpose of the drills is to increase speed and accuracy, and expand your knowledge of terminology.

# Timed Writings

### Timed Writing 1

                                                                        Words

This gentleman was admitted with a heaviness in his central chest. His CK rose to          15

approximately seven or eight times normal and in concert he developed the evolving EKG      29

pattern of an anterior myocardial infarction. He returned home continuing to complain of chest   43

discomfort reminiscent of his infarct and was transferred urgently to Toronto for heart      56

catheterization. I cannot remember the details of catheterization, but it is my understanding   69

that the gist of the study was that the major damage if not all damage which could be predicted   88

from the coronary anatomy had occurred, and the patient was not at risk of any subsequent    104

substantial infarct. Thereafter he returned to full activity without complaints of shortness of   117

breath, syncope, palpitation or peripheral edema and no further chest discomfort.        128

This gentleman has had one week of a bloating sensation in his stomach associated with    143

cramping and nausea. He has had no diarrhea, vomiting, or blood per rectum. Twenty-four   157

hours ago he experienced malaise and weakness and came to the Emergency for assessment.   171

He had also developed a nickel-size area of burning in the lower central midline and a slight   188

sensation of dyspnea.       191

Initially his complaints appeared to be totally non-cardiac and after completing an EKG the   205

patient was scheduled for discharge home. He complained of an ache in his left jaw. Repeat   221

EKG was done and because of apparent ischemia on the cardiogram the patient was held for   237

observation. In retrospect the patient notes that he has had three or four one-half hour episodes   253

of left jaw pain in recent months.       260

The gentleman has no established upper gut pathology. He denies significant chronic    272

obstructive pulmonary disease. There is no significant history of arthritis.    282

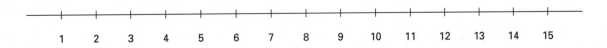

1    2    3    4    5    6    7    8    9    10    11    12    13    14    15

**Timed Writing 2**

|  | Words |
|---|---|
| Under general anaesthesia the abdomen was prepared with Betadine solution and draped. The | 13 |
| previous upper midline incision was opened. On opening the peritoneum, there was air and a | 28 |
| large amount of bile-stained fluid throughout the abdomen with exudate on the small bowel. | 42 |
| This was tediously suctioned off. There was omental fat over what turned out to be the | 58 |
| gastroenterostomy. This was lifted up and dissected and we came upon the perforation, an | 72 |
| opening about 3 to 4 mm in size. There was induration around it. It was the gastroenterostomy. | 89 |
| This was closed with three interrupted sutures of 00 chromic. Then, we carefully placed | 103 |
| sutures around the periphery to bring down the omental fat and this seemed to create quite an | 120 |
| effective seal. We then irrigated the peritoneal cavity with copious amounts of warm saline. | 134 |
| After this was suctioned off several times and we were satisfied that we had it as clean as | 152 |
| possible, a Penrose drain was brought through a stab in the left upper quadrant and left down | 169 |
| close to the area of perforation. Similarly, an intracath was brought through the epigastrium and | 184 |
| left in the same area. The linea alba edges were then brought together with interrupted figure- | 199 |
| of-eight sutures of 3-0 stainless-steel wire. The subcutaneous wound was irrigated out with | 212 |
| Tis-u-sol. A continuous suture of 3-0 vicryl was used in the subcutaneous wound edges and | 227 |
| the skin edges were brought together with a continuous vertical mattress suture of 3-0 prolene. | 242 |
| The intracath was sutured to the skin with 00 silk. The drain was sutured to the skin. A safety | 261 |
| pin was placed through it. Dry gauze dressings were applied, held in place with Montgomery | 276 |
| tapes. | 277 |
| We had considered doing a vagotomy but in view of the gross contamination and the | 292 |
| patient's liver is heavy with a rounded edge, we felt that we should not open up any further | 310 |
| tissue planes in such an ill man. | 317 |

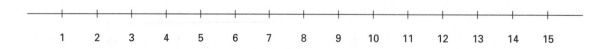

**Timed Writing 3**

|  | Words |
|---|---|
| This patient was seen in the emergency department at St. Joseph's Hospital for | 13 |
| assessment of a painful swollen elbow. His history dates back to yesterday morning when he | 28 |
| was sitting at the table and noticed that his elbow felt somewhat different than it had. Looking | 45 |
| at it he noticed that it was red and swollen. There was some slight discomfort in the elbow as | 64 |
| well. During the day his discomfort became worse and the swelling became worse as well. In | 80 |
| fact, by nightfall it was almost unbearable despite the fact that he was taking Tylenol #2 two | 97 |
| tablets q4h. Around midnight he was unable to sleep and he was up most of the night with the | 116 |
| pain. The swelling persisted and became worse again in the morning and he therefore came to | 132 |
| the emergency department at approximately 1010 hours. He was assessed by Dr. Smith and | 146 |
| was referred on the suspicion that he has suffered from cellulitis. | 157 |
| On functional inquiry he states that he has otherwise been remarkably well. He does not | 172 |
| recall any trauma to his left elbow. He has not broken or punctured his skin in any way. He has | 192 |
| not had a similar problem elsewhere and in fact he has never had this problem in the left elbow. | 211 |
| He did have gout in his right elbow but it presented much more slowly and the swelling was | 229 |
| much less, approximately a year or two ago. There has been no symptoms of DVT elsewhere, | 245 |
| nor of any shortness of breath or pulmonary embolism. He has had no recent angina. He walks | 262 |
| with a walker as he has for some time. He denies any cough, phlegm or wheezing or any | 280 |
| shortness of breath. He has had no chest pain, no palpitations, no nausea, no sweating, no | 296 |
| disphoresis. He has had no gastrointestinal or genitourinary problems. He recalls no clotting or | 310 |
| bleeding diatheses. He can swallow uneventfully. His weight is stable at 175 pounds, or slightly | 325 |
| higher than that. He is 5'6" tall. | 332 |

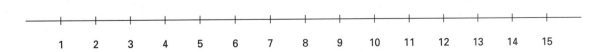

1    2    3    4    5    6    7    8    9    10    11    12    13    14    15

**Timed Writing 4**

|  | Words |
|---|---|
| This man first had a diffuse bladder tumour resected by myself from the left side of the | 17 |
| bladder. This was a fairly extensive tumour but a low grade, low stage tumour. He had a further | 35 |
| recurrence in the same area fulgurized in May. That has been his only recurrence. He has been | 52 |
| cystoscoped on a regular basis ever since his initial resection. He was last scoped in September | 68 |
| of this year. On talking to me today prior to this procedure he continues to deny any urinary tract | 87 |
| difficulties. | 88 |
| Using Xylocaine gel as a topical anaesthetic the bladder was examined using the 17 French | 103 |
| cystourethroscope. There is no overt evidence of recurrent tumour. There is scarring on the left | 118 |
| hand side of the base of the bladder just lateral to the left ureteral orifice. At the upper limit of | 138 |
| this scarring, at about three o'clock, well back from the bladder neck is one small area of | 155 |
| erythema, although this does not have the appearance at least at this time of recurrent tumour. | 171 |
| The rest of the bladder showed no abnormality at all. | 181 |
| I suggested to him that he should be scoped again in three months' time just to keep an eye | 200 |
| on this area in the left side. | 207 |
| He informed me that he and his wife were planning to travel south for the winter, | 223 |
| approximately the next five months. I have informed him that there is no real necessity for the | 240 |
| scope to be done in exactly three months and that when he returns from his holiday in the | 258 |
| south, he should contact me and we can then make arrangements for his examination. | 272 |
| I also recommended that if he experiences any discomfort while on his vacation, he should | 287 |
| attend at the emergency department of the nearest hospital to seek treatment. | 299 |

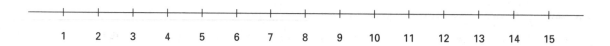

1   2   3   4   5   6   7   8   9   10   11   12   13   14   15

**Timed Writing 5**

Words

Under general anaesthetic the patient was prepped and draped with iodine and alcohol. The     14

lateral incision was made. Scope was inserted via distal lateral portal. Exploration revealed     27

grade II chondromalacia of the central medial portion of the patella. The medial compartment     41

revealed a bucket handle tear, shredded, of the medial meniscus. The lateral compartment was     55

normal. The intercondylar groove is normal. Through a medial portal a Beaver blade was     69

inserted and the anterior pole detached. A large fragment of the meniscus was removed. The     84

posterior bucket portion was then flipped in the intercondylar groove and through a second     98

portal just along the medial margin of the patellar tendon the Beaver blade was inserted and     114

with traction applied, the posterior horn was clipped, and the second major fragment then     128

removed. The remnant of the meniscus was debrided using the muncher. The undersurface of     142

the patella was then shaved. The knee was flushed. The portals were closed with vicryl. A     158

Jones bandage was applied. The patient was returned to the recovery room in good condition.     173

The patient was sedated before coming to the operating room and this was further     187

supplemented with Demerol 60 mg and Valium 7 mg IV. The throat was sprayed with     202

Xylocaine. An 18 Levin tube was inserted and only a few cc's of saliva-like material were     218

aspirated. The scope was then introduced without difficulty down through the esophagus.     230

There is a mild reddening in the esophagus but no ulceration. The lower esophageal sphincter     245

was located at 37-38 cm. There seems to be some polypid change at the lower     260

esophagogastric area and lesser curvature was obtained. I think these are all within normal     274

limits. The scope was then introduced down through a normal appearing antrum and into the     289

first and second parts of the duodenum. There is no duodenitis, ulceration, or other abnormality     304

there. The scope was withdrawn.     309

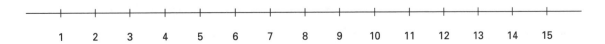

1    2    3    4    5    6    7    8    9    10    11    12    13    14    15

**Timed Writing 6**

|  | Words |
|---|---|
| Under general anaesthesia the McIvor mouth gag was inserted. Using the adenoid curette a | 14 |
| large amount of adenoid tissue was removed. Tonsillectomy was done by dissection. | 26 |
| Large, chronically inflamed tonsils were removed. Bleeding controlled using coagulation | 36 |
| diathermy. Ears were examined. The old Teflon tubes were lying in the canal. They were | 51 |
| removed. There was a large amount of debris and wax around the Teflon tubes. They were | 67 |
| removed. | 68 |
| The right Teflon tube was attached firmly to the tympanic membrane and this was | 82 |
| removed. I elected to remove the Teflon tube because in February, another month, it will be two | 99 |
| years since she has had the Teflon tubes attached to the tympanic membranes. | 112 |
| The perforation where the Teflon tube was attached was freshened so as to stimulate | 126 |
| healing. I expect the perforation to close over the next two or three weeks provided she does | 143 |
| not get water in her ears. | 149 |
| This lady, who is a known diabetic, may have been hypoglycemic, and slipped and fell at | 165 |
| home, injuring her pelvis. | 169 |
| She now complains of some pain in her right groin and X-rays revealed mildly displaced | 184 |
| fractures to the right superior and inferior pubic rami. | 193 |
| No specific treatment beyond bedrest and gradual mobilization when the discomfort settles | 205 |
| down is required. I don't anticipate any significant residual problems. | 215 |
| Thank you for asking me to see her. I will continue to follow her with interest. | 231 |

```
  ┬   ┬   ┬   ┬   ┬   ┬   ┬   ┬   ┬   ┬   ┬   ┬   ┬   ┬   ┬
  1   2   3   4   5   6   7   8   9   10  11  12  13  14  15
```

**Timed Writing 7**

| | Words |
|---|---|
| This young girl presents with recurrent biliary colic and documented cholelithiasis. Ultrasound | 12 |
| demonstrates no dilatation of the biliary tree. The patient has not been jaundiced and has not | 28 |
| had pancreatitis. | 30 |
|     With the patient under general anaesthesia, the abdomen is prepped and draped and a right | 45 |
| subcostal incision used to enter the peritoneal cavity. The gallbladder is mildly edematous but | 59 |
| there is no evidence of chronic cholecystitis. The stomach is somewhat distended with air. A | 74 |
| nasogastric tube was inserted. The duodenum is normal. By palpation large and small bowel | 88 |
| plus internal genitalia are normal. Both ovaries are of normal size. The right kidney is perhaps in | 105 |
| the upper limit for normal in size, but feels of normal consistency. The liver is normal. | 121 |
|     With suitable exposure the cholecystohepatoduodenal ligament is opened. The cystic | 131 |
| artery runs inferior and anterior to the cystic duct. It is ligated proximally with silk, distally | 147 |
| clipped and divided. The cystic duct is dissected back to what appears to be a common bile | 164 |
| duct which is small in size but within normal limits. Palpation of the common bile duct and the | 182 |
| head of the pancreas are normal. The cystic duct was ligated leaving about a ½ cm stump with | 200 |
| 0 silk. The cystic duct was divided distal to the suture and the gallbladder removed from below | 217 |
| upwards. Gallbladder hemostatis was secured with electrocautery. | 224 |
|     A suction drain is left to the area of the gallbladder bed. With instrument and sponge count | 241 |
| correct, the wound was closed using running #1 vicryl for posterior sheath and peritoneum and | 256 |
| again for the anterior sheath. 3-0 vicryl subcutaneously and then subcuticular 3-0 vicryl and | 270 |
| steri-strips are used to complete wound closure. The patient was then awakened and returned | 284 |
| to the recovery room having been stable throughout the procedure. | 294 |

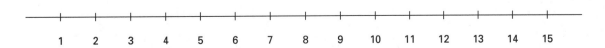

1   2   3   4   5   6   7   8   9   10   11   12   13   14   15

**Timed Writing 8**

|  | Words |
|---|---|

This woman presents with an equivocal lesion just above the right areola. Clinically and     14

radiologically this is benign. The patient however has returned on three occasions, concerned     27

that there is increased size to the lesion and at this point the patient is brought to the operating     46

room for excisional biopsy to ensure that this is in fact benign disease.     59

With the patient under general anaesthesia the right breast is prepped and draped. With the     74

patient under anaesthesia there is concern as there appears to be a bit of retraction of the skin     92

just at the areolar margin at 1130. A circumareolar incision is performed. The palpable lesion     107

appears merely to be a lipoma which is removed with its capsule intact. This did not, however,     124

explain the appearance of retraction. There is a good deal of caseous-like material in the ducts     140

present in this area. A fairly large amount of breast tissue extending under the areola out a short     158

distance beyond it and down to the chest wall is removed in attempts to make sure that there     176

could be no possible malignant lesion to explain this apparent retraction of skin.     189

On closely inspecting the area, no such disease can be appreciated. The material is sent for     205

istologic examination and on quick section no malignant disease is found.     216

Hemostatis is with snap and tie and electrocautery. Any attempts to close the breast tissue     231

resulted in retraction of skin and there were no deep sutures placed. The skin is closed with     248

interrupted 5-0 Prolene and Steri-strips.     253

The patient is then returned to the recovery room having been stable throughout the     267

procedure.     268

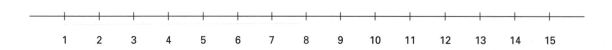

1    2    3    4    5    6    7    8    9    10    11    12    13    14    15

## Speed, Accuracy, and Terminology Development Exercises

### Exercise 1

(Average Word Strokes 5.61)

|  | Strokes |
|---|---|
| The patient's trochanteric bursae were injected on December 4 and the 72 hours | 78 |
| following that she had marked improvement in her ability to ambulate. She was | 156 |
| seen in consultation by Dr. Parker who as before discussed with Mrs. Jones | 230 |
| the probable cause in the near future of hip replacement. At this time, Mrs. | 307 |
| Jones feels able to function at home with Home Care assistance, and she thus | 383 |
| will be discharged today on Feldene 20 mg p.o., q.q.m., Tylenol No. 3 up to | 458 |
| q.i.d., p.r.n. | 472 |

### Exercise 2

(A.W.S. 6.27)

|  | Strokes |
|---|---|
| Complete eburnation of the whole medial compartment was noted right down to | 75 |
| subchondral bone in the femoral condyle. Medical meniscus, however, was intact. | 153 |
| It was very slightly fibrillated along its inner border but there were no | 227 |
| tears in the meniscus and no loose bodies in the medial compartment. There | 301 |
| were very small intercondylar osteophytes only and the anterior cruciate was | 376 |
| intact. | 384 |

## Exercise 3

(A.W.S. 6.29)

|  | Strokes |
|---|---|
| Under general anaesthesia with endotracheal intubation, the right eye area | 74 |
| was prepped and draped. A superior rectus bridle suture was placed and tied | 150 |
| to the head drape. A fornix-based conjunctival flap was raised and the | 220 |
| bleeding points cauterized. The anterior chamber was entered with a Graefe | 295 |
| knife and extended right and left with corneal scissors. Two peripheral | 367 |
| iridectomies were done at 10 o'clock and 2 o'clock positions. Catarase | 438 |
| was injected into the posterior chamber and allowed to remain for two minutes. | 516 |

## Exercise 4

(A.W.S. 6.54)

|  | Strokes |
|---|---|
| Nearby coronary arteries become wider and develop tiny new branches which | 73 |
| deliver blood to the surrounding muscle. This is called "collateral | 141 |
| circulation." The time required for recovery normally takes three to | 211 |
| four weeks depending on the extent of the damage, rate of healing, and | 281 |
| whether or not there are complications. It is reassuring to know that | 352 |
| most patients survive their heart attack. Your restrictions and your | 421 |
| limitations are generally only temporary. Most patients are able to | 489 |
| resume their normal lifestyle. Remember, healing takes time! | 550 |

# Exercise 5

(A.W.S. 6.37)

|  | Strokes |
|---|---|
| The heart has great recuperative powers. Yet, some people become very | 71 |
| fearful after a heart attack. They become overly concerned and make life | 144 |
| difficult for themselves and others. Some withdraw from society and | 212 |
| begin to enjoy their ill health. Others accept a heart attack as a challenge | 289 |
| to do everything against their rehabilitation. Some even deny their health | 364 |
| problem. | 372 |
| In some individuals, feelings of anxiety, anger, denial, depression, and | 444 |
| even hostility may be experienced following a heart attack. Do not be | 514 |
| surprised if you behave strangely. | 548 |

# Exercise 6

(A.W.S. 6.53)

|  | Strokes |
|---|---|
| On examination, the bladder was smooth-walled and clean. There is no | 69 |
| trabeculation, no evidence of stone or tumour. Both ureteral orifices were | 144 |
| visualized and functioned normally. Within the posterior urethra he had | 216 |
| only an early degree of benign prostatic hypertrophy. | 269 |

# Exercise 7
(A.W.S. 5.5)

|  | Strokes |
|---|---:|
| The patient's main problem was his chronic obstructive lung disease. He was | 75 |
| likely having a recurrent atrial arrhythmias accounting for his rapid heart | 151 |
| rate. He likely had some cor pulmonale. He had been on Digoxin 0.125 mg per | 228 |
| day and this will be continued. A Digoxin level was performed and this showed | 306 |
| the Digoxin level to be the upper limits of normal. Thyroid function tests | 381 |
| were also normal. It was felt that the patient should continue on his Digoxin | 458 |
| as well as on Synthroid 0.2 mg per day and Sulfisoxazole 500 mg t.i.d. He | 532 |
| will be seen in the office by Dr. Scott for a follow-up period and advised to | 608 |
| have a Holter monitor to see what arrhythmias the patient is having as an | 681 |
| outpatient. | 692 |

# Exercise 8
(A.W.S. 5.5)

|  | Strokes |
|---|---:|
| This eighteen-year-old girl was admitted to hospital on November 16, 1995, | 74 |
| with gastrointestinal bleeding. In hospital, she required nine units of blood. | 153 |
| She had a G.I. series, which showed a filling defect in the antral area of the | 231 |
| anterior wall, about 4 mm in diameter. She had esophagoscopy done, and no | 305 |
| evidence of gastritis was noted. A good deal of blood was noted within the | 380 |
| body of the stomach, possibly covering an ulceration, however, no specific | 454 |
| bleeding point was noted when this was done by Dr. Smith. It was felt that | 529 |
| the patient might have had a mucosal tear as a cause of her bleeding. | 598 |

# Exercise 9

(A.W.S. 6.04)

|  | Strokes |
|---|---|
| After G.A. was induced by crash intubation while the patient was awake, the | 76 |
| pneumatic tourniquet was applied high on the right arm. The hand and forearm | 153 |
| were cleaned with Savlon after the tourniquet had been inflated, and the wound | 231 |
| irrigated well with normal saline. It was explored and he was found to have | 307 |
| severed the brachioradials, flexor capri radialis, extensor carpi radialis -- | 384 |
| longus and brevis, the radial artery, as well as two mucocutaneous nerves. It | 462 |
| missed the median nerve as well as the flexor tendons. The dorsal branch of | 538 |
| the radial nerve was partially lacerated. | 579 |

# Exercise 10

(A.W.S. 6.07)

|  | Strokes |
|---|---|
| The muscle elements were sutured with 4-0 plain catgut and the tendons with | 75 |
| 4-0 white Mersilene. The radial artery was approximated, using microvascular | 152 |
| technique with 8-0 virgin silk, and the nerves approximated with 8-0 silk; | 226 |
| after ligation of several of the veins with 5-0 plain catgut, the tourniquet | 302 |
| was released and after ten minutes the wound was explored. He appeared to have | 381 |
| good pulsation of the radial artery and had good distal pulsation. The anasto- | 460 |
| mosis was patent. Hemostasis was again obtained, by ligation of several veins | 538 |
| with 5-0 plain catgut and the wound margin closed with 5-0 Ethilon and a dressing | 620 |
| of Bactigras, fluff gauze and Kling was applied, as well as a full cast. Patient | 701 |
| tolerated the procedure well and returned to the recovery in good condition. | 777 |

# Exercise 11

(A.W.S. 5.17)

|  | Strokes |
|---|---|
| The sudden admission of a family member to hospital with a heart attack is, | 75 |
| to say the least, a very upsetting experience. We want you to know that | 147 |
| even though we are terribly busy and perhaps can't take as much time as we | 221 |
| would like to show it, we understand that you, too, are very upset and | 291 |
| worried. | 299 |
| The well-being of our patients is very important to us. We know that one | 372 |
| of the things that will contribute to that well-being is an understanding | 445 |
| and supportive family. We consider you a very important part of the team | 518 |
| that is going to help your spouse to recover. | 563 |

# Exercise 12

**(A.W.S. 5.86)**

| | Strokes |
|---|---:|
| Several heart attack patients and their families were asked to describe | 71 |
| the thoughts and fears that they had as they progressed through the various | 146 |
| stages of recovery, from admission, to Intensive Care, to the convalescent | 220 |
| ward, back home, and finally back to work. They hope that their sharing | 292 |
| will increase your understanding. | 325 |
|     When a person suffers a heart attack, the symptoms vary. Some have severe | 399 |
| crushing chest pain, which may spread into their neck, arm or jaw. Others | 473 |
| may feel a burning sensation similar to indigestion. Whatever the symptoms, | 549 |
| the patient arrives at the Emergency Department in a very anxious and fear- | 624 |
| ful state. He, and his family, may suspect that he has had a heart attack, | 699 |
| but hope that it is not true. It comes as quite a blow when the physician | 773 |
| confirms their worst suspicions and orders a transfer to Intensive Care. | 845 |

# Exercise 13

**(A.W.S. 5.51)**

| | Strokes |
|---|---:|
| Once the pain has gone, the patient starts to feel quite well. Some of | 71 |
| the patients who were interviewed said that they felt so well that they | 142 |
| tried to convince themselves that they had not really had a heart attack. | 215 |
| They became bored with bedrest and tried to do things that they were told | 288 |
| they shouldn't be doing. They had little to do but look at their monitors | 360 |
| and worry about their pulse and blood pressure. Others said that they | 432 |
| were aware that they were overly sensitive and over-reacting to everything. | 507 |

# Exercise 14

(A.W.S. 5.61)

| | Strokes |
|---|---:|
| They snapped at their families, complained about everything, and blamed every- | 78 |
| one and everything for causing the heart attack. The nurses are well able | 152 |
| to tolerate this behaviour since they understand the anxiety of the patient. | 228 |
| They realize that in most cases, these are 40- to 50-year-old males who are | 305 |
| used to being in charge of everything and all of a sudden, they are expected | 381 |
| to submit to the orders of 20- to 30-year-old females. The resulting feelings | 461 |
| of helplessness and frustration are not too well understood by the patient | 535 |
| at the time and so can lead to reactions of anger and discontent. | 600 |

# Exercise 15

(A.W.S. 5.61)

| | Strokes |
|---|---:|
| Some patients said that they didn't want to talk to anyone -- family included. | 76 |
| This is very hard for the family to cope with. The patients said that | 146 |
| looking back at this time, they realize that there were so many thoughts | 218 |
| going on in their minds and they needed time to sort them out. They were | 291 |
| worried about their future, job, family, and whether they would be able to | 365 |
| function adequately again. In a way, they were grieving -- for their lost | 437 |
| self image, of being strong, confident and invulnerable. | 493 |

# Exercise 16

**(A.W.S. 5.95)**

|  | Strokes |
|---|---:|
| It is important that the family listen, encourage and above all, be patient. | 76 |
| They must ignore and forget unkind things that the patient may have said. | 153 |
| He is voicing general frustration and not specific grievances against the | 226 |
| family. Frequently, due to medication for pain, he has no recollection of | 300 |
| these things later. The family frequently has feelings of guilt. They | 372 |
| must not blame themselves for having caused the heart attack. The causes | 445 |
| of heart attacks are not fully understood. We do know that they result from | 521 |
| arteriosclerosis (hardening of the arteries) which is a disease process that | 597 |
| has been going on for years and is the biggest health problem of our present | 673 |
| time. | 678 |

# Exercise 17

**(A.W.S. 5.97)**

|  | Strokes |
|---|---:|
| The patient, a 53-year-old Caucasian female, had a right total condylar knee | 76 |
| replacement in July. She has been doing reasonably well since that time with | 153 |
| no significant evidence of activation of her rheumatoid disease. However, two | 231 |
| weeks prior to this admission she had gradual onset over a week of soreness in | 309 |
| both inguinal regions anterolateral thighs, initially eased by lying or sitting, | 389 |
| worsened in the heel-strike phase of step. | 431 |

# Exercise 18

(A.W.S. 6.33)

|  | Strokes |
|---|---|
| Investigation -- hip X-rays again showed the marked joint space narrowing | 73 |
| with sclerosis and early protrusio acetabuli on the left side, but no | 143 |
| major changes. Pelvis at S.I. joints -- no active disease. Lumbar spine | 216 |
| showed L5-S1 disc narrowing with sclerosis of margins and degenerative | 286 |
| change in posterior joints. Bone scan showed slight increased uptake in | 358 |
| both hip and knee areas. | 382 |

# Exercise 19

(A.W.S. 6.6)

|  | Strokes |
|---|---|
| Her other appendicular joints have not been a significant problem. She | 71 |
| was taking Feldene 20 mg p.o. q.a.m., multivitamins, but no cortico- | 141 |
| steroids. She was bedrested for hours, with repeat examination at that | 214 |
| time showing improved hip movements with lessened groin and anterolateral | 287 |
| thigh pain, but with marked soreness to pressure over both trochanteric | 358 |
| bursae and aggravation of that by external rotation, and hip adduction. | 429 |

# Exercise 20

(A.W.S. 5.95)

| | Strokes |
|---|---:|
| Once you are discharged from hospital, you should continue to add activities | 76 |
| according to your physician's advice. It would be helpful to yourself if you | 153 |
| established realistic weekly goals of activity or other alternatives of life- | 230 |
| style which are important for your heart's health. For example, make a contract | 310 |
| with a family member that you will lose one kilo each week for a month, or | 386 |
| you will walk a set distance every day, reduce cigarette consumption by one | 461 |
| cigarette per day until you stop. | 494 |

# Exercise 21

(A.W.S. 5.92)

| | Strokes |
|---|---:|
| This 64-year-old man was admitted with acute pulmonary edema to Ottawa Civic | 76 |
| Hospital in the early morning hours of December 5, 1995. He had apparently | 151 |
| been well up until the night of his admission, went to bed and then awoke | 224 |
| with acute orthopnea. He was brought over to the Emergency Department where | 300 |
| he was assessed initially by Dr. T. Kellie who felt that he was in acute | 372 |
| pulmonary edema, and treated him with intravenous Furosemide. By the time | 446 |
| I saw him at 0800 hours the following morning, he had settled down. He was | 521 |
| breathing comfortably, but his temperature was elevated at 38.6°. A chest | 595 |
| X-ray performed showed evidence of an active bronchopneumonia with consoli- | 670 |
| dation in the right mid-lung field. | 705 |

# Exercise 22
(A.W.S. 6.56)

|  | Strokes |
|---|---|
| Under general anaesthesia, the left chest was suitably prepared and draped. | 75 |
| Through an elliptical incision, including the biopsy site, modified radical | 150 |
| mastectomy was performed. There were some very florid-looking nodes in the | 225 |
| axilla which were excised in continuity with the specimen and which were | 297 |
| felt to be highly suspicious of malignancy. The wound was sluiced out with | 372 |
| water, patted dry, sprayed with Polybactrin spray. Hemovac was inserted | 443 |
| through two separate stabs and the wound was closed with multiple inter- | 510 |
| rupted silk sutures. Suitable dressings were applied. The patient with- | 581 |
| stood the procedure well and returned to the recovery room in good condition. | 662 |

# Exercise 23
(A.W.S. 6.05)

|  | Strokes |
|---|---|
| The pain that results from the lack of oxygen (ischemia) is called "angina." | 75 |
| It is described by most people as a heavy, tight constriction in the middle | 149 |
| of the chest which occasionally may spread to other areas such as the arms, | 224 |
| neck, jaw, or upper back. It usually follows activity, emotional excitement | 300 |
| or exertion after eating. Anginal episodes are usually brief -- a matter | 371 |
| of a few minutes. When medications like nitroglycerin are taken, the pain | 446 |
| is promptly relieved. These drugs tend to enlarge the coronary arteries, | 519 |
| allowing blood to be delivered more effectively to the heart muscle. | 587 |

# Exercise 24

(A.W.S. 6.00)

| | Strokes |
|---|---:|
| Under general anaesthesia, with the patient in the lithotomy position, | 70 |
| perianal skin was shaved and then the sigmoidoscope was introduced into | 142 |
| a well prepared bowel to the hilt of the instrument. No evidence of any | 214 |
| pathology was noted. The patient had a very tight anal sphincter even | 285 |
| under deep general anaesthesia. A manual dilatation of the anal sphincter | 359 |
| was performed, dilating it up to four fingers easily. One could feel | 428 |
| subcutaneous fibres of anal sphincter snapping and popping at the time | 498 |
| of the dilatation. There was a posterior anal skin tag, which I thought | 570 |
| might be the site of a tiny fistula in ano; however, there was no evidence | 644 |
| whatever of any external opening within this skin tag. The skin tag was | 716 |
| excised and suitable dressings were applied. The patient withstood the | 785 |
| procedure well and was returned to the recovery room in good condition. | 854 |

# Exercise 25

(A.W.S. 5.93)

| | Strokes |
|---|---:|
| This 66-year-old-man has recurrent basal cell carcinoma of the top of his | 73 |
| nose. He presents for further excision. Under general anaesthesia, the | 143 |
| face was prepped and draped. The lesion was excised with a margin of | 213 |
| normal skin and down to the cartilage at the tip of the nose. Hemostasis | 285 |
| obtained. The defect was closed with a full thickness skin graft obtained | 359 |
| from the right supraclavicular area. Graft sutured in place and immobilized | 435 |
| with a tie-over dressing. The donor defect closed by suturing. Dressings | 509 |
| applied. | 517 |

# Exercise 26

**(A.W.S. 6.61)**

|  | Strokes |
|---|---|
| Femoral head and neck were then reemed and tapped, lateral cortex expanded | 76 |
| and four-inch Howmedica screw inserted. The four-holed, 135° side plate | 150 |
| was secured to the screw and lateral cortex of the femur. Traction was | 223 |
| released, fracture impacted and interfragmentary compression achieved. | 294 |
| The wound was copiously irrigated with Saline, closed in layers | 366 |
| over two Hemovac drains. Vicryl was used for the deep layers and 3-0 steel | 443 |
| subcuticular wire for the skin. Sterile dry dressing was then applied, | 516 |
| and the patient returned to the recovery room in satisfactory condition. | 589 |

# Exercise 27

**(A.W.S. 5.96)**

|  | Strokes |
|---|---|
| Thank you for referring this 33-year-old lady for reassessment of left | 72 |
| upper thoracic chest pain. As per her discharge summary, she was admitted | 147 |
| here from October 13 to October 17 with similar pain and was tentatively | 214 |
| diagnosed as suffering from pleurodynia. Investigations at the time | 285 |
| did not reveal a specific cause; her ECG being normal, her chest X-ray | 357 |
| being normal; and her lungs showing no evidence of pulmonary emboli. | 427 |
| Several viral and mycoplasm titers have apparently been sent but are not | 502 |
| reported yet in the old chart and are therefore not helpful at the moment. | 578 |

# Exercise 28

(A.W.S. 5.88)

| | Strokes |
|---|---|
| The patients remember continuing to be overly sensitive at home and that | 72 |
| they frequently felt best when left alone. As the weeks passed, they | 141 |
| gradually became more confident and stronger and their attitude improved. | 214 |
| They all reported occasional set-backs but these became less and less. | 284 |
| Some patients said they had a great fear of having a second heart attack. | 357 |
| There is a danger that this fear may cause them to become completely dependent | 435 |
| on others. It is felt that this fear is a natural reaction to the situation | 511 |
| and will disappear as they gain more confidence. It is important for the | 584 |
| family to be aware that they can become over-protective and that this can be | 660 |
| crippling and delay recovery. It is not necessary to severely restrict | 731 |
| family activity. Regular rest periods are important and during this time, | 805 |
| household activity should be at a minimum. Gradual return to activity is | 878 |
| encouraged as it improves the patient physically and psychologically. | 947 |

# Exercise 29

(A.W.S. 5.77)

|  | Strokes |
|---|---:|
| Vague chest pains are normal during this time. However, if the pain | 68 |
| should become severe and persist, the patient should loosen clothing | 136 |
| and rest, and take medication if prescribed. If it remains severe for | 206 |
| longer than one-half hour, notify the physician, call an ambulance | 272 |
| and try to remain calm and supportive. | 310 |
| As the days pass and the patient continues his new lifestyle, his heart | 381 |
| muscle frequently becomes stronger than it has been for many years. | 448 |
| Patients frequently say that life has taken on a new meaning and that | 518 |
| they feel better and more appreciative than they have in years. They | 588 |
| have a new sense of what is truly important in life. | 641 |

## Exercise 30

(A.W.S. 5.39)

|  | Strokes |
|---|---|
| Most patients were anxious to return to work, even though they enjoyed | 70 |
| their days of leisure. Some were discouraged at first and felt that they | 143 |
| did not improve fast enough and tired easily. A few had worked in areas | 215 |
| where a lot of heavy manual labour was required and so had to adjust to | 287 |
| a new area. Most of them found it took at least six months before they | 359 |
| felt they were performing adequately. | 396 |
| All patients agreed that in each step of recovery, the understanding, | 465 |
| patience, and support of the family and hospital personnel were vital. | 534 |
| Everyone agreed that the end result was well worth all the team effort | 604 |
| that was required. | 622 |
| Remember that there are a lot of people who are available and prepared | 692 |
| to help -- ask for help if you need it. | 729 |

# Exercise 31

(A.W.S. 6.65)

|  | Strokes |
|---|---|
| In the majority of cases, angina is caused by a process called "arterio- | 76 |
| sclerosis" (commonly known as "hardening of the arteries"). Arteriosclerosis | 153 |
| has become the major health problem in North America. Its effects are seen | 228 |
| in many disease processes -- e.g., high blood pressure (hypertension), | 296 |
| cardiovascular accident (C.V.A. -- or stroke), peripheral vascular disease | 368 |
| (disease of circulation to legs and arms causing leg ulcers, etc.), and | 438 |
| "myocardial infarction" (heart attack). | 477 |
| Arteriosclerosis is a slowly evolving process. This occurs as the arteries | 552 |
| become progressively more narrowed. Sticky, fatty material becomes overly | 626 |
| concentrated in the blood. As this develops early in life, all of us have | 700 |
| it to some degree by the time we reach middle age. There is considerable | 773 |
| evidence that the causes of hardening of the arteries are mostly due to the | 848 |
| modern, affluent way of life -- e.g., physical inactivity, obesity, cigarette | 923 |
| smoking, and high animal fat intake. | 959 |

# Appendix E: Computerized Requisition Forms

Illustration AE.1   Microbiology Test Requisition

---

**PETERBOROUGH HOSPITALS LABORATORY MEDICINE**
## MICROBIOLOGY TEST REQUISITION

☐ PCH  ☐ SJHC  ☐ Haliburton  ☐ Minden  ☐ Other_____

☐ In-patient  ☐ Out-patient     ☐ Referred-In

Date Ordered:m\d\yr_____

Ordering Physician:._____

Nurse:_____

Specimen collected by:_____

Collection Date:m\d\yr_____Time:_____

☐ Repeat Specimen  ☐ Physician Requested  ☐ Laboratory Requested

**☐ Emergent**      **☐ Urgent**      **☐ Routine**      **☐ Timed**

O.R. Date: m\d\yr_____O.R.Time:_____

Specimen Type/Anatomic Site:_____

RelevantClinical Information/Symptoms_____

Special Instructions:_____

Antibiotic given: _____Antibiotic preferred:_____

✓ test requested below

| | | | | | |
|---|---|---|---|---|---|
| ☐ | Routine Culture 5095 | ‖‖‖‖‖ | ☐ Fungus/Yeast Culture 5070 | ‖‖‖‖‖ | ☐ Clostridium difficile toxin 5085 ‖‖‖‖‖ |
| ☐ | TB Culture 5055 | ‖‖‖‖‖ | ☐ Parasitology 5080 | ‖‖‖‖‖ | |
| ☐ | G.C. Culture 5145 | ‖‖‖‖‖ | ☐ Chlamydia 5060 | ‖‖‖‖‖ | |

☐ **Other:**_____

☐ **Other:**_____

---

**PETERBOROUGH CIVIC HOSPITAL**
One Hospital Drive, Peterborough, Ont., K9J 7C6

**Illustration AE.2    Blood Testing Requisition**

## PETERBOROUGH HOSPITALS LABORATORY MEDICINE
## BLOOD TESTING REQUISITION

☐ PCH  ☐ SJHC  ☐ Haliburton  ☐ Minden  ☐ Other_____     ☐ **Emergent**

☐ In-patient        ☐ Out-patient        ☐ Referred-In

Collection Date:m\d\yr_____Time:_____     ☐ **Urgent**

O.R. Date:_____Time:_____

Relevant Clinical Information/Special Instructions:                    ☐ **Routine**

_____

Ordering Physician:._____     ☐ **Timed** ____

Nurse:_____

| ✓ | HAEMATOLOGY | | ✓ | CHEMISTRY | | ✓ | CHEMISTRY | | ✓ | SEROLOGY | |
|---|---|---|---|---|---|---|---|---|---|---|---|
| | CBC 2000 | ▮▮▮ | | SODIUM 3040 | ▮▮▮ | | GGTP 3190 | ▮▮▮ | | ANA 5200 | ▮▮▮ |
| | CBC/DIFF 2010 | ▮▮▮ | | POTASSIUM 3050 | ▮▮▮ | | UREA 3020 | ▮▮▮ | | ANTI-DNA 5220 | ▮▮▮ |
| | CELL MORPH. 2030 | ▮▮▮ | | CHLORIDE 3060 | ▮▮▮ | | TSH 3600 | ▮▮▮ | | | |
| | RETIC 2040 | ▮▮▮ | | GLUCOSE FASTING 3003 | ▮▮▮ | | FREE T4 3610 | ▮▮▮ | | | |
| | MONO SCREEN 2060 | ▮▮▮ | | GLUCOSE RANDOM 3010 | ▮▮▮ | | VITAMIN B12 3625 | ▮▮▮ | ✓ | DRUGS / MISC | |
| | ESR 2050 | ▮▮▮ | | GLUCOSE AC 3003 | ▮▮▮ | | RBC FOLATE 3630 | ▮▮▮ | | ACETAMINO-PHEN 3380 | ▮▮▮ |
| ✓ | COAGULATION | | | GLUCOSE PC 3014 | ▮▮▮ | | FERRITIN 3340 | ▮▮▮ | | BARBITURATE SCREEN 3390 | ▮▮▮ |
| | INR 2500 | ▮▮▮ | | CREATININE 3030 | ▮▮▮ | | IRON 3310 | ▮▮▮ | | SALICYLATE 3470 | ▮▮▮ |
| | A.P.T.T. 2510 | ▮▮▮ | | TOTAL BILIRUBIN 3220 | ▮▮▮ | | TIBC 3320 | ▮▮▮ | | ETHANOL 3430 | ▮▮▮ |
| | BLEEDING TIME 2520 | ▮▮▮ | | MICRO-BILIRUBIN 3120 | ▮▮▮ | | IRON SATURATION | | | DIGOXIN 3410 | ▮▮▮ |
| | D-DIMER 2540 | ▮▮▮ | | CALCIUM 3100 | ▮▮▮ | | CORTISOL A.M.  P.M. | | | PHENYTOIN 3420 | ▮▮▮ |
| | FIBRINOGEN SCREEN 2560 | ▮▮▮ | | PHOSPHATE 3200 | ▮▮▮ | | BLOOD GASES ART   3489 | ▮▮▮ | | PHENOBARB 3460 | ▮▮▮ |
| ✓ | TRANSFUSION SERVICES | | | MAGNESIUM 3110 | ▮▮▮ | | BLOOD GASES CAP   3519 | ▮▮▮ | | CARBA-   3400 MAZEPINE | ▮▮▮ |
| | TYPE & SCREEN 1900 | ▮▮▮ | | URATE 3210 | ▮▮▮ | | BLOOD GASES VEN   3504 | ▮▮▮ | | THEOPHYLLINE 3480 | ▮▮▮ |
| | SUPPLY | _____ RBC | | TOTAL PROTEIN 3240 | ▮▮▮ | | CHOLESTEROL 3270 | ▮▮▮ | | GENTAMICIN PRE   3440 | ▮▮▮ |
| | SUPPLY | _____ ml FFP | | ALBUMIN 3250 | ▮▮▮ | | TRIGLYCERIDES 3280 | ▮▮▮ | | GENTAMICIN POST  3445 | ▮▮▮ |
| | SUPPLY | _____ PLTS. | | AST 3160 | ▮▮▮ | | HDL-C 3290 | ▮▮▮ | | LITHIUM 3450 | ▮▮▮ |
| | OTHER _____ | *check LAB/NURSING manual for product availability | | LDH 3170 | ▮▮▮ | | LDL (CALC) | | ✓ | MISC | |
| | ADULT DIRECT ANTIGLOBIN | | | CK 3070 | ▮▮▮ | | HbA1C GLYCATED PROTIEN 3350 | ▮▮▮ | | | |
| | CHECK FOR RhIG | | | CK-2 3080 | ▮▮▮ | | SPC 3580 | ▮▮▮ | | BLOOD CULTURE X | ▮▮▮ |
| | COLD AGGLUTININS | | | ALK   3180 PHOSPHATASE | ▮▮▮ | | IMMUNO- 3540 GLOBULINS | ▮▮▮ | | ANTIBIOTIC GIVEN 5000 | |
| | TRANSFUSION REACTION INVESTIGATION | | | ACID   3260 PHOSPHATASE | ▮▮▮ | | | | | | |
| | | | | AMYLASE 3090 | ▮▮▮ | | | | | | |

Form # JF 5046
July/96

**Illustration AE.3    Urinalysis Requisition**

## PETERBOROUGH HOSPITALS LABORATORY MEDICINE
## URINALYSIS/OTHER BODY FLUIDS

☐ PCH  ☐ SJHC  ☐ Haliburton  ☐ Minden  ☐ Other_____

☐ In-patient    ☐ Out-patient        ☐ Referred-In

Date Ordered:m\d\yr_____

Ordering Physician:._____

Nurse:_____

Specimen collected by:_____

Collection Date:m\d\yr_____Time:_____

☐ Random Urine        ☐ 24 Hour Urine

☐ **Emergent**        ☐ **Urgent**        ☐ **Routine**        ☐ **Timed**

O.R. Date: m\d\yr_____O.R.Time:_____

Clinical Information:_____

Special Instructions:_____

NOTE: USE MICROBIOLOGY TEST REQUISITION FOR ALL CULTURE REQUESTS

| TESTS ON URINE | |
|---|---|
| ROUTINE URINALYSIS 3655 | ‖‖‖‖‖‖ |
| MICROSCOPIC URINALYSIS | |
| PROTEIN 3241 | ‖‖‖‖‖‖ |
| SODIUM 3045 | ‖‖‖‖‖‖ |
| POTASSIUM 3055 | ‖‖‖‖‖‖ |
| AMYLASE 3092 | ‖‖‖‖‖‖ |
| URATE 3210 | ‖‖‖‖‖‖ |
| CALCIUM 3105 | ‖‖‖‖‖‖ |
| OSMOLALITY 3142 | ‖‖‖‖‖‖ |
| PREGNANCY TEST 3640 | ‖‖‖‖‖‖ |
| CREATININE 3035 | ‖‖‖‖‖‖ |
| CREATININE 3037 CLEARANCE (NOTE.SERUM CREATININE ALSO REQUIRED) | ‖‖‖‖‖‖ |
| PATIENT - HT. | |
| WT. | |
| OTHER | |

| OTHER TESTS | |
|---|---|
| SWEAT CHLORIDES | |

| STOOL | |
|---|---|
| OCCULT BLOOD 3635 | ‖‖‖‖‖‖ |
| OTHER | |
| OTHER | |

| STONES | |
|---|---|
| STONE ANALYSIS | |
| OTHER | |

### BODY FLUID TESTING

☐ CSF   ☐ JOINT   ☐ PLEURAL

☐ OTHER _____

| | |
|---|---|
| GLUCOSE | |
| PROTEIN | |
| CELLS | |
| CRYSTALS | |
| PHOSPHATE | |
| OTHER | |
| OTHER | |

**\*FOR LAB USE ONLY:**     Specimen Volume:_____mL        Surface Area:_____"

☐ **PETERBOROUGH CIVIC HOSPITAL**        ☐ **ST. JOSEPH'S HEALTH CENTRE**

One Hospital Drive, Peterborough, Ont., K9J 7C6        384 Rogers St., Peterborough, Ont., K9H 7B

Form # JF 5047                                                    June/96

# Index

# Reader Reply Card

We are interested in your reaction to *Procedures for the Medical Administrative Assistant*, Third Edition, by Lorna Plunkett. With your comments, we can improve this book in future editions. Please help us by completing this questionnaire.

1. What was your reason for using this book?
   - ☐ university course    ☐ college course
   - ☐ continuing education course    ☐ personal interest
   - ☐ other (specify)

2. If you used this text for a program, what was the name of that program?

   _____

3. Which school do you attend?

   _____

4. Approximately how much of the book did you use?

   ☐ ¼    ☐ ½    ☐ ¾    ☐ all

5. Which chapters or sections were omitted from your course?

   _____

6. Did you find the depiction of the forms realistic?

   _____

7. Were there enough sample forms, too many, or not enough?

   _____

8. Was the writing style easy to follow?

   _____

9. Does the text provide sufficient explanations of procedures?

   _____

10. Did the assignments help you to better understand procedures and concepts?

    _____

11. Did you find the appendices useful?

    _____

12. What is the best aspect of this book?

    _____

13. What did you like least about this book?

    _____

14. Is there anything that should be improved?

    _____

15. Please add any comments or suggestions.

    _____

(fold here and tape shut)

------------------------------------------------------------------------------------------

**MAIL ▶ POSTE**

Canada Post Corporation / Société canadienne des postes

**Postage paid**
If mailed in Canada

**Port payé**
si posté au Canada

**Business
Reply**

**Réponse
d'affaires**

0116870399          01

0116870399-M8Z4X6-BR01

Heather McWhinney
Director of Product Development
HARCOURT BRACE & COMPANY, CANADA
55 HORNER AVENUE
TORONTO, ONTARIO
M8Z 9Z9

# Getting straight "A"s
# doesn't have to be a mystery...

these practical, concise, and affordable study guides will tell you how!

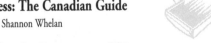